Social Engineering

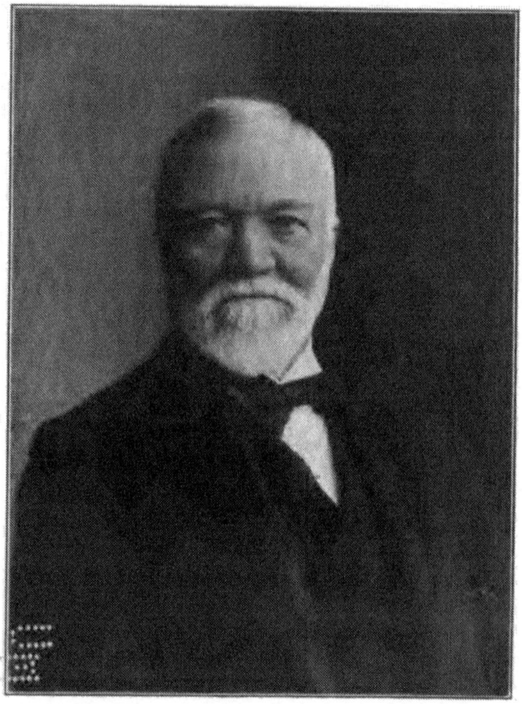

Andrew Carnegie

FOUNDER OF THE CARNEGIE INSTITUTION, WASHINGTON, THROUGH WHICH THESE STUDIES WERE MADE.

OCIAL ENGINEERING

A RECORD OF THINGS DONE BY AMERICAN INDUSTRIALISTS EMPLOYING UPWARDS OF ONE AND ONE-HALF MILLION OF PEOPLE

BY

WILLIAM H. TOLMAN, PH.D.

SOCIAL ENGINEER

Director American Museum of Safety; Secretary American Section, International Congress of Improved Dwellings; Corresponding Member Imperial Technological Museum, Vienna; Member International Committee Les Assurances Sociales; Corresponding Member Société des Habitations à Bon Marché, Paris

WITH AN INTRODUCTION

BY

ANDREW CARNEGIE

FIRST EDITION

SECOND IMPRESSION

McGRAW-HILL BOOK COMPANY

239 WEST 39TH STREET, NEW YORK

6 BOUVERIE STREET, LONDON, E.C.

1909

PREFACE

In my studies of social and industrial problems during the last fifteen years, I was impressed with the extent and the variety of efforts that were being made to promote better relations between capital and labor. At first there was no name for this kind of work. In 1898, for lack of a better term, I called it industrial betterment, a phrase which passed quickly into current use and literature. At that time industrial betterment was scarcely comprehended, but to-day the changes are being rung on betterment—industrial, social, civic and religious. Several years later, the National Civic Federation organized a department of betterment, and called it "welfare work."

Industrial betterment is more comprehensive, inasmuch as it concerns the efficiency promotion of the worker as well as the plant, in other words, this betterment of the labor element is a cold business proposition and is undertaken commonly to get the best results out of labor. Welfare work concerns the improvement of the personal conditions of the laborer; this is often offensive to him and is resented by him, savoring as it does of paternalism and charity.

Recognizing the inadequacy of both terms, industrial betterment and welfare work, to express the relations of interdependence between capital and labor and the sympathy which should exist between these two elements in the successful promotion of a business, I am convinced that the ideal relationship is best expressed by the term mutuality.

During the last decade mutuality has made steady progress and is manifesting itself in a great variety of efforts; because of this the relations between capital and labor have become more sympathetic. The awakened interest in this subject shows that the time has come for treating these problems of life and labor scientifically; museums of safety, social insurance, pensions, coöperation, profit-sharing, housing, recreation and affiliated questions are receiving the earnest consideration of some of the ablest men and are therefore the live questions of the day. There is an increasing number of industrialists who are desirous of promoting mutuality in their business. "Social Engineering" will serve as a handbook of suggestion and guidance for the practical application of the experience of others.

Acknowledgment is hereby made of aid received from the Carnegie Institution of Washington, through its Department of Economics and Sociology, in the preparation of this book.

INTRODUCTORY

HAVING read the following pages with deep interest, I have no hesitation in recommending them to all interested in the welfare of their fellows, especially of the workers. The hearts of those will be touched who have the welfare of their fellows at heart, and the heads of those will be convinced who wish the condition of the laboring people improved; I believe that they can be and are being so, rapidly and generally, at least thruout the bounds of the Republic.

It is cheering to know that our country is in the van, altho some European countries are moving in the same direction.

It is by the efforts of individual firms that the right solution of the problem will be furnished, and not thru Socialism, which can only talk speculatively, while individuals can work practically, curing evils that Socialists point out. This is the right division between the Individualist and the Socialist. There is quite a large domain in which the latter can point out defects and shortcomings. Let us thank them for this, and let us not forget that it is our duty to labor for the cure of defects.

I write this at Christmas and the book has come to me as a most appropriate gift for the season. I take pleasure in commending it to all those who would do their part in life to make the world a little better than they found it.

Andrew Carnegie

NEW YORK, *Christmas Day*, 1908.

CONTENTS

SOCIAL ENGINEERING

CHAPTER I

EFFICIENCY PROMOTION

The essential characteristic of the industrial conditions of to-day is the substitution of mechanical for muscular power, whether the source of energy for the machine be supplied by water, steam, electricity or air. Accordingly, inventive genius has lavished its powers on the perfection of the inanimate machine, the inert mass of iron or steel, awaiting only the application of the energizing force of nature to make it perform the complicated wishes of the inventor.

In recent years it has been slowly dawning upon the mind of the employer that his human machine—his hands as he sometimes calls them—needs attention, needs rest, needs the best environment for the production of the best results.

Some employers have improved the conditions under which their men work, because they felt that they owed their operatives something more than wages; they felt that their employés had done the labor share in the production of wealth, and that recognition of some kind was due them for that. Others again improved the condition of their operatives because it paid in actual dollars and cents, and another class has been influenced by genuine altruism.

Whatever may be the motives of the employer, whether he be influenced by the most sordid selfishness or the noblest altruism, the writer claims that the employé has been the gainer by any improvement in his industrial environment. Especially is this so where the wage earner has had the economic foresight to seize these advantages to perfect himself, whereby he makes himself of greater commercial worth to his employer. His wage earning capacity has been increased, and the tendency is towards a recognition of this fact in advancement or a feeling of security in his present position. The individual who improves his own condition cannot fail to be of greater worth to the industry, to his own home and to the community, facts which are positive assets in industrial, social and civic stability. Industrial betterment gives the individual this opportunity.

In modern business there is little room for sentiment; the ordinary employer demands a cash equivalent for each dollar paid out. The situation is reflected by the commercial proverb, "Business is business." But here and there employers are beginning to realize that investment in manhood pays; that improved men for improved machines have economic value, because a more vigorous man can do more work, a more intelligent man will do more intelligent work, and a more conscientious man will do more conscientious work.

"I want machines so simple in their operation that any fool can run them," remarked an employer the other day. The fool machines may be run by the fool workman, but the employer will have the monopoly of the folly of such an industrial policy. Improved machines demand improved men to run them.

"What more than wages?" is an industrial question that is being asked by men, some of whom feel that the labor share of their wealth production should have a larger reward than the mere payment of wages; other employers are sufficiently far-sighted to recognize that whatever makes the worker more human, more contented, more skilled, is a positive industrial asset in the business and is a large factor in industrial stability.

There are factories where the men as well as the machines must be "hand picked." For example, in the Weston Electrical Instrument Company[1] galvanometer measurements can be shown where the deflections are obtained with a current of five-billionths of an ampere. A current of the strength of half an ampere suffices to illuminate the standard sixteen-candle-power incandescent lamp. This work demands the finest technique, the clearest heads and directing intelligence.

Every employer wants the best workmen he can get; by best

[1] Weston Electrical Instrument Co., Newark, N. J. Manufacturing Electrical Measuring Instruments. Organized 1888. Number Employés, 368.

he means those that will earn the wages he pays, and so perfect themselves that he must advance them. "I go over my pay roll every Saturday night," said a manufacturer, "to see whose salary I can raise. My men are no more anxious for advancement than I am to promote them."

Mutuality should be the guiding principle in business, which can be conducted on this plane; mutuality means sympathy. In a New England department store the work began at 8:30 A.M. and closed at 5:30 P.M. It was the custom of other firms to begin at nine and close at six, the half hour before nine o'clock bringing very little trade and the half hour before six a fairly steady flow. This firm believed in mutuality, and showed their sympathy in a great variety of ways, thinking that the more closely they could manage their business on democratic lines, the greater would be their success. A meeting of the employés was called, and the question of changing the hours was left to their decision. Bear in mind that the half hour before six was very highly valued by the women and girls, as it gave them opportunity for comfortably preparing for home before the rush on trains and cars, and evening entertainments. Although they realized what closing at six would mean to them, several said at the meeting that they did not want their firm to lose the half hour's business, which otherwise would go to the rival stores. When the vote was taken it was found that a decided majority were in favor of closing at six. Mutuality is a commercial asset; it makes for industrial peace.

Employers are admitting that they ought to improve the conditions of the employed, but they are fearful lest in so doing they may make a mistake, they may not do the right thing, their efforts will be looked on with suspicion, they will not be appreciated. This recognition on the part of the employer that he owes his staff something more than wages, has created a new professional calling, that of the Social Engineer, who can tell the employer how he may establish a desired point of contact between himself, his immediate staff, and the rank and file of his industrial army.

There is a direct relation between capital, labor and management, the three essential elements necessary to every enterprise. Consider how useless is capital without management, which directs its resources, and in turn how both capital and management are dependent on the willing hands of labor to execute their will. For example, capital should conscientiously do all in its power to improve the condition of the workers. On the other hand, labor should not view with cold suspicion the overtures of capital, but should meet them in a friendly spirit, with a mind open and ready to coöperate. Many employers have told me that their efforts for industrial betterment have been met with surly looks, suspicion and indifference.

It is not fair to expect the employer to do all. America stands before the world as the land of opportunity and fair play. The capitalist should not be regarded as a thief and a robber, but labor should recognize the sincerity of his motives, and give him a chance to prove his sincerity by working with and not against him.

Not from the churches, not from the universities and colleges, not from the common schools, but from the hands of the great captains of industry who are recognizing and providing for an all-round development, the character of the plain people is being moulded and shaped along lines of civic and social usefulness. Never before in the history of the world has the employer had such colossal opportunities for guiding and uplifting the thousands of men and women, who spend at least a third of each working day in his employ. If employers realized that they hold within their grasp the possibilities of industrial contentment, social stability and communal welfare, they would plan and scheme how to improve the conditions of their employés with the same zeal as they now devote to promoting the efficiency of their business, extending its operations and reaching out for the acquisition of new commercial territory.

This volume on industrial betterment will be a study of what employers are doing to improve the conditions of their operatives, and the opportunities they are offering, whether in the industry in question or in their homes or in the community.

I shall approach the subject with the central thought that the factory, mill or workshop is the industrial home of the employé, where he must spend at least one-third of each working day. Money is spent lavishly, if need be, on the improvement and perfection of inanimate machinery, and its housing, and employers are beginning to realize that it will pay them to improve and perfect their animate machines, so that they are affording opportunities to the individual to become an improved man for the improved machine.

Setting aside any consideration of altruism or philanthropy, it is good business to provide the best light, pure air and water, the essentials of health for factory and workshop. That there is a response is evident when the increased production is shown at the end of the month. Attention to hygiene and sanitation is a large element in efficiency.

Within the year the Cleveland Hardware Company[1] has built a new factory building, and from its past experience decided it would pay to put into this building the very finest sanitary arrangements it could find. This plan was followed out to the very best of its ability and experience.

It employs a large number of girls in its factory, and has fitted up an ample and well-lighted dressing room for their convenience, giving each girl an expanded metal locker. A woman is in charge of this room, who has under her care a well-stocked medicine chest, so that she can take care of the girls' wants. There is a department in connection with this room which is furnished with tables and chairs for a lunch room.

This is not done on an elaborate scale, but perhaps is elaborate, considering the people dealt with, as the majority of these girls are Polish, and are probably as rough and coarse as any working class. Since they have had good washing facilities, however, the fact has been noticeable that they appreciate and take advantage of these opportunities.

Each floor of the factory has been fitted up with arrangements of this kind for the use of the men, all of whom have been given private lockers. In this building all closets are ventilated by the exhaust fan system, which has made sanitary conditions practically perfect.

Sanitary drinking fountains were also put into this building,

[1] The Cleveland Hardware Co., Cleveland, Ohio. Vehicle Hardware. Organized 1881. Number Employés, 1200.

and after trial were considered so satisfactory that they were established throughout the entire factory.

Too often an industrialist thinks that any old thing will do for a water closet, inconvenient in its location and uncared for. Under such conditions it is no wonder that the men are careless and dirty. This is more the rule than the exception. Invariably in questioning why such conditions exist the answer is, "It doesn't pay to make better accommodations because the men abuse them." That this is not always the case finds illustration at the works of the Weston Electrical Instrument Company, where the water closets are ample in number, and so distributed as to be convenient of access from any part of the works; connected with each group is a lavatory. When the works were planned, some of the directors doubted the wisdom of so expensive a system; they feared the motive might not be appreciated or the property respected, and cited the fact that the water closets in the old works had met the customary fate. The president replied that in the old establishment there had been nothing to appeal to the personal self-respect of the men, or their respect for the property, and that he believed the proposed new departure would be received with favor by the employés; "Anyway," said he, "I am going to investigate this question myself," and he did. He went into all sections of New York City, from Carnegie Hall to the slums; and his report was that wherever he found superior water closets he found them respected. Consequently the company proceeded along the lines recommended, and the result is entirely satisfactory to every one concerned.

Although the subject of dining or lunch rooms for the workers is treated at length in the chapter on Hygiene, yet the provision of well-cooked, wholesome, appetizing food has a direct bearing on efficiency. The ill-effects of indigestion are well known by the educated and wealthy who can choose their food and the time for eating it; indigestion due to luncheons eaten cold at work benches or bolted at home during the short noon hour is an item which cannot be figured on cost tickets, but it exists nevertheless in every American factory. "I consider that the cost of maintaining our dining hall is more than made up by the increased efficiency of the men and women lunching there," is the testimony of the employer of some 3,500 people.

It may be that an employé leaves home without breakfast, or with scanty preparation for the day, or is unable to do justice to lunch. Instead of growing faint with hunger because of accident or the whims of an appetite, a bite to eat may be had even during working hours. At such a time the employés of the Acme White Lead and Color Works[1] have the privilege of a restaurant, which furnishes good coffee and tea with milk and sugar, at one cent a cup; soup is three cents a plate; hot meat and potatoes eight cents a portion, and desserts three cents.

As a stimulus to daily promptness and regularity in attendance, the Curtis Publishing Company[2] in making up the vacation list gives preference to those clerks who have the best record for attendance and punctuality. Each absence counts two points, and each lateness of less than one hour, one point, against the record of any clerk. The employés having the least number of points against them have first choice in the selection of vacation time. Points against employés of less than a year's engagement will be computed in proportion to their length of service. Employés who have been connected with the company for at least six months are entitled to a vacation at a convenient time, between June first and September first in each year, on the basis of one week-day for each month's service within the year; but no vacation in any case exceeds two weeks, unless at the expense of such employé and with the approval of the proper bureau manager or officer.

James R. Keiser[3] gives one week's vacation to all the time employés of one year's standing. In addition, he adds one day for each additional year of service till the vacation period

[1] Acme White Lead and Color Works, Detroit, Mich. Manufacturers Paints, Enamels, Stains, Varnishes. Organized 1884. Number Employés, about 500.

[2] The Curtis Publishing Co., Philadelphia, Pa. Magazine Publishers. Organized July 1, 1891. Number Employés, 1000.

[3] J. R. Keiser, Inc., New York City. Manufacturers Neckwear and Women's Belts. Organized January, 1892. Number Employés, 400.

reaches two weeks for those of six years' service. The fines for tardiness go to the fund for needy employés.

The C. Howard Hunt Pen Company[1] allows each operative who is regular in attendance every day of any calendar month one day's vacation with pay, so that operatives who have been fortunate enough to have worked every working day in the year, have two weeks' vacation with full pay for the time. The hours of labor have been reduced from ten to eight per day, and certain machinery formerly in use that caused considerable injury to operatives, has been replaced by modern types, which cause no further trouble of that kind.

A description of libraries would naturally come under the head of Education, but one industrialist has so widened the scope of the conventionalized library that it is a large factor in the increased efficiency of his plant.

"Whatever will help my employés to earn more money, will please me, because I well know that they are then in a position to be advanced to the next higher position," said an industrialist to me. This principle finds local application in a large factory, where through the widened use of the library it is possible to trace an almost direct line from the library to the suggestion box.

The men and women of this factory are coming to realize more and more that in the books in the cases on the first floor of Building No. 1, and on the shelves of the traveling libraries, lie the means to gain an education which may be denied them through adverse circumstances, or to ripen and extend the knowledge they already may possess. The means are right at hand, easy of access every working day in the year.

Means have been adopted whereby this information may be most conveniently distributed. For instance, should a skilled mechanic encounter a problem upon which he is not fully informed, and has not the time to look up the information, if he will notify the librarian, the information will be located and the proper book sent at the hour one of the traveling libraries visits his particular building.

[1] C. Howard Hunt Pen Co., Camden, N. J. Manufacturers Round-pointed Pens. Organized 1901. Number Employés, 175.

While it is desirable for the workmen to live near their business, there are many thousands for whom this is impossible. If an arrangement can be made for them to go and come from their work at the desired time, it is good administration for an employer to concern himself with this problem. At the present time the problem of transportation is a much-vexed question. The over-population of the industrial centres is forcing the workmen to seek homes in the suburbs.

One company whose factory is located about ten miles from Boston, induced the railroad to run a special train, stopping at all way-stations and bringing the employés directly into the yard. In consideration of a half fare, the company guaranteed the road $35 a day; but there has been no accounting with the railway company since the first month. It is estimated that the train is easily earning $50 to $60 a day, and carries between 500 and 600 of the employés. Other large industries arrange with the local trolley companies to send enough cars within their grounds so as to accommodate every one immediately on dismissal. In one instance, where it is impossible to come into the yard, the women are dismissed ten minutes earlier than the men, so that they may be sure to have seats.

The Illinois Central Railroad Company has an arrangement for operating special service from Du Quoin to the Davis, Forrester and Majestic Mines,[1] which are distant from Du Quoin two, two and one-half and four miles, respectively. Round trip service is operated daily except Sunday. Tickets are sold twice each month, containing 28 rides at $1.25 each, which makes the round-trip rate nine cents per day.

The Chicago and Northwestern Railway Company furnishes the Emerson Manufacturing Company a train morning and evening, for which the firm guarantees a certain amount to them. They furnish tickets to the employés at the rate of 54 rides for $1.50, or 26 rides for 75 cents. The distance is about a mile and a half. The service has been very satisfactory indeed. The cars are kept clean, and are heated and lighted in winter time.

[1] Majestic Coal and Coke Co., Du Quoin, Ill. Engaged in Coal Mining. Organized 1904. Number Employés, 350.

At an Ohio factory the women leave ten minutes before the men, and come an hour later in the morning to insure their having seats in the street cars. In the same establishment the elevators start ten minutes before work begins in the morning, and run ten minutes after work stops at night.

Marshall Field & Company [1] have established within the last year what is known as the "Beginners' Room" or school. When a salesman is employed he is first sent to this room, where he receives a day's instruction on their system, policy and methods. He is tested at the close of the day, and if unable to pass, is required to remain in the room another day. If at the end of the second day's instruction he is not qualified, the firm feels that he is not fitted for a position as salesman.

At the same store there is a new system for the employment of junior help, by means of which every one of the three thousand young people receives individual attention. This means that any young man or young woman employed to-day will be looked after for the next three months, so as to know how he or she is getting along. If not successful, it may be because unfitted for that particular line of work or department, in which case a transfer will be made, but if the person is progressing, he or she is called to the office and with a few words of encouragement given a raise of salary—this being done without request on the part of the employé. This system requires a large part of the time of one superintendent, but is resultful in that employés are made to feel that some one is really interested as to whether or not they make a success of life.

A trained nurse can be an important factor in efficiency, as instanced by the report from this department at the Waltham Watch Company,[2] where it is not simply an added expense but a real economy.

[1] Marshall Field & Co., Chicago, Ill. Dealing in and Manufacturing Merchandise. Organized March 7, 1901. Number Employés, 11,000.

[2] Waltham Watch Co., Waltham, Mass. Manufacturers Watch Movements and Watch Materials. Organized 1854. Number Employés, 4131.

"It is almost impossible to estimate the ground which has been gained in preventing absences from work, prevention of contagion and infection, especially at times when there is a prevalence of disease or possibly a threatened epidemic. During the recent epidemic of grip, six to eight cases were visited daily at the Adams House; these with outside calls making a total of thirteen daily; many of the girls were showing acute symptoms, all of them were anxious and worried and afraid of serious illness; some of these girls in attic rooms of lodging houses had been sick one or two days with no care except what could be given by a friend between working hours; these conditions were bettered—the faithful friend relieved of the care and anxious patients and friends encouraged and reassured. Simple cases responded to nursing treatment, others were referred to a physician; many of these girls recovered and were at work again within a week.

Although the work is largely medical, surgical and contagious cases have been attended and also several nervous cases, two cases of reported sore throat returned diphtheritic cultures and were immediately isolated at the contagious ward; these cases made a speedy recovery.

The service shows itself to be an avenue through which people may be protected against poor medical advice and provided with proper care; and also a provision which will ensure the proper using of the company's valuable supply of free beds at the hospital.

The gratitude of the lodging house people is touching, and those who suffer illness in their homes are also our strong friends. The service enables these incidents to take place at home, thus strengthening family ties, calling forth sympathy and devotion and placing responsibility where it belongs."

Comfort can be an efficiency promoter. In some processes it is possible for the operator to sit at her work while she may attend several machines; in some cases where the machines are some distance apart this would be impossible. To do this the Waltham Watch Company has provided chairs, with grooved rails at the bottom, so that they can slide along a little track, thus allowing the operative to tend the machines comfortably. They have nearly 150 of these special chairs that are fitted up at a cost of $3 each, in addition to the original cost of the chair. The foot rests are so planned as to be adjusted to any desired height. The general superintendent informs me that these chairs are used only in those cases where one operative attends two or more machines which necessitates moving from one to another. They are very much appreciated in his factory, and under similar conditions he thinks that they would prove of great advantage to operatives elsewhere. A somewhat similar system is used in another factory where high-backed stools are provided for the women at work. Where one woman supervises several pieces of machinery a gentle push slides the stool back and forth along the floor on a miniature railroad, saving steps and strength. Where intense, concentrated light is necessary, as in handling some of the microscopically minute parts of the instruments, the operator is provided with a conveniently adjustable and properly shaded incandescent lamp.

A business man appreciates the loss of a few minutes; with that end in view he insists that the employé shall begin the day on time, and exacts penalties for lateness. Slight physical ills if taken in time, yield at once to treatment, with benefit to employer and employé.

A physician in the employ of one store is at his office in the building from nine until twelve each morning, and all employés are free to consult him in case of need. His work includes all hygienic and sanitary questions and an examination, not unlike that which is common in questions of life insurance, for all the people entering the employ of the house. There is no expense to the employés in this consultation, which often saves a patient from going home and losing a day.

Seeing how other people do the same thing is a valuable experience, if the observer be a skilled worker and keen to note differences. The National Cash Register Company[1] recognizes the wisdom of observation as a proficiency promoter by organizing a policy of educational trips. The first was in 1902, a trip to New York, Boston, Philadelphia, Washington

[1] National Cash Register Co., Dayton, Ohio. Manufacturers Cash Registering Devices. Organized 1884. Number Employés, 3765.

and Pittsburg. There were two such trips in 1902 and one in 1903. Since then there have been frequent trips to Cincinnati, Chicago, New York, Boston and other eastern points, and also several western.

A recent announcement by this company indicates the mutuality of this plan:

"For the purpose of comparing our work with that of other factories, and also for the purpose of becoming acquainted with newer and better methods for producing work, this company is willing to send the following representatives, accompanied by their wives, on an educational trip through the East:

Two men from the No. 79 Assembling Department.

Two men from the No. 35 Assembling Department.

One man from Nos. 135, 172 and 400 departments.

One man from the Detail-Adding Department.

One man from the Tool Room.

One man from the Machine Room.

One man from the Mill Division Woodworking Department.

One man from the Cabinet Division Woodworking Department.

The men in these different departments are to select the men for these trips; that is, it will be left to a vote of the men in the departments as to whom they shall send. We hope this is only the beginning of educational trips for our workmen.

We want these men to look carefully into conditions in other places, and to inquire into their ways of doing work, prices paid for the work, and make a general report to the men upon their return. We want these men to make a fair and impartial report of their investigations to the men.

We want to do the best work in every department in this factory, and if any one else is doing better work than we are, or is doing things for his men that cause better work than we are doing, we want to know it.

We shall be glad to have the different departments take up this question as soon as possible and notify us as soon as selections have been made, and before November 23rd."

In the complexity of the relations of modern business, especially when there are literally thousands of workers in the same establishment, it is impossible for individual treatment of new workers in showing or telling them their duties, and yet they must know what they are, and what is expected of them. With that end in view some industrialists publish a book of general rules, which is given to each new employé. As typical, I have selected the general rules to be observed by employés of the First National Bank of Chicago:[1]

"Employés must be at their desks not later than 8:30 A.M. Saturdays, and 9:00 A.M. other days, and as much earlier as their work requires, and enter office through gate at timekeeper's desk. They will remain until their work is finished, and will not leave the office during business hours without the permission of the assistant cashier.

Absence from the office without permission must be avoided, but in the event of detention, either by sickness or accident, an early notice must be sent to the bank.

Employés must not use the telephone for private purposes during business hours except for matters of great importance; will defer all personal business until they have finished their day's work, and must not encourage their friends to visit them at the bank.

Smoking before 3:15 P. M. is strictly prohibited. Saturdays, 12:15.

Orderly and gentlemanly demeanor and invariable courtesy toward the public and fellow employés must be observed.

Discussion during business hours of matters not relating to the affairs of the bank is not permitted.

Neatness and order in care of books, desks and office furniture should be observed.

Secure a copy of the rules of the department in which you work, and read them carefully.

Every employé is expected to give his best efforts to the affairs of the bank, and to protect its interests in every way. A waste of time, stationery or other material will not be tolerated.

[1] First National Bank of Chicago, Chicago, Ill. Engaged in Banking. Organized June, 1863. Number Employés, 550.

Clerks are not permitted to traffic among their fellow employés for themselves, nor in the interests of persons outside of the bank.

While in the service of the bank employés are cautioned not to enter into outside business enterprises. Speculation, betting or gambling in any form will not be tolerated.

Avoid getting into debt. If financial assistance is needed however, state your case to the assistant cashier. Borrowing money at usurious rates of interest is forbidden.

Late hours and the habitual use of intoxicating drinks, and the frequenting of saloons and places of questionable resort will be deemed a sufficient cause for dismissal.

Employés must keep in strict confidence whatever knowledge they may acquire of the affairs of the bank and refer all questions addressed to them upon such matters to the officers for reply.

When employés are promoted, or their duties changed, they must see that their successors understand the work of the desk vacated, and if after a reasonable trial, the successor seems unqualified, the assistant cashier or department manager must be notified.

It is the duty of employés to submit to the assistant cashier any facts of which they may become possessed concerning a fellow clerk, and the credit department concerning a customer, in cases where the knowledge of such facts would tend to protect or advance the interests of the bank.

Employés must look at the bulletin board daily for any new rules, instructions or notices that may be posted. Ignorance of rules or instructions will not be considered sufficient excuse for failure to comply with same.

Employés will take luncheon in the bank dining room, where not to exceed twenty minutes will be allowed. Smoking is not permitted in the dining room.

The senior clerks should be particular in the observance of the rules of the bank as an example to the younger employés.

All employés over 18 years of age must be members of the Bank Pension Fund. Copies of rules and regulations of the pension fund may be had upon application to the assistant cashier.

Attention is called to the Clerks' Savings Association, which allows interest on savings accounts.

Employés are invited to make use of the bank library, in which will be found standard works on banking, finance, economics, commercial law and various other subjects relating to banking. Those wishing to take books home for a limited time may do so by first having them registered.

The officers will be glad to extend a considerate hearing to any employé who may desire to confer with them upon any matter, either of private or official nature.

A reliable character and intelligent and faithful discharge of duty are the best recommendations for advancement."

The rule book at Marshall Field & Company contains 111 pages and fits comfortably into a man's pocket. The type is large and the spaces are wide. The reason for the book is concisely set forth in the introduction, which states that:

"The important part of any rule is the spirit of it. This is gained by understanding the wisdom and necessity of the rule, and not by mere obedience because it is a rule. No rule seems hard when you see that it is wise—worked out from experience, made necessary by existing conditions.

The object of a rule is not to abridge the rights of any one, but to point out the path which experience has taught is the wise one to follow. The traveler making his way over unaccustomed roads is grateful for the guide posts which tell him the way to his destination—he never complains when the sign at the crossing tells him to go the up-hill way, for he is glad the sign is there, and obeys cheerfully because he knows he is on the right road.

The aim of these rules is to conduct this great institution in the most harmonious manner; to give to our employés the benefit of long experience, to save them retracing unguided steps, to enable them to grow in the knowledge of sound business principles and become a credit to themselves and the house.

Keep close to the Rule Book; follow out the spirit as well as the letter of its advice, and you will find yourself on the right road to satisfactory and praiseworthy service."

The opening rules are simple:

"Become thoroughly informed regarding the stock in which you are placed. Learn the names of the goods, where they are kept in stock, their qualities, sizes, prices, for what they are used, etc.

Learn from the manager of your section, or his assistant, what is expected of you, and as quickly as possible, make your actions correspond with these duties.

Do not hesitate to ask for information upon any point of business which requires explanation, either of the manager of your section, his assistant, the floormen, the division superintendent, or of the office of the general management.

The strictest propriety and greatest courtesy are rigorously required under all circumstances and upon all matters, whether customers wish to purchase, or have finished and request the final care of purchase tickets; whether to exchange merchandise or return the same for credit; to inform themselves regarding the article on sale, or simply to visit the different sections. Negligence in manner or in speech will not be allowed under any circumstances.

We must have the best efforts of all salespeople and others toward removing from the minds of all any feeling that our employés are sometimes independent, indifferent or lacking in intelligent attention. Attention consists of good manners carefully directed to satisfy customers' wishes. It means showing goods politely, introducing them in a gentlemanly or ladylike manner. Whether customers buy or not, whether they are acquaintances or strangers, whether richly dressed or poorly dressed, or whether the goods are being paid for or charged, we must insist that absolutely no difference be shown."

William Filene's Sons Company,[1] Boston, print on the outside of their small book of rules:

"Ignorance of rules is no excuse. Know the rules and live up to them. You have the power to change these rules at any

[1] Wm. Filene's Sons Co., Boston, Mass. Manufacturers Women's, Misses' and Children's Ready-to-Wear Apparel. Organized 1851. Number Employés, 600.

time if you can get a majority of your fellow employés to vote with you at the meeting of The Filene Coöperative Association."

It takes a workman some days to familiarize himself with a new factory or workshop, especially if there are large numbers of employés. It is therefore essential that the new worker should be promptly informed of the conditions and requirements of his new work. For that object, the Baldwin Locomotive Works[1] posts this notice:

"ORDER

Cleanliness and good order must be observed throughout the works.

Each workman is required to keep his bench, vise, lathe, forge, machine, or whatever tool and place at which he is employed, cleaned and free from rubbish.

Machines must be kept clean at all times.

Particular care must be taken to put all combustible matter, such as oily waste, etc., in a safe place to prevent any chance of fire.

All obsolete or imperfect castings, forgings, lumber, etc., must be removed to the proper place at once.

All castings and forgings, as soon as ready, must be delivered to the proper department for finishing.

All work, as soon as completed at one machine, must be delivered to the next succeeding machine.

LABORERS

A workman will not be allowed to call a laborer to perform any part of his work that can be done by himself.

Laborers are not employed to wait upon workmen, but to assist where more than one man is required.

BEHAVIOR

Smoking, reading or loitering during working hours are positively prohibited.

[1] Burnham, Williams & Co., Philadelphia, Pa. Baldwin Locomotive Works. Locomotives, Electric Locomotives, Electric Trucks. Organized 1831. Number Employés, 18,500.

Abusive, vulgar or profane language, quarreling and fighting will result in immediate dismissal.

WORKING TIME

Each workman is required to be at his place and commence work when the signal is given, and will be fined one hour for preparing to quit before the stop signal is given. He must report himself to the time office and his foreman when late.

Strict account will be kept of late time, and those coming in after 7:00 A.M. and 1:00 P.M. will be fined one hour.

Those habitually late, and those absenting themselves without notice of such intention to their foreman, will not be retained in employ.

Those leaving the works before 12 M. and 6 P.M. must report to their foreman and the time office to secure their time for the day.

The week of labor will close at 6 P.M. on Saturday, and payment of wages for the same will be made on the regular pay day in the following week, at a fixed rate per hour or piece.

Work necessary to be done before or after the regular hours on Saturday, will be rated at time and a quarter. Regular night workmen will be paid for single time only.

TIMEKEEPING AND PAYING

Workmen are required to report to the timekeepers as follows: Number of hours per day; name of job and machine or engine; time employed on it; when commenced and when finished. Piece workmen are required to return and charge all their completed work in the week in which it is finished. They should see personally that timekeepers get their correct time daily, and must also enter, on their slates, each evening before leaving the works, their time for the day. No time or pay will be allowed unless these particulars are complied with.

Those expecting to be absent on Monday should report their time for the week to the foreman and time office before leaving the works on Saturday, and those absent on Monday without having so reported, should send their preceding week's time to the time office on that date.

On entering the service, each employé is required to record

his name in the paymaster's register. Unless so registered, he cannot draw pay.

Wages will be paid on the regular pay day, after signal to quit work is given.

Application for payment of wages will be made in person to the paymaster.

Personally report to the paymaster before leaving the works on pay day, any errors in wages paid.

In case of deficiency, the balance due will be enclosed in the envelope for the following week.

Those expecting to be absent on pay day and wishing to arrange for any member of their families to draw their pay, must personally notify the paymaster.

A workman running two machines on piece work will not be paid day work for time lost by machine on account of break-down or while waiting for work.

WORK

Each workman must know, before commencing a piece of work, that it will finish to the sizes marked on the sketch or card given him, whether the work is to be completed by him or others.

Spoiled or defective work must be immediately reported to the foreman.

The damage for spoiled work will be charged to the workman, unless occurring from a reasonable cause, and being made known at once to the foreman.

A workman accepting a piece of work from another to finish, will be held responsible for any errors in work that have been made by preceding workman.

Work must be kept neatly piled and properly marked, and each succeeding workman must see that the mark is continued on work finished by him.

TOOLS

Tools of a general character, such as drills, reamers, taps, etc., must be returned to their proper places, in good order, or if damaged must be reported at once. Careless damage will be charged to the workman.

Workmen are not allowed to make any new tools without the

consent of their foreman, or use the tools of others without the consent of the workman or foreman.

Each employé is responsible for the tools placed in his charge on commencing work, and upon leaving the employ he must deliver the key of his box or drawer, and satisfy the foreman that his stock of tools is complete and in proper order before a settlement will be made.

Economy in the use of material of all kinds, oil, waste, emery, files, etc., is strictly enjoined on every workman.

New material must not be cut when pieces can be had that will answer, and all surplus material must be immediately returned to the proper place.

When a new file is needed the old one must be returned."

All suggestions at the National Cash Register Company are written on duplicate machines. The original is kept by the employé, while the duplicate goes to the company. It acknowledges all suggestions, which are then sent to the foreman or supervisor of the department to which it pertains for investigation, opinion or comment. The suggestions with the comments go before the committee, where it is decided to adopt or reject them. If adopted the employé is notified and paid one dollar.

In this way suggestions go direct from an employé to the management, where an unbiased investigation is made. Those received from factory employés are handled by a committee of factory officials best qualified to pass on the merits of the same, and those received from office employés go to the committee of officers of the company and heads of departments. Each of these committees has eight members and a secretary, whose duty it is to receive and investigate all suggestions before bringing them before the committee for decision.

All suggestions are numbered and entered in a book. The secretary then refers it to the head of the department to which the maker of the suggestion belongs, or to the party most directly interested, not disclosing the name of the suggester. It frequently happens that a suggestion concerns more than one department, when it is investigated in a similar manner through all of them, and its bearing on all considered. The original suggestion is never sent with the correspondence during the investigation, but is retained in the office of the committee, and a copy is made for investigation purposes, or the subject-matter embodied in the correspondence.

The regular meeting date for the committee is the first Friday in each month, at which time all suggestions are taken up separately and decided upon.

In case the committee does not agree with the reports of the various departments upon a suggestion, a further investigation is ordered, or the suggestion is adopted or rejected, according to the views of the committee.

If a suggestion is rejected and the employé thinks the committee has not understood its import he may give a further explanation, and ask for another investigation, which is cheerfully granted. Also, if a suggestion is rejected, and later on its adoption is found advisable, the employé first making the suggestion receives the credit.

Every three months, or at the end of each quarter, the best suggestions are selected from those adopted during the quarter and a joint meeting of the committees handling factory and office suggestions is held for the purpose of awarding quarterly prizes.

In addition to the quarterly prize which is paid in gold, each employé receiving such prize is presented with a diploma and a bronze medal of suitable design. These quarterly prizes, diplomas and medals are distributed at a special meeting at which all employés are invited to be present. Talks are given by the various officers of the company, outlining the value of the suggestion system, thanking employés for the interest shown and encouraging them further to increase their efforts in this direction.

In reply to my inquiry, how he came to adopt the suggestion system at his factory, Mr. Patterson said: "A weigh-master who used to be with me in the coal business was working over there in the factory cleaning castings, and in a talk with him one day I asked him why he was working in that position, and why he didn't bring himself to the attention of his foreman and earn promotion through suggesting some changes. I asked him if there were no things over there which he could see could be changed, and he said, 'Lots of them, but,' he said, 'there's no use in making any suggestions, for the foreman would only take all the credit for them, and would think I was trying to get his job.' I thought to myself, 'There's sense in what this workman says,' and I decided then and there to try to get some plan whereby these suggestions could be brought directly to the attention of the management.

"The suggestion scheme has become an established thing in the factory now, and we would not think of abandoning it. Of the 6000 suggestions received each year, we are able to use, in whole or part, about one-third, so that we are well repaid for the time and expense given toward the proper carrying out of this idea."

Despite the fact that the factory methods and machines have been under the closest scrutiny for years, the net saving on suggestions made during the first six months of 1906 amounted to nearly $15,000. Besides suggestions which save money, there are hundreds offered and adopted whose money value can not be reckoned.

The following notice was freely circulated among the employés:

"Any employé making a suggestion regarding work or modifying instructions which he has no authority to change, is entitled to a prize of $1 for the suggestion if adopted.

Suggestions lead to promotion and increased salaries. They show an interest in our work and organization and a capacity for greater responsibilities.

We invite suggestions upon mechanical improvements, suggestions which will increase sales, increase profits, increase cash on hand, decrease competition, decrease opposition to our methods, or which will improve the work in any department.

Suggestions which will effect a saving on the pay roll and the cost of manufacture will be particularly appreciated. When requested, suggestions will be regarded as confidential.

QUARTERLY PRIZES

Twenty-eight additional prizes, until further notice, will be awarded at the end of each quarter for the most valuable suggestions received during that period.

First Prize ....$	50.00	
Second Prize	30.00	
Five Prizes, $20 each	100.00	
Eight Prizes, $15 each	120.00	
Ten Prizes, $10 each	100.00	
	———	$400.00

FOREMEN'S PRIZES

Heads and assistant heads of departments and office managers will not receive the one dollar award or compete for the above quarterly prizes, but can compete for the following prizes offered for the best suggestions adopted:

First Prize ....$	50.00	
Second Prize	30.00	
Third Prize	20.00	
	———	$100.00
		———
		$500.00

Members of the board of directors, the factory committee and district managers are not included in the above."

A favorite method of efficiency promotion, whether in business or other lines of human activity, is the offer of some kind of prize. For example, the Pennsylvania Railroad Company has had a system of premiums for the best line and surface at the time of inspection, which is held annually.

1. A premium of $1200; $800 to the supervisor and $400 to the assistant supervisor having the best line and surface between Pittsburg and Jersey City and between Philadelphia and Washington during the entire year since the last annual inspection.

2. Four premiums of $800 each—$600 to the supervisor and $200 to the assistant supervisor having the best line and surface on each of the main line Superintendents' Divisions between Pittsburg and Jersey City and between Philadelphia and Washington during the year since the last annual inspection.

3. A premium of $1000—$700 to the supervisor and $300

to the assistant supervisor, of that supervisor's division which has shown the greatest improvement in line and surface during the year on the main line between Pittsburg and Jersey City and between Philadelphia and Washington.

4. A premium of $100 is awarded to the supervisor for the best main line yard, both with reference to line and surface and general appearance of the yard, between Pittsburg and Jersey City and Philadelphia and Washington at the date of the annual inspection.

The award of the above premiums is the result of periodical inspections which are made during the year between Pittsburg and Jersey City and between Philadelphia and Washington by a committee consisting of the Chief Engineer of Maintenance of Way (who is chairman), the Engineer of Maintenance of Way, and three Division Superintendents; the results are announced at the termination of a general inspection which is made usually in the early part of October by the operating officers over the main line. On the Superintendents' Divisions the award to the foremen is made upon the recommendation of the Assistant Engineer of the Division.

This system of awarding premiums annually has had a stimulating effect and has proven a success.

The A. B. Chase Company,[1] Norwalk, Ohio, offer four annual prizes for the best suggestions for improvement on their instruments without increasing the cost; the best suggestions for improvement that can be utilized regardless of cost; and the best suggestions for reducing the cost, or for economy in production without detriment to the quality of the work; and fourth, for the best suggestions not included in the other three classes for improving the business or the condition of the employés.

After they had continued their suggestion department for some three or four years, the firm found that some of the foremen objected, and made it unpleasant for the men who made suggestions, and caused a little friction. Now the men are paid $5 or $10 for any suggestions that they may make that can be utilized, and send them direct to the office so that the

[1] The A. B. Chase Co., Norwalk, Ohio. Manufacturers of Pianos and Player Pianos. Organized September 1, 1875. Number of Employés, 165.

foreman need not know who is making the suggestion. He only knows that the firm wants certain things done.

If any of the workmen invents anything new worthy of a patent, the company gets it patented and gives him a half interest in it, and in this way they are able to keep the men always interested in improvements and the advancement of their work, and their hearty coöperation in everything that is done.

A premium of five per cent. is paid on the weekly earnings of all engaged in the actual manufacture of goods, for turning out work which is neat, and which does not require any alteration or mending, in the establishment of H. S. Peters.[1] There is also a limited form of profit sharing, where those admitted to participation in it are all employés who fill responsible positions. The amount allotted to each is dependent on the importance of the position occupied by him in the business. This plan has not yet been worked out to include all employés, because the firm is doubtful as to the wisdom of such a course.

A system of premiums for regular and faithful work in the sizing department, where the roving habits of the workmen, many of whom were of foreign birth, had become a source of serious annoyance and inconvenience to the management, was introduced in 1897 by the John B. Stetson Company.[2] To remedy these conditions it was decided to offer to the men who worked steadily throughout the year an amount equal to five per cent. of the total wages earned, this amount to be presented to such employés in the form of a Christmas gift. Under the operation of this plan 35 per cent. of the sizers employed in 1897 remained until the end of the year. For the three succeeding years the premium was increased to ten per cent., with the result that the number of steady workers increased from 50 to 80 per cent. of the entire number. In 1901 and 1902 with 15 per cent. premium paid, the percentage reached 88, while during the later years, from 90 to 99 per cent. of the total force

[1] H. S. Peters, Dover, N. J. Manufacturer Overalls. Organized January 1, 1891. Number Employés, 76.

[2] John B. Stetson Co., Philadelphia, Pa. Manufacturers Hats, felt, stiff and soft. Organized 1891. Number Employés, 4709.

in the sizing department received 20 per cent. increase on their wages as a reward for faithful service.

At a meeting of the stockholders in the fall of 1902, it was decided by the John B. Stetson Company to place at the disposal of the president and the board of directors 5000 shares of the increased common capital stock, of a par value of $100 each, to be used by them for distribution among the company's employés under such terms and conditions as they deemed proper. The plan as adopted differs from the usual form of profit sharing in that the allotment of stock to an employé is not conditional upon his age or upon the length of time he has been in the company's employ, nor is the amount of stock allotted to him dependent on the salary he receives. Moreover, the stock eventually becomes the absolute property of the employé without any expense to him whatever. The following statement concerning the operations of the plan has been furnished by the company:

"Certificates for the allotted stock are issued in the name of five trustees, and the certificates are not transferred to the names of the individuals until the expiration of fifteen years, except in the event of the death of the employé or his severing his connection with the company.

As dividends on the allotted stock are declared and paid, each individual is credited with his proportion of the dividends less five per cent. on the balance due on the stock at the close of the year. When the accumulation of dividends less the interest charge amounts to the par value of the stock, the employé is then paid the full amount of the dividends that are declared each year, but, as stated above, he cannot come into possession of the certificate itself until fifteen years have elapsed. The object of this provision is at once apparent—it insures a steady income for the employé so long as he is in their employ, by preventing him from disposing of his stock.

The employé has the privilege of drawing from the dividends declared each year an amount equal to five per cent. of the par value of the stock. If he avails himself of this privilege the stock is not paid for as quickly as if he were to allow all the dividends to accumulate.

In the event of death, there is handed to the executors a

certificate of stock of the par value of the amount that stands to the employé's credit on the books. If the employment of the individual is terminated because of his physical or mental condition preventing him discharging his duties, settlement is made in the same way as in the event of death; but if the employé is discharged for cause, there is handed him a check for the amount at that time to his credit on the books. That the difference of paying by check and by certificate may be understood, it is necessary to state that at this time the stock is selling on the market for $350. While the market value of the stock fluctuates, it has been allotted the employés at par, $100 per share."

The presentation of life insurance policies to employés is another form of reward adopted by this company. These policies are mainly on the 20 and 25 year endowment plan, the premiums being paid by the company, and the accumulated dividends turned over to the beneficiary when the policy becomes due. At the present time there are in force 20 policies of insurance, two of which are for $10,000 and the remainder $5000 each. Since the adoption of the plan nine policies, aggregating $200,000, have matured.

December 24, 1907, the tenth semi-annual bonus payment at the Remington Typewriter[1] factory was made in the Factory Hall, when $13,800 in gold was distributed among 276 selected workmen, including 2 thirty-year; 13 twenty-five-year; 4 twenty-year; 84 fifteen-year, and 137 ten-year men.

The 1700 employés in general are paid strictly according to ability and industry irrespective of length of service. In addition badges are given to all over ten years in continuous employment. A bonus of $100 in gold per year is paid semi-annually to those only with ten years' service or more, who are more than ordinarily efficient, diligent and loyal during every six months as measured by their history and labor cards, which are carefully posted during each half year.

In the first bonus distribution, June, 1903, 240 employés participated; in the tenth distribution, December, 1907, 149 of these were still participating, while 127 new names had, in

[1] The Remington Typewriter Works, Ilion, Ill. Manufacturers Remington Typewriter. Organized 1873. Number Employés, 1700.

the interval, reached the 10-year service group and qualified in other respects.

BONUS PAYMENTS

Bonus men and period of Continuous Service

Date	10 yr.	15 yr.	20 yr.	25 yr.	30 yr.	Total	Amount
June '03	156	55	20	6	3	240	$12,000
Dec. '03	167	57	21	6	3	254	12,700
June '04	148	77	25	4	5	259	12,950
Dec. '04	133	83	26	3	5	250	12,500
June '05	95	101	28	2	3	229	11,450
Dec. '05	103	103	28	8	3	245	12,250
June '06	130	90	35	6	3	264	13,200
Dec. '06	131	91	38	6	3	269	13,450
June '07	145	94	36	11	3	289	14,450
Dec. '07	137	84	40	13	2	276	13,800
Total	1350	885	297	60	33	2575	$128,750
			Total extra bonus and prizes				2,200
			Total bonus and prizes .				$130,950

ANALYSIS OF 240 BONUS EMPLOYÉS AT FIRST DISTRIBUTION, JUNE, 1903, AND OF STATUS OF SAME MEN AT TENTH DISTRIBUTION IN DECEMBER, 1907

Description	Groups					
	30 yr.	25 yr.	20 yr.	15 yr.	10 yr.	Total
Employés receiving bonus June, 1903	3	6	20	55	156	240
June, 1903, bonus employés still on bonus list at December, 1907	..	3	14	40	92	149
Reasons why 91 June, 1903, bonus employés are not on December, 1907, bonus list:						
Left and returned . . .	..	..	..	6	5	11
Efficiency reduced . . .	..	..	..	1	4	5
Transferred to branches . .	..	..	..	..	4	4
Left for other employment .	..	..	1	1	7	8
Resigned and retired . .	..	1	..	1	9	11
Resigned to engage in own business	..	..	1	1	8	10
Resigned owing to illness .	2	1	2	4	16	25
Died	1	1	2	2	11	17
Employés receiving bonus at December, 1907 . . .	2	13	40	84	137	276

The C. Howard Hunt Pen Company has placed a certain amount of stock in the name of the heads of every department in the works, and also its leading salesmen. The stock is to be paid for by dividends earned, with the only restriction that, if the holder should die, the company reserves the privilege of buying the stock at whatever amount has been paid for it, plus an equal share of any surplus that should have accrued to the stock.

Early in 1904 the business of the Gibson Iron Company[1] was incorporated; out of a capital of $60,000, $5000 worth of stock was divided among ten of the leading employés who were thought worthy of receiving it. The recipients of the stock were not asked to pay for it, their long and faithful service as employés entitling them, in the judgment of the company, to receive it without cost. However, no stock of the company is sold outside of the corporation, nor would a single share of it be sold at any price. With employés who receive the stock, the company has made the provision, by agreement, that for the consideration of one-half of its face value in spot cash, the stock shall revert back to the company at the expiration of active service in its employment, or at the death of the holder; so that under no conditions can the stock go to anyone outside of the present corporation. The company has also pledged itself that merit and quality in the conduct and work of its employés shall continue to be recognized by further gifts of stock.

Parke, Davis & Company[2] have set aside 4000 shares of treasury stock, par value $100,000, to be sold at book value, which is one-half of the selling market value, to traveling salesmen, department chiefs and other employés whom they desire to retain permanently in their service. Six years ago they did the same thing, setting aside 4000 shares of capital stock for the benefit of their best talent. At that time the money was borrowed for the purchasers, who were charged five per cent. interest.

The American Swiss File and Tool Company[3] allots stock

[1] Gibson Iron Works Co., Jersey City, N. J. Iron Foundry, Pattern and Machine Shop. Organized 1881. Number of Employés, 50.

[2] Parke, Davis & Co., Detroit, Mich. Manufacturing Pharmacists, Chemists and Biologists. Organized 1866. Number Employés, between 3500 and 4000.

[3] American Swiss File and Tool Co., Elizabeth, N. J. Manufacturers High Class Files. Organized July 17, 1899. Number Employés, 102.

to energetic and intelligent employés. The stock is given fully paid up, and a part of the profits of the business are set aside to pay for it.

The company does all in its power to encourage its employés to become members of building and loan associations, and the workmen generally show a disposition to follow the advice given them in this respect. The company also contributes liberally to the maintenance of local hospitals, to which employés have the right of admission and treatment free of charge.

The families of deserving men are looked after in case of sickness, and in many instances half the ordinary wages of workmen suffering through a long period of sickness has been paid to their families. In such cases the money paid has been regarded as an advance in anticipation of future earnings, and a small percentage of the wages which accrue after recovery is deducted until the money is returned. This course is followed in accordance with the known and expressed wishes of the employés who have been so assisted. They seem to feel that self-respect requires that they should not be under an obligation which they have the ability to repay.

At the Patton Paint Company [1] there are two councils, composed of the heads of the various office and factory departments, meeting once a week. All matters for the improvement of business methods and the comfort and betterment of the employés are considered by these councils. The councils' recommendations are submitted to the active head of the company, who approves or disapproves pretty much as does the Governor of the State.

The Pilgrim Steam Laundry Company [2] is another concern to adopt the cabinet form of industrial government. A semimonthly conference of heads of firm and overseeing help is held with a view to the adoption of new plans and the rectification of wrong policies. A factory committee composed of employés elected from each department to look after details concerning the work and workers, holds a weekly meeting.

[1] Patton Paint Co., Milwaukee, Wis. Paint Manufacturers. Organized August, 1900. Number Employés, 350.

[2] The Pilgrim Steam Laundry Co., Brooklyn, N. Y. Organized 1894. Number Employés, 200.

In asking a large industrialist, who was among the first to see the value of a stated factory publication, what was his opinion of such a periodical, and whether it was good business, he replied: "Our publications are sent to every member of the selling force throughout the world, to every employé, and to a selected list of non-employés who are especially interested in us. It is difficult to express or measure the value we place upon it, but we believe it to be one of the most essential publications we get out, and are constantly striving to improve it. We cannot, as we would like to do, have conventions and personal meetings with our selling force every week or two, but our monthly fills the gap, disseminating the latest information of what we are doing and what we are trying to accomplish, and keeps all parts of our great organization in close touch. It does keep us in close touch with our employés; that is its principal function. It tells the selling force on the one hand what the making and recording forces are doing, and on the other hand keeps the latter informed of what the selling force is doing. Not only that, but it keeps the agents in one part of the country informed of what those in other districts are doing, and creates a healthy stimulus or competition among them. It is one of the best channels for maintaining enthusiasm and interest among employés, and this can be demonstrated by noting the eagerness among the employés when the publication is distributed, and the anxious inquiry if some individual fails to receive his copy."

This company has issued such publications as:

N. C. R.—first issue 1892.

Woman's Welfare—first issue September, 1902.

Men's Welfare—first issue July, 1904.

Bulletin—first issue June 24, 1904.

Factory News—first issue November 22, 1905.

In 1898 the first number of the *Chameleon* appeared, a pamphlet published on the 15th of each month by the Sherwin-Williams Company [1] in the interest and for the benefit of their staff. It is attractively printed, full of illustrations, and is among the best publications for employés.

The staff publication of the T. B. Laycock Manufacturing

[1] Sherwin-Williams Co., Cleveland, Ohio. Paint and Varnish Makers. Organized 1866. Number Employés, 2000.

Company,[1] *Factory News*, has this on its title page: "It's right because it is our factory motto, and our motto is right in principle, precept and practice. It's right to accord employés that full measure of courtesy and respect which is expected from them; and the management that fails to see and appreciate this needs more light."

The first issue was November, 1899, and it has been most successful in promoting a closer and more sympathetic touch, as well as a mutual feeling of good will, between employers, officers, heads of departments and employés.

The H. J. Heinz Company[2] started *The 57* in January, 1899, as a means of bringing their employés in touch with one another, and teaching them the higher principles of life that lead to happiness and success. It is published under the supervision of the firm, who report that its purpose is being fulfilled and results in much good to both employer and employé through the interest which each manifests on behalf of the other.

The *Little Blue Flag* first appeared in April, 1901, as a periodical of the Lowe Bros. Company,[3] of Dayton, Ohio. Its object is a closer and more frequent touch with the agents, and a means of interesting the employés, who read it generally. The firm reports that it is accomplishing the object for which it was published.

Burt's Box Bulletin[4] appeared in April, 1903, for the mutual good of the employés and the more rapid and correct filling of orders. The circulation is 2000 copies.

The Colorado Fuel and Iron Company[5] found that they must have some medium through which their thousands of employés, scattered over hundreds of miles of territory, could be reached.

[1] The T. B. Laycock Manufacturing Co., Indianapolis, Ind. Manufacturers Metallic Bedsteads, Davenports, Spring Beds, etc. Organized 1890. Number Employés, 400.

[2] H. J. Heinz Co., Pittsburg, Pa. Manufacturers Food Products. Organized 1869. Number Employés, 4346.

[3] The Lowe Bros. Co., Dayton, Ohio. Paint and Varnish Makers. Organized 1862. Number Employés, 200.

[4] F. N. Burt Co., Buffalo, N. Y. Paper Box Specialists. Incorporated September 1, 1906. Number Employés, 1800.

[5] The Colorado Fuel and Iron Co., Denver, Colo. Dealers in Coal, Coke, Iron and Steel. Organized 1892. Number Employés, 15,000.

For this purpose, a weekly magazine, *Camp and Plant*, was established, which has proved an invaluable aid to the company in bringing the various camps and works in closer touch, and in furnishing a medium through which the people can be reached.

On account of the expense, the weekly magazine has been discontinued, and its place taken by *Bulletin, Sanitary and Sociological*, published monthly by the medical and sociological departments of the Colorado Fuel and Iron Company for distribution among the employés of the company. Each bulletin contains practical suggestions and useful information upon vital health and life problems. Scientific names are eliminated and unfamiliar terms avoided as far as expedient. It is hoped the bulletins will be found of interest and widely read. School teachers are urged and requested to study these bulletins and impart the information therein contained to their pupils, and the local doctors are asked to communicate the same to the adults.

The Steel Works Club Library Bulletin was issued in 1904 to enable the members of the club, which is composed of the employés of the Illinois Steel Company,[1] to keep posted on matters pertaining to the library.

The personnel of the First National Bank of Chicago consists of 550 employés. Among so large a force it seems desirable that there should be some means of intercommunication, in order that it might not be all work and no play for Jack. This desire expressed itself in a paper called *The Review*, which is published monthly by the employés of the bank. The salutatory in the first number, May 1, 1904, stated that this bank, up to the present time, had taken the lead, not only in the amount of its total deposits, not only as a powerful economic force in performing the banking operations of thousands of individuals, firms and other banks, but also in its internal management. Here a liberal and far-sighted policy has always been one of its chief characteristics.

"To enumerate: The First National Bank has at this writing its own library, its own printing office, its own dining room, its own savings fund association, and last but not by

[1] Illinois Steel Co., Joliet, Ill. Manufacturers Steel and Steel Products. Organized May 2, 1889. Number Employés, 20,000.

any means the least, its own pension fund. As some one has so aptly expressed it 'we are a community by ourselves.' What is more natural, then, than that we should have our own newspaper?"

Strawbridge & Clothier's *Store Chat*, edited by and in the interest of the employés of Strawbridge & Clothier,[1] is published for them occasionally, in the hope of promoting the general welfare and bringing each into closer relations with all. The leading article stated that "it is—an experiment. Its success even in its continued existence will depend upon the interest with which it is received by the fellow employés."

Thought and Work, a monthly journal of mutual interest and information, is issued by the employés of the Siegel-Cooper Company,[2] the first number appearing April 1, 1903. In the salutatory it was stated, "It will be the aim of the journal to be self-supporting, hence a price of three cents a copy has been made. As life in a large store typifies the countless variations of mercantile endeavor, and as its ramifications extend socially in many directions, this journal should prove interesting and uplifting to the 4000 workers on the pay roll of this establishment."

The Monaghan Mills,[3] Greenville, S. C., began in 1904 the publication of a semi-monthly, *Men of Monaghan*, as a medium of communication between the executive and the rest of the force. It is edited by the secretary of the factory Y. M. C. A., and is generally read.

Its name has been changed to *The Monaghan*, but as the editorial states, "This does not mean that the policy has been changed, but as it is a paper gotten out for all the people of the village and not the men only it has been thought best to eliminate the 'Men' part of the name in order that there may be no misunderstanding the purpose. We propose to print all the interesting things about the churches, school, lodges, the two associations and everything that happens in the village

[1] Strawbridge & Clothier, Philadelphia, Pa. Dealers in General Merchandise, Wholesale and Retail. Organized July 1, 1868. Number Employés, 5500.

[2] Siegel-Cooper Co., New York City. Dealers in General Merchandise. Organized 1896. Number Employés, 3300.

[3] Monaghan Mills, Greenville, S. C. Manufacturers Cotton Goods. Organized 1900. Number Employés, 700.

which we think will interest the people, always giving one page to news items."

The F. C. A. Echo is issued monthly by the Filene Coöperative Association, Boston, Mass., at 60 cents per year, 5 cents a copy. The Filene Coöperative Association is an organization of all the employés of the William Filene's Sons Company.

The company is in no way responsible for articles appearing in the columns, as it assumes no voice in the management of the paper, and does not see the publication until it is printed.

The editors announce that the paper is open to all for contributions of news items, stories, poems, or sketches of any kind, and that they aim to make it a newspaper with educational features rather than an educational paper with news features.

Among Ourselves is a monthly magazine devoted to the interests of the employés of Montgomery Ward & Company,[1] Chicago, and was organized in 1905.

Store Topics was started in 1906, as a paper "for the store people, of the store people, and by the store people" of Jordan, Marsh & Company. Its intended mission is to present each month, in as interesting and readable a way as possible, personal items and happenings of general interest to the army of employés in the store; to be a medium for exchanging ideas and imparting information that relates to practical storekeeping and might tend to increase the usefulness of each and all; to establish a closer bond of good-fellowship and coöperation among the many workers who are enrolled under the Jordan-Marsh business banner. That was its object when first launched—it is its fixed aim to-day.

The Met is published the first and third Wednesdays of each month by the publication committee of the employés of the Metropolitan Trust and Savings Bank,[2] Chicago.

In a circular issued October 17, 1907, Paul Foerster of the publication committee states:

"*The Met* is not an advertisement of, for or by the bank. It is a newspaper of the bank—just as the *Chicago Daily News* or *Evening Post* or *American* are newspapers of the city."

[1] Montgomery Ward & Co., Chicago, Ill. Catalogue or Mail Order House. Organized 1872. Number Employés, 5250.

[2] Metropolitan Trust and Savings Bank, Chicago. Organized November, 1892. Number Employés, 53.

If it were more generally understood that the workmen have very few places where they can go for wholesome recreation or social gatherings after working hours, employers would appreciate the situation and provide places, in some instances allowing them the privilege, under certain restrictions, of meeting in the factory, setting aside a special room. A notable illustration is the club room provided in the Sherwin-Williams paint factory in Cleveland, Ohio; while the H. J. Heinz Company has devoted two stories in one of its new buildings to a hall with accommodations for 1500 people. While this auditorium is intended primarily for the employés, its use may be extended to the citizens of the city.

At the Westinghouse Electric and Manufacturing Company [1] no special movement is in force to lessen intoxication, excepting the discharge of an employé for habitual drunkenness and loss of time on that account. The company uses its influence to regulate the number and character of saloons in the immediate vicinity.

The fixed policy of the Tide Water Oil Company [2] is to promote men from the ranks to the position of foreman and to other posts requiring skill. In making selections to fill places of this kind that become vacant, men who are known to have the drinking habit are not considered eligible. A premium is thus placed on temperance, industry and skill, which has a very happy influence on the conduct of the men. Sobriety is the rule among them, and a large number are regular depositors in savings banks and building loan societies; 102 workmen, 8 per cent. of the total number employed, own their own houses, and have paid for them out of the savings from their wages.

The factory building of Carter, Howe & Company [3] has a thoroughly modern system of ventilation by means of exhaust fans. It is also supplied with drinking water from a driven

[1] Westinghouse Electric and Manufacturing Co., Pittsburg, Pa. Manufacturers of Electrical Apparatus. Organized 1886. Number of Employés, 17,000.

[2] Tide Water Oil Co., Bayonne, N. J. Refining and Marketing Petroleum. Organized 1888. Number Employés, 1200.

[3] Carter, Howe & Co., Newark, N. J. Manufacturers Fine Gold Jewelry and Chains. Organized 1841. Number Employés, 325 to 350.

well, direct pipes from which, with faucets, are on each floor. The water has been analyzed, and been pronounced wholesome and good. Thus breathing untainted air and drinking perfectly pure water of even temperature the year round, there is not the former craving for stimulants, and but little trouble has occurred from excessive drinking on the part of employés. By these means the firm has brought about what it regards as a condition of practical temperance.

The rule of the Boston Elevated Railway Co.[1] requires a man who applies for a position to subscribe to certain statements. One of them is that he does not use intoxicating liquors. If he is unable to make oath to this statement, the superintendent of employment has no authority to employ him.

If a man in their service is known to be intoxicated, he is discharged forthwith. If he enters a liquor store in uniform, for the first time he is severely disciplined; the second time he is discharged.

In a mining community, celebrations take place on a small scale every pay day. Prohibition was first tried and proved a failure. Drunkenness became more frequent than when the saloons were allowed to run. Drink was sold at "blind pigs," in the rear of stores and bunkhouses, or distributed from "wet bread wagons."

In preparation for the approaching Fourth of July, 1901, eight barrels of beer, four kegs of whiskey and a proportionately large amount of wine was shipped into the one camp of Coalbasin. The glorious Fourth was followed by a suspension of work in the mine for several days.

After consultation with the sociological department, Mr. Osgood, then chairman of the board of directors, decided that Coalbasin was a good place to test a plan for the partial solution of the liquor problem by a bar where liquors might be sold under restrictions imposed by the men themselves.

Now the Colorado Fuel and Iron Company is trying four experiments: The regulated saloon, the restricted club, the soft-drinks club and the open reform saloon.

The plan of the regulated saloon is this: In some camps the

[1] Boston Elevated Railway Co., Boston, Mass. Organized 1852. Number Employés, 8000.

monopoly of the liquor trade is given to a responsible person, no other saloons being permitted. This person is held responsible for the decency and sobriety of the place. This plan has not been found to be an entire success.

The restricted club is being given a trial in two of the camps. It is self-supporting, the monthly due being 50 cents. The building is a one-story frame structure of four rooms. There is a bar, a billiard and pool room, a card and game room and a reading room. Two evenings every month the club is given over to the wives and daughters and to visiting friends of the members. One of these clubs also has a theater. These clubs have a monopoly of the sale of liquor in the camps, but no treating is allowed.

The soft-drinks club will shortly be given a trial at another camp. There will be billiard and pool tables, and apparatus for serving coffee and light lunches. It will be entirely self-supporting, and no alcoholic liquors of any kind will be allowed on the premises.

During the year an experiment with the open reform saloon will be made. At these saloons there will be pure liquors for sale, but "soft drinks," such as milk, tea, coffee, chocolate, together with sandwiches and bakery lunches, will be dispensed. The card and billiard room will be made more attractive with games and music than the barroom.

Instruction in cooking and sewing by special teachers is added, it being argued that cooking has an important bearing on the liquor problem. To quote the words of the chief surgeon of the company: "To a hungry man a home's attractiveness begins at the table. But if he comes home to a supper of tasteless, indigestible food, served without any attempt at making it inviting, or the table attractive, is there any wonder that he seeks the saloon for stimulants?"

Club houses intended as a check to the drink habit so prevalent among the men by furnishing a place where intoxicants can be purchased only under certain well-defined regulations, and where various forms of wholesome amusement are provided to take the place of the debasing and demoralizing features of the saloon, are provided by the Colorado Fuel and Iron Co. The club house at Primero, where liquors of all kinds can be had, but where no drunkenness or disorder is allowed, is the only place in the village where intoxicants are sold. At the Floresta anthracite mine two rooms in the boarding house have been fitted up with billiard and card tables, and provided with periodicals and writing material for the accommodation of the miners. The Coalbasin club house is a one-story frame building of four rooms and cellar, with a front veranda. The bar is located immediately in the rear of the porch, and is furnished in a very plain and unattractive manner, no display of bottles, pictures, or other suggestions to drink being permitted. To the right as one enters is the billiard and pool room, while to the left is a room for cards and games. On the extreme left is a reading room equipped with the latest magazines, newspapers and periodicals. The furniture and furnishings are plain, but neat, and everything is conducted in a quiet and orderly manner. The following rules show how the affairs of the club are regulated:

"1. The club house will be open for the use of members from 9 A.M. to 10 P.M., daily, except Saturdays, when it will remain open until 11 o'clock P.M.

2. Members whose occupations are such as to require special working clothes are requested not to remain in the club rooms in their working clothes.

3. No credit will be given to members or visitors. All charges must be paid at the time they are incurred.

4. No gambling will be allowed in the club, but playing games of cards for small stakes will be permitted, the stakes in no event to exceed the following limits:

Poker—penny ante and twenty-five cents limit.

Billiards—twenty-five cents per cue.

Pool—ten cents per cue.

5. Women or children residing in or near Coalbasin will not be allowed to visit the club rooms except at such time as may be specified by the board of directors.

6. Strangers, including women and children, will be permitted to visit the club rooms for the purposes of inspection between 9 A.M. and 5 P.M, except Sundays and holidays, if provided with a permit from the board of directors.

7. No books or papers shall be taken from the club rooms.

8. Members will be charged for any damage done to the fur-

niture or fixtures of the club due to their carelessness or design.

9. No subscription paper shall be circulated nor any article exposed for sale in the club house without the authority of the board of directors.

10. Notices shall not be posted on the bulletin board except upon the authority of the board of directors.

11. All talking in the reading room is prohibited.

12. No member shall use the billiard or pool tables for more than three successive games to the exclusion of others desiring to play.

'NO TREATING' RULE:

In order to promote the temperate use of wine, beer and liquors which may be sold in the club house, no member or visitor shall be permitted to pay for a drink or drinks of any other member or visitor.

Membership in the club may be active or associate; only active members having the right to vote. Associate members are charged only half the dues paid by active members."

At the Interborough Company[1] drinking any beer, wine, liquor, or intoxicating drinks, or entering any drinking place during hours of duty, or the carrying of any intoxicating drinks about the person, or bringing of same on the premises of the company, while on duty, is cause for discharge.

The constant frequenting of drinking places, or the indulgence to excess in intoxicating liquors when off duty, is cause for discharge.

Mrs. Sidney P. Laughlin, mother, and George A. Laughlin, son, had heard so often that the saloon was the only club house for the working man that they were determined that this should not apply to the workmen of a company wherein the management was under their control. Accordingly they built a club house for the use of the employés of the Cleveland Axle Manufacturing Company[2] and the Cleveland Canton Springs

[1] The Interborough Rapid Transit Co., New York City. Organized May, 1902. 9500 Employés.

[2] Cleveland Axle Manufacturing Co., Canton, Ohio. Manufacturers Wagon and Carriage Axles. Organized 1858. Number Employés, 200.

Company, at Canton, Ohio. The maintenance, running expenses, janitor and repairs of the club are paid by these companies, making the club absolutely free to the men. Although it is primarily intended for the use of their own employés, members are at liberty to bring any of their friends for whom they can vouch.

The club is arranged to contain baths, a writing room, library or recreation room, billiard room, bowling alley, auditorium and game room, chess, dominoes, but no cards. The officers of the club are selected by the employés, who have the entire control of its management. The club has been in existence some five years and still maintains its popularity, although not so largely attended as at first. One evening each month is termed Ladies' Night, and frequently a ball is given.

One industrialist in Indiana tried to counteract the drinking habit among his men by a preaching service conducted by the different ministers in the city once a week in the factory. After a trial of six months he abandoned it, telling me that he was doubtful of its success.

The by-laws of the Curtis Mutual Benefit Society provide that no benefit shall be paid for any sickness, injury or disability arising from intemperance, or from any immoral act on the part of a member, nor shall any money for funeral expenses be allowed in such cases.

Westinghouse Electrical Benefit Association pays no benefits to members who may have received injury while intoxicated, or through other wilful or immoral conduct on their part.

As a penalty for intoxication, the Solvay Mutual Benefit Society[1] provides that any member whose disability is occasioned by the use of intoxicating liquors, or who becomes intoxicated while on the sick list, is liable to suspension from the society for a period determined by the trustees.

Some industrialists are coming to realize that the usefulness and efficiency of their plant can be increased by using it at night and not allowing it to lie idle. In this way a social by-product is obtained.

[1] The Solvay Process Co., Syracuse, N. Y. Manufacturers Alkalies and Allied Products. Organized September 20, 1881. Number Employés, 2500-3000.

A night school at John Wanamaker's Philadelphia store is composed of nearly 300 of the older boys, who stay two evenings each week, having free supper in the store, and afterwards reporting to the school rooms. The corps of 22 teachers is of high grade, and the work done compares most favorably with that in many regular schools. The branches taught are reading, writing, English, arithmetic, stenography, correspondence, bookkeeping, commercial geography, commercial law and business methods.

A drum and bugle corps of 31 members, a military band of 50 members, an orchestra of 17, a uniformed cadet battalion of 210, a minstrel troupe of 17, and a literary club, which includes all the members of the school and gives training in recitation and public speaking, are another part of the school life. The boys of the morning class and the girls recite before their respective classes. The boys of the evening school speak before their entire school, and in the senior class prepare and deliver original speeches. The boys of the cadet battalion elect from among themselves their military officers, except the chief, and these officers become successful disciplinarians.

A monthly report of the standing and progress of each pupil is made to the parents, and each of the three branches of the school has its separate annual commencement.

All the schools are trained in singing. An unusual thing is the singing together in the four voices, of 280 boys of the evening school. There is, also, a junior savings fund in which 1427 accounts have been opened. The school's physical work includes calisthenics, United States Army setting-up drill and military drill, and also regular gymnasium work. These are seen to have marked effect on the bearing and physical development of the young people. The school Alumni association has 120 members and the Alumnæ 300 members.

On the arrival of summer this social educational work is maintained through a summer camp at Island Heights, N. J., for which five acres of land have been acquired, and a good-sized house erected as headquarters. The boys live in tents during their camp of two weeks. The rest of the summer the headquarters house is in use by the women and men of the establishment.

A fact made clear in the practical outworking of these plans is that this variety of interests, of training and recreation, entering into the lives of the young people, in addition to their work in the business of the store proper, distinctly raises their standard in morals, ethics, mental ability and physical strength; makes their work more easy and more effective, and makes them men and women fitted to fill higher positions, with broad outlook and large income.

Intimately connected with the problem of efficiency promotion, is the opportunity for the industrialist to have some central bureau or office where he may obtain suggestions and experience which he can apply to the conduct of his own business along lines of industrial betterment.

One of the first organized movements in the United States which had for its object the collection of information regarding every phase of industrial betterment, was the American Institute of Social Service,[1] organized in New York in 1898 under the presidency of Dr. Josiah Strong and W. H. Tolman, director. In the promotion of its object it became a clearing house of practical effort for the great variety of methods for improving conditions, giving to this new form of socio-industrial effort the new term, "Industrial Betterment," by which are meant the various phases of improvement in the promotion of better relations between employer and employé; arbitration, trades unions, employers' associations, trusts, wages, hours of labor, housing, education and recreation and other movements.

One organization, the National Civic Federation, has adopted this idea by opening an entire department so as to promote still further the principles of industrial betterment, calling it, however, "Welfare Work."

The Institute disseminates information by means of its own publications, special reports and personal and written consultations. It has given hundreds of lectures, illustrated and other, on betterment subjects, to universities, colleges, theological seminaries, institutes, schools, churches, chambers of commerce, boards of trade, labor unions, clubs, summer assemblies and drawing room meetings. In the winter of 1901 the Director presented, through 59 illustrated lectures, the principles

[1] American Institute of Social Service, 80 Bible House, New York.

of industrial betterment, in a tour including St. Paul on the north, San Francisco on the west, New Orleans on the south. Among the results was a movement for civic improvement in Montgomery, Richmond and New Orleans. One woman was prompted to see how her stablemen and grooms were cared for. She found that her horses were better cared for than they; so she gave orders that comfortable bedrooms should be made, a bath added and a sitting room. One manufacturer added a social secretary to his staff. These are some of the concrete results, but it is impossible to estimate the activities resulting from this inspiration to industrial betterment.

By means of collaborators in the leading foreign countries, it drew upon the sources of information in socio-industrial problems. These collaborators were distinguished social economists, men of affairs, statesmen and publicists, among whom are Koegler, Director of Workingmen's Insurance, and Exner, of Vienna; Francotte, former Minister of Labor and Industry, Lepreux, Director of National Bank, Dubois, Director General Labor Department, Brussels; Siegfried, former Minister of Commerce, Levasseur, Administrator of the College of France, Senator Constant, Member of the Hague Court, Paris; Dr. Zacher, Chief of the Department of Social Statistics, and Prof. Dr. Hartmann, Imperial Insurance Department, Berlin; Wetzler, Director Social Museum, Frankfort; Dr. Dunbar, Director Hygienic Museum, Hamburg; Baron Kaneko, Member of the Imperial Privy Council, Tokio; Earl of Meath, President British Institute of Social Service, Rt. Hon. James Bryce, Rt. Hon. John Burns, President Local Government Board, Dr. John B. Paton, London; Count Tornielli, Ambassador from Italy to France; Bodio, Chief of the Statistical Department, Luzzatti, ex-Minister of the Treasury, Rome; Sir Horace Plunkett, Dublin; Prof. Louis Wuarin, University of Geneva; Prof. J. G. Mandello, Budapest.

Its international standing has been recognized by the award of the Grand Prix by the International Jury at Paris, 1900; St. Louis, 1904; Liège, 1905, and Milan, 1906.

Another organized movement for the express purpose of promoting industrial betterment is in a class all by itself, because it was the first association of business men to start this policy.

The Cleveland Chamber of Commerce[1] appointed its Industrial Committee in 1900 in recognition of the growing breach between capital and labor, and the belief that anything which tended toward more intimate relations and a more kindly feeling between these two classes would result in a better understanding and a nearer approach to mutual coöperation.

The committee has insisted from the first that the primary basis of any improvement must be found first in reasonable hours, fair wages and healthful surroundings for employés. Of the two thousand members of the Chamber, four hundred and fifty are employers of labor. At the inception of the committee's work, twenty-five of these were engaged in some definite form of industrial betterment. When a year ago the committee took a census of this, the result showed that approximately two hundred employers were interested in some form of it.

The most gratifying progress, however, is evidenced in the general inclination of employers toward the provisions of light, well-ventilated, comfortable and wholesome stores and factories, and of other means for securing the health and comfort of employés—features which were originally considered extraneous to business and classed as distinctive betterment work, but which are now provided as a matter of course.

Hardly a factory is now built without provision for rest, recreation and lunch rooms, and the general tendency toward improvement is shown in the fact that the building code recently adopted by the city lays especial emphasis upon sufficient light, air and toilet facilities.

Gratifying instances have been reported of a voluntary and substantial increase in the wages of employés, which have accompanied faithful service and a prosperous development of business.

The committee has laid special emphasis upon placing the responsibility for improvements upon employment organizations. Instead of providing for employés, the tendency now is to make provision for employés to help themselves. The management of the lunch room, of entertainments, the development of insurance features is left with the employé, the firm standing ready to assist and to provide adequate facilities for operation. This plan has resulted in greater interest and independ-

[1] Communicated by Howard J. Strong, Assistant Secretary.

ence among employés, the lack of paternalism on the part of employers and freedom from suspicion of any ulterior motive.

Two recent instances of the attitude of employers will be of interest. One concern is in the process of erecting a new factory. This factory is to contain eighty thousand square feet of floor space, forty thousand of which is to be devoted exclusively to industrial betterment; the manager of this company says that this kind of work is the only thing which saved his business from collapse. In another instance, the manager of a concern which was planning a new factory gave instructions of this kind to his architect: "I want you to build a beautiful building, one which will be an ornament to the neighborhood in which it is placed, and which will make the neighbors glad that we came; a building which will be an inspiration to our workers. After the building is completed we will adapt it as far as possible to the manufacture of cloaks." The result is a building which looks like a university or a public library.

CHAPTER II

THE SOCIAL SECRETARY—A NEW PROFESSION

IN the changed industrial and economic conditions of to-day, the great concentration of capital and the massing of thousands of the employed have brought about new problems. In the old times master and man lived and worked together; there was a daily point of contact, a continuous personal touch. To-day all is changed. The employer in many cases is as much an absentee as were the nobles of France in the latter part of the 18th century and the landlords of some of the worst tenements in slumdom to-day.

It is an industrial condition that naturally followed the organization of great capital into syndicates and trusts. With an industrial army of thousands of employés, it became necessary, for the best administration and efficiency, that they be grouped into sub-divisions, in charge of responsible leaders, in order that this working machine should respond to the directing control of the commander-in-chief; in other words, the day has passed when the employer is able to individualize those who work for him; not knowing them by name or even by sight, the personal touch, the point of contact has been lost.

With the growing intelligence on the part of the workers, evidencing itself in a dissatisfaction with their social and economic surroundings, they are slowly learning how to crystallize their incoherent wants and their smothered discontents into definite propositions for an improvement of their conditions.

As is clearly recognized, the personal touch between employer and employé has been largely lost, and it is not desirable, even if it were possible, to return to the earlier days. But for the successful conduct of the business man to-day, a point of contact must be established in some way. From a wide observation in this and other countries, I find that the business man strives for the highest efficiency in the making, selling and advertising part of his factory, mill or store; no detail is too trifling, nor can too great care be exercised; but all the while the labor end of his business, the human part of it, is taking care of itself, or left to the professional care-taker, who is not in the employ of the firm, nor is he always "in business for his health." However, our American industrialists are beginning to realize that an intelligent regard and a tactful care for the labor part of the business is not only right, but a large factor in industrial peace and contentment.

The social economist foresaw this tendency, and knew that the industrialist must establish a connection between himself, his immediate staff and the rank and file of his industrial army, if commercial peace and prosperity were to characterize his establishment. Every man of affairs earnestly desired this, but did not know how to obtain it.

This idea of the Social Secretary I brought to the United States in 1900, as a result of my studies in social economy in that section of the Paris Exposition of that year. I found that the idea had originated in France, where it had been carefully elaborated by Cheysson of Paris and Van Marken of Delft; but the credit of its application to the practical affairs of business is due to our country. Soon after the announcement of this new profession through the American Institute of Social Service, of which I was the Director, it received many inquiries, one from a New England woman who said she wanted to be a social secretary; how could she do it? The necessary information was given and every possible help afforded. She quickly grasped the idea and went to the largest department store in her own city, telling the proprietor that he ought to have a social secretary, and that she wanted the position. It was the first time he had ever heard of any such thing or knew that he wanted one, but the woman convinced him that it would be one of the best things he could do for his people. He was favorably impressed and added her to his staff. He remarked on a recent occasion that she was worth to the store more than he had ever paid her in salary.

The problem which confronts the social secretary is how to improve the conditions of life and labor for the individual, not only in the factory and workshop where he spends the greater part of his working day but in his home and all other relations in which he meets his fellowmen. The first requisites are sympathy, infinite tact and patience. Not only is the social secretary to promote whatever will improve the conditions of the laborer but he is there to check whatever is detrimental to the business through carelessness or indifference on the part of the workers.

The fact that the social secretary himself is a paid employé, subject to discipline and holding his position during good behavior, is of the utmost importance and far-reaching benefit in establishing a fellow feeling, for is he not one of them? The social secretary does not treat the laborers en masse, but maintains his individuality so that the employé feels that he is part of the directing intelligence and not a mere cog in the wheel. In many a business, particularly where there is a large amount of comparatively unskilled labor, the social secretary, being free to get a knowledge of all the departments, should engage the workers, thus better maintaining a uniform standard of requirements and character. The social secretary, not being identified with any one department, lessens the chances of favoritism so that an employé dismissed from one department, cannot be employed by another where the manager may be less particular. In a factory or department store, for example, the social secretary should meet the applicants for work and establish from the very first sympathetic relations. When a girl begins work in a big factory or store, the strangeness of the new life, the timidity that comes with the forming of new relationships and the unusual fatigue, frequently bring depression and discouragement. Then, too, the fact that the employés have some one to whom they can take their grievances without the fear that they will be discharged on the spot or misconstrued, but can be sure of sympathy and confident that their case will receive attention, is a source of great satisfaction. This kind of treatment creates a better feeling between employer and employé because the workers realize that it is fair treatment, and no one responds more quickly to fair play than the working man. Besides all this, the tactful sympathy of the social secretary often wins the confidence of the girls, who are led to entrust to her their home troubles and their personal private affairs.

The social secretary in a department store is practically a house mother to a great big family, and there is ample need for all the mothering she can spare. The great majority of immigrants are very illiterate; their children after a few years' schooling seek work, perhaps in a department store. Not having the guidance of a mother capable of instructing them intelligently, they are drawn to the social secretary, who, by her thorough knowledge of what they need, advises them intelligently and helpfully.

The social secretary is to act as the representative of the employés and, as such, to bring to the firm or the heads of departments any grievances that affect the employés individually or collectively. It is her business to establish the most cordial and friendly relations with the foremen, for the sake of securing their intelligent coöperation and support for all agencies that will make the employés happy and comfortable in their work, and in every way to encourage them to take a real interest in the workers under them. Not only that, but each employé has an opportunity to make any suggestion looking towards an improvement in the work rooms.

In industries where the social secretaries are men they could most advantageously engage all the men, except the skilled workers and the clerks; they have the receipt of suggestions and adoption of improvements in the work rooms; the responsible headship of the recreative and educational work; they visit the sick and promote good-fellowship; they arrange transfers from a department where the work is slack, to another where there is too much, and they also make promotions, in consultation with the heads of departments.

What and how the industrial army eats is of the first importance to them. The social secretary organizes the factory dining room, takes charge of the staff, buys the provisions, arranges the daily menu, thus insuring the best foodstuffs. Valuable social service is rendered by encouraging the more delicate girls to drink milk instead of tea. During the noon hour the social secretary has the finest opportunity for helpfulness. He sees that the girls are quietly served, looks to it that the tables are left tidy and keeps the girls happy and reasonably quiet. Two or three times during the winter, concerts may be given at the noon hour. At the noon hour the girls are at hand willing to be interested or amused, but they will not be preached or lectured to. This break in the routine of the work day must be packed with brightness and happiness.

In studying the life and labor in a great factory it might seem that the routine during work hours was of the first importance, but none the less important to them and their employer is the way the girls use their free time at home, on the streets and during their periods of recreation and education. So many girls have no idea of wholesome recreation; they want a pleasant time, but do not know how to get it. They walk the streets at night, ogling the men, picking up acquaintances, who lead them to dance halls, where they get their first lessons in drink; after that, the downward career is begun. The desire for a good time is perfectly legitimate, but in the absence of wise direction, finds its satisfaction in vicious surroundings, with the tendency ever downward. The social secretary organizes study classes. Membership in the classes should be limited to employés at the factory, 30 the upper limit, with fees from two to four cents a night, whether the girl is present or not. The social secretary is the administrative head, but the teachers are experts. The classes are not self-supporting. This educational work to be successful must recognize that girls hard at work all day do not care to learn too much or study too hard. The classroom must be bright and cheery; entertaining books may be read to the girls while sewing; there is music and the girls can talk to each other all they wish. Choral classes composed of men and women can be recruited from the office staff, thus holding the interest of the clerks, many of whom are hall bedroomers. "What," I asked the social secretary in a large department store, "from your point of view, is your work?" After a moment's thought she said, "I think I would state it like this: to advise, to uplift, to inspire with courage and ambition, to censure judiciously and to try to point out the best course in each individual case."

The social secretary can exert a powerful influence within the business itself and for her employés after hours, but there is a social service even wider than this that can be performed. Many a bit of human experience in sorrow and suffering comes dangerously near the tragic, and, but for the word of hope and cheer, all grip on the present might be lost. Every individual who is saved for himself is saved for society; instead of becoming a dependent, he not only stands alone, but is the means of helping another.

Dealing with human beings at every step of his way, the social secretary must inform himself of the various social phenomena while referring each manifestation to the underlying principle, thus acquiring a store of practical experience which will enable him to meet the emergency. In many cases the local conditions and requirements must be studied carefully so that the necessary adaptation may be made at once, for a brilliant success in one instance may be a dismal failure in another of apparently the same kind, because the local environment was ignored.

In seeking an opinion on the work of the social secretary in a large publishing house, I wrote one of the employés, who replied:

"I will endeavor to answer your letter asking my opinion regarding the work of the social secretary in our establishment.

"For several years this work has been going on here with so much satisfaction that it now seems like one of the indispensable industrial betterments. Our secretary keeps in touch in all departments, always ready to give attention wherever and whenever it is needed. We are encouraged to make suggestions for the betterment of our health or improvement in the system, and prizes are offered for practicable suggestions. We have a fire brigade of our own with a very efficient fire marshal. The buildings are supplied with readily accessible fire escapes and red lights at the exits mark the way. By having fire drills it has been shown that the building can be emptied in from two to three minutes.

"Much more could be said in detail about the work the social secretary has done and is doing in the interest of the employés, and I can testify to the fact that we have very many comforts and advantages, and that they are appreciated by the employés, which come directly or indirectly through the social secretary's efforts."

Another young lady writes:

"We have . . . in fact, almost everything essential to the bodily comfort, health, pleasure and protection of the employé; these are some of the improvements wherein lies some of the work of the social secretary. I am an employé of the company for over ten years. I have always received excellent wages for my services, but until this 'betterment condition,' which is in existence upwards of four years, I was in a way unknown; now I am a member of committees. My opinion is asked (and those of my fellow employés); I have the privilege of making suggestions on any lines. Naturally this is very complimentary to the employé, and is one of the results of our 'betterment system.'"

The H. J. Heinz Company for the last seven years has employed two social secretaries. The firm says, "The system is very satisfactory." These two officials are not known as social secretaries among the employés. They have some other nominal duties and their employés for the most part consider that they are engaged to perform those duties, but as a matter of fact, their important work with this house is along the social secretary lines. It is the experience of this company that the plan is much more satisfactory than to have them known exclusively as social secretaries.

The Colorado Fuel and Iron Company, through the sociological department, employs one social secretary, known as Welfare Manager, R. W. Corwin, M.D. It also employs a corps of workers to give their whole time to this work, under the direct superintendence of Mr. Walter Merritt, a specialist in such work, who gives his whole time. Dr. Corwin writes, "We have had such a secretary for eight years and have no intention of discontinuing the position, as we feel it an essential part of the administration of a great concern like ours."

This sociological department was organized in 1901, for coördinating and directing of "all matters pertaining to education and sanitary conditions and any other matters which should assist in bettering the conditions under which our men live," said Dr. Corwin.

An idea of the complexity of conditions and the different

elements in this proposition may be gained from the fact that there are 32 nationalities speaking 27 languages in the different mining camps and other properties of the company, and that these camps are scattered over an expanse of territory more than 1000 miles in extent. Many of the company's employés are drawn from the lower classes of foreign immigrants, Italians, Austrians, Germans and Mexicans predominating, whose primitive ideas of living and ignorance of hygienic laws render the department's work along the line of improved housing facilities and instruction in domestic economy of the utmost importance. Dr. Corwin states that it is the aim of this department not only to aid the company, but to benefit the employés and their families, by means of educating the younger generation, of improving the home relations, and furthering the interests of the men, making them better citizens and more contented with their work. It makes its influence felt in the public schools, where it urges that good buildings and equipment be provided, competent teachers chosen and free text books and supplies furnished to pupils.

The work of the social secretary in the case of this company takes on a very wide extent of service and social utility.

In 1903 a general plan was proposed by the International Harvester Company[1] requiring a social secretary at each works, through whose activities industrial betterment might be promoted uniformly. The pressure of active business organization put this plan to one side, and the temporary sociological committee did not become a permanent department. Recently, however, a bureau has been established in the general manager's office at Chicago, and a permanent head appointed, with a view to promoting the humane and healthful features of factory and office life among its employés. No publicity has been desired or sought for what this company has been doing for a number of years in a somewhat incidental manner, but along rational lines, and with a purpose and spirit of permanency and progress.

At the twine mills and foundry core rooms, matrons have been placed to assist in looking after the young women; and

[1] International Harvester Co. Manufacturers Agricultural Machinery. Organized 1902. About 30,000 Employés.

these matrons assist in many ways—visiting the sick, promoting a harmonious social spirit and directing the lunch room.

Industrial betterment work has been so largely a matter of general growth and improvement, rather than a specific departure, that the question of cost and financial return has been absorbed in the business without a special tabulation.

In 1904 a social secretary was employed by the Ludlow Manufacturing Associates;[1] she is no longer in the employ of the Associates, but is engaged by the Athletic and Recreative Society, an organization of the men and women of the village of Ludlow. It was organized in 1896, for the purpose of encouraging and maintaining places for indoor games, reading rooms and social meetings.

The society is the home for cooking, dressmaking, millinery, laundry, physical culture, swimming and dancing classes; the dramatic, orchestral, choral, football and baseball clubs; it has a bowling alley and a pool room. More and more the community is carrying the responsibility of the work as a social obligation.

The work which centers about the social secretary is purely communal. The company is coöperating by a building which will include among other things a doctor's office and waiting room; a parlor and bedroom for the social secretary; a kindergarten and day nursery; a hospital containing two four-bed wards, two double wards, one single ward; an operating room, with separate rooms for anesthesia and sterilizing; a sun room, bathroom, toilet arrangements, doctor's dressing room; and a large pantry connected by dumb-waiter with the kitchen in the basement of the boarding house.

At Joseph Bancroft & Sons Company[2] the social secretary acts as the representative of the employés, and as such brings before the firm or the heads of the departments any grievances that affect the employés individually or collectively.

Cases of illness and accident are reported to her, and she confers with the physician in attendance, thus keeping in touch

[1] Ludlow Manufacturing Associates, Ludlow, Mass. Dealers in Jute and Hemp Products. Organized 1848. Number Employés, 3000.

[2] Joseph Bancroft & Sons Co., Wilmington, Del. Manufacturing, Bleaching, Dyeing and Finishing Cotton Piece Goods. Organized 1889. Number Employés, 1450.

with the cases. Homes wherein there is distress are visited by her, and if there is need of financial aid, she brings the matter to the attention of the firm.

In accordance with the Child Labor Law, she sees that no child under the required age is employed in the works, looking after the age certificates and affidavits necessary. There are under her supervision (a trained teacher in charge) classes in domestic science for the girls employed throughout the works. A branch of the Wilmington Institute Free Library has been established, and books, which in her judgment are proper for the employés to read, are selected by her. The dining room where the employés are served with lunch at the noon hour is under her care, she taking charge of the cooks, buying the provisions, arranging the daily menu and supervising the other details.

The secretary of the firm reports, January 9, 1908, "We consider that the lady in question has been most useful and is now practically indispensable as a point of contact between our company and its employés."

The social secretary at the Pilgrim Steam Laundry Company has the supervision and initiative of the traveling library of selected books, circulating between 200 and 300 volumes a month; weekly talks of 15 minutes by president, welfare manager, or invited guests; literature class during winter; question box; distribution of pamphlets, verses, etc., where most helpful; the free and careful use of the medicine chest; prescriptions and advice given to workers free—50 to 70 a month; hot luncheon at noon, a simple menu—corn beef hash, double portion, 8 cents; potato salad, half portion, 3 cents; banana, one cent; tea, cream and sugar, 2 cents; ice water during summer months; trips to various points of interest on Saturday afternoons; theater parties when possible; tickets for special occasions; mutual aid society for benefits in case of illness or death; Penny Provident for saving pennies; bringing odds and ends to give to others less fortunate.

R. H. Macy & Co.[1] have what is practically a social secretary; she is a trained nurse, who is known as the store matron, whose duty it is to look after the health and general welfare of the

[1] R. H. Macy & Co., New York. Department Store. Organized 1858. 5000 Employés.

employés, and assist them whenever she deems it advisable and necessary. "We have had such a person in our employ for about ten months and have found her work very satisfactory," the firm reports.

Welfare Cottage, as it is called, is one of the regular six-room houses rented by the Proximity Mills [1] to their employés at Greensboro, N. C. It is the social center for the social secretary employed by the firm to do all the good in all the ways she can; it thus becomes a daily object lesson of simplicity and neatness. Most of the furniture is home made, and nothing too expensive for even the poorest to afford.

The social secretary visits the people and takes a personal interest in their yards and homes, and whenever it seems fitting, a helpful suggestion is given. She is always received cordially, but an unusually bright smile passes over a tired mother's face when the secretary enters her home and says, "We are going to have a little party at the cottage Tuesday afternoon, and we wish you to come." These meetings are held every week for the housekeepers and mothers. Interesting subjects are discussed and the secretary finds opportunities to present matters in which she wishes the coöperation of the home-makers. Refreshments are served, and some little souvenir is given, such as a "Perry picture" mounted on cardboard. In order to avoid large crowds, invitations are given according to streets or sections; in this way, no one is slighted, and each set has a party about every two months. The mill girls have their club meetings Saturday afternoon. Here they make hats, baskets and picture frames, have stories read to them, or play games. The sick are visited and often taken cut flowers, pictures, fruit, or some dainty prepared by a member of the cooking class. If necessary, more substantial aid is given.

A bit of communal betterment is the work of village and roadside improvement. In order to encourage the residents to make their surroundings more attractive, the company offers cash prizes for the neatest and prettiest premises, and aids them by plowing the yards, if desired, hauling off rubbish, and furnishing grass seeds and flowers. Last spring a thousand shade trees were set out, two being planted in front of

[1] Proximity Manufacturing Co., Greensboro, N. C. Manufacturers Cotton Goods. Number Employés, 2500.

each dwelling. A few years ago prizes were offered for the best suggestions for improving and beautifying the homes and the general appearance of the village. By this means the company found out what the majority most desired, and as far as practical is carrying out these suggestions. The company takes special pains in looking after the dwellings. A force of carpenters and glaziers is constantly on hand to keep the buildings in repair. The health of the village is exceptionally good. A force of men is kept constantly employed in cleaning ditches, removing weeds and rubbish from the streets and keeping the roads and sidewalks in repair.

CHAPTER III

HYGIENE

The industrialist of to-day in building a new factory is usually willing to plan for the most complete system of hygiene and sanitation. Steel and iron construction allow the maximum space for windows, which are wide and may extend from within a few inches of the floor to within a few inches from the ceiling. In this way the rooms are flooded with light so that the employé can watch every process in his work without straining his eyes. Incidentally the light, doing away with dark and dingy corners, reveals any dirt and litter which may collect—sunshine is the best microbe killer. The large windows permit an abundance of fresh air in summer, when it is so much needed. In winter, when the windows must be closed, a ventilating system of exhausts and forced air draws off the vitiated and forces in the pure. Special attention is paid to the location and installation of sanitary water closets, wash rooms and baths.

Ample provision is made for lunch rooms, rest rooms for the girls and women to be used at the lunch hour and rooms for a hospital and first aid to the injured. The Weston Electrical Instrument Company before planning its new works employed two mechanical and engineering experts to visit the most notable manufacturing establishments in the United States, studying problems of construction, machinery and physical conditions. Another expert traveled through the country for a year to learn what American employers were doing for their employés outside the question of wages. When the present plant was erected the company reserved the most desirable portions of the premises for several commodious halls, furnished them as recreation room, library, kitchen, dining room, gymnasium, natatorium, bicycle depot and hospital. At an inauguration reception, May 22, 1903, the entire club outfit, with the working capital of $1000 contributed by a director, was formally transferred to the employés, who, electing their own committee on plan and scope, soon completed the formation and incorporation of the Weston Employés Club of Newark, New Jersey.

The provision of the most improved sanitary and hygienic conditions is the very A B C of industrial betterment; it is not charity or welfare work; it is good business, because it enables the worker to labor under such conditions as will allow him to fulfil to the utmost his part of the wage contract.

Enough modern factories are being built to demonstrate the wisdom of this industrial philosophy and convince manufacturers of the future that their very first plans must include this kind of industrial betterment if their business is to be a success.

Many an industrialist is hampered by factory and workshop conditions which existed before there was any thought of industrial betterment. When a man is obliged to work in a dark and dingy room without ventilation, with narrow unwashed windows, he is unconsciously affected by his gloomy surroundings, even if he has never been accustomed to anything better; he cannot fail to be antagonistic to an employer who gives so little heed to healthful surroundings in which he must work.

At the Plymouth Cordage Company's [1] works a modern system of ventilation was installed. In winter when the windows must necessarily be closed, fresh air is supplied by means of large fans which draw the air from the outside and force it through a system of heating pipes into the various buildings at the same time the foul cool air is drawn off the floors. Thus there is a complete change of air throughout, every fifteen minutes. This apparatus is regulated by an inspector who constantly watches the thermometers in the various departments to see that an even temperature is maintained.

The United Shoe Machinery Company's [2] buildings and workrooms are exceptionally well lighted and ventilated. About 90 per cent. of the wall area is glass. All windows can be opened to admit fresh air, and a very thorough system of ven-

[1] Plymouth Cordage Co., North Plymouth, Mass. Manufacturers of Cordage. Organized 1824. Number Employés, 1220.

[2] United Shoe Machinery Co., Boston, Mass. Manufacturers Shoe Machinery. Organized February, 1899. Number Employés, 4000.

tilation is in use, forcing fresh air into the rooms, and exhausting the impure air. This forced ventilation is especially appreciated in the toilet rooms. The employés are provided with lockers, individual wash basins and shower baths; and in addition for female employés, bath tubs and a cosy rest room —all in charge of a matron.

Illness in the members of the staff may cause serious trouble or loss, so careful thought is given by the Fifth Avenue Bank,[1] New York, to everything that will promote good health. All the water used in the building must pass through a large filtering plant before entering the service pipes. An electric exhaust fan draws out the impure air. Facilities are provided for invigorating shower baths before or after work. A room convenient of access is especially fitted with racks for bicycles. Books and periodicals on banking subjects are circulated.

The employés of Parke, Davis & Company are of a high degree of intelligence, and their social condition is far above the average of that of many wage earners in the more densely populated cities of the country. In a long experience, the company says that it has found that good wages and short hours are preferred by the people to elaborately furnished toilet rooms, baths, gymnasia and similar devices for the betterment of the industrial worker. At the same time they have made every necessary provision for sanitary installation for their employés, including the equipment of dressing and toilet rooms for men and women in every building, adequate ventilating arrangements where necessary, including the use of dust collectors and blowers; respirators and eye-shields for the protection of employés working in the milling rooms and machine shops; an ample supply of drinking water in every department, and hot tea at the noon hour; safeguards on dangerous machinery to prevent the maiming of hands. The factory and administration buildings are of modern construction, and well adapted to their various uses.

The Weston Electrical Instrument Works are equipped with a steam heating plant, embracing a number of original ideas and controlled by centrifugal pumps, designed to permit easy and certain government of temperature. Automatic recording

[1] Fifth Avenue Bank, New York City. Organized 1875. Number Employés, 115.

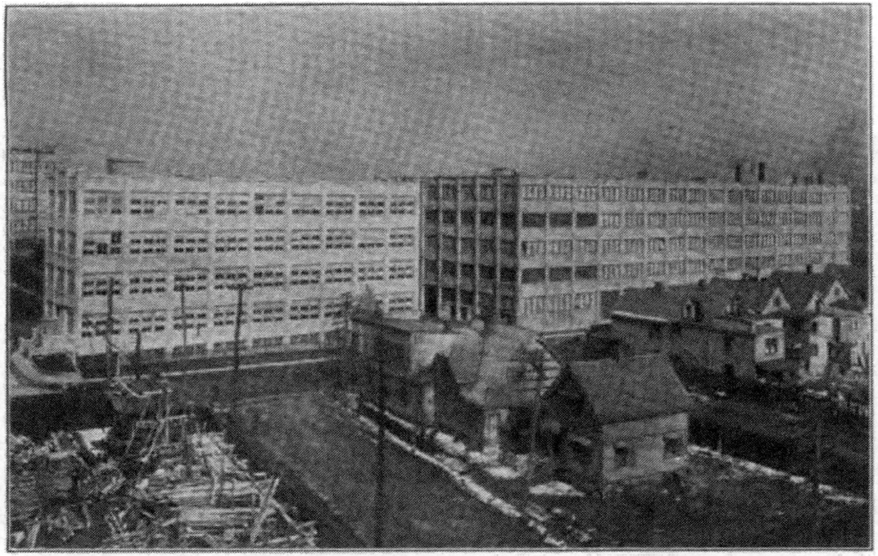

Illustration Showing the Extensive Space for Light and Air in the Edison Laboratory and Factories, Orange, N. J.

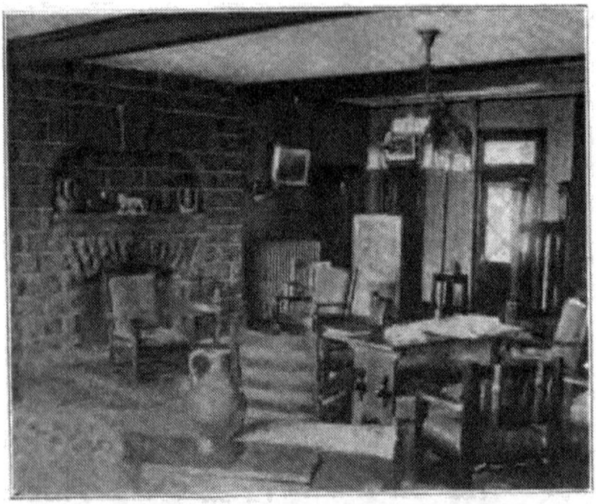

Sitting Room at the Colorado Fuel and Iron Company's Men's Club at Redstone.

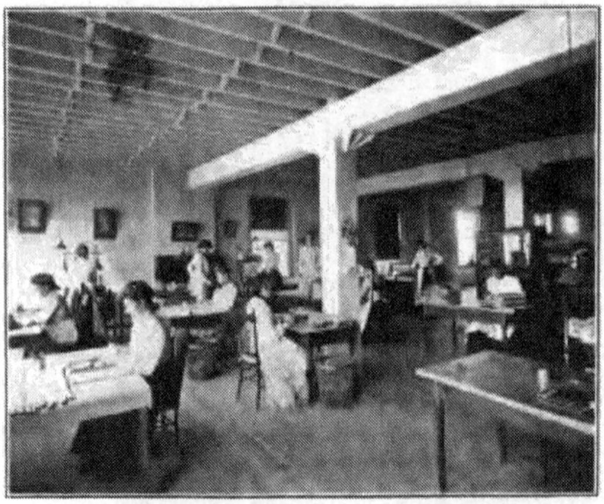

One of the Work Rooms at the Lowe Brothers Company. Light, Clean, Well Heated by Steam, Backs Provided for Chairs, Toilet and Lavatory Conveniences on Each Floor.

thermometers are placed in various parts of the factory, and the engineers are directed to maintain in the colder months a temperature of 70 to 72 degrees. The company has put in cooling systems in the forge and rolling mills and most of the departments have put the men on eight hours a day during the summer season. They find that this is not only a benefit to the employé, but also a benefit directly to the company. After putting in these cooling systems and working the men eight hours it was discovered that a piece worker turned out practically the same amount as under the ten and twelve hour system.

The cooling system includes a large fan drawing air from the outside of the building, and distributing it through the building in large galvanized pipes, openings from which are placed as nearly as possible over each man working at a fire or a set of tools.

In the blacksmith shop special efforts were made to get good light as well as good ventilation. At first large skylights were put in the roof of the blacksmith shop, but were impracticable on account of their getting covered with soot and grease, thus making it practically impossible to get any light through them. Then the glass was removed from the skylights, which were covered with sliding doors, so that they can be opened and closed at will from the inside of the shop. These openings to an extent act as a flue, the hot air and sulphur smoke from the fires is almost entirely carried out of the building, and in addition to this, almost absolutely unobstructed daylight is secured. "I do not believe that anything we have ever done for our employés was appreciated as much by them as this was, and we feel that the company is a very great gainer by having these departments so thoroughly well lighted and ventilated," remarked the president of the company.

It may be a satisfaction to the employés of Strawbridge & Clothier's Philadelphia store in the delivery basement to know that the air in the entire basement is taken out every 12 minutes by the tubes in the cashier's room and never returns. The air supplied to take the place of this is pure, fresh air from above the roof brought down by a modern ventilating system. The basement contains about 180,000 cubic feet; the tubes take out 15,200 cubic feet every minute, and in 12 minutes every foot of air in the basement is changed. This means a change of air six times an hour during a working day. It should be an important factor in the agreeable, prompt and pleasant manner of fulfilling duties. The air space allowed each employé is about seven times that required by the most progressive modern hospital practice; this allowance is based on the work rooms being manned to their fullest capacity. Ventilation is secured by sliding shutters in the roof of each bay, by a series of towers which may be opened in full, or in part, and by a large power-blower. From the fact that the buildings are either detached or semi-detached, the dividing lanes and alleys insure a constant circulation of air.

Each Ferris[1] workshop is the size of an entire floor, so that the light comes from four sides through very large windows. White curtains at every window give the factory a homelike appearance which is still further brightened by potted plants furnished and cared for by the girls.

In another factory, for all windows but those with a northern exposure there are white curtains which keep out the direct rays of the sun without sacrificing any of the light.

The International Harvester Company continues the industrial betterment work promoted by the individual works, and steadily broadens the activities which tend to improve the working and living conditions of its employés, numbering over 30,000. At the largest plants resident physicians are stationed to look after the health of the employés and to furnish aid in case of accidents, and a visiting nurse covers a large district under the direction of one of the works' physicians. No employés are accepted under 16 years of age, and of the entire roll perhaps 1000 are young women.

Ventilation, sanitation and pure drinking water are all subjects of careful thought and attention, and devices for removing dust and gases and safeguarding dangerous machinery are constantly being improved and applied at all works. Lockers and lavatories are numerous and modern, and rest rooms for the women employed in foundries and twine mills are comfortable and cleanly, and serve for both rest and recreation.

[1] The Ferris Brothers Co., Newark, N. J. Manufacturers Corset Waists. Number Employés, 400.

The windows at the Natural Food Company[1] are not only provided with double panes of glass to exclude any possible dust, but the fresh air enters the building through a series of fine wire screens and is passed over heated pipes in winter and over cold pipes in summer, and is entirely changed in the factory every fifteen minutes. Not a particle of dust or smoke mingles with the fresh air that circulates freely through the building, and which floods every part of the great structure. As a large tract has been laid out in beautiful lawns by the company, it will be impossible for any kind of nuisance to interfere with the purity of the air.

Next to pure air, cleanliness is of importance; in fact the purity of the air is largely determined by the presence or absence of dirt. Immaculate cleanliness, essential to the fine work done by the Weston Company, demands an atmosphere not only free from dirt and grit, but as near dustproof as possible. The health of employés and the requirements of business are best served by identical conditions.

At the National Cash Register Company absolute cleanliness is demanded throughout the factory. All offices and work rooms are swept each morning before their occupants begin work. The floors are scrubbed once a week. The factory windows are kept as speckless as the smartest office building. Eighty janitors are employed to keep the twenty-three acres of floor space clean. The floors are always kept well shellaced, this process especially preventing disease germs from spreading.

The Machinist Press of New York City paint their printing presses with white enamel paint, the men calling them the "White Squadron."

Instead of painting the trusses and structural iron work inside the buildings the conventional "foundry red," the color is a light buff at a Massachusetts foundry. The roof is painted inside with water paint.

The first attempt at industrial betterment at the Cleveland Hardware Company concerned the matter of cleanliness. Garbage cans were placed at convenient intervals around the fac-

[1] The Natural Food Co., Niagara Falls, N. Y. Manufacturers Shredded Whole Wheat Products. Organized December, 1900. Number Employés, 400.

tory, and the men were given good washing facilities. The firm went to considerable trouble to keep the entire plant in order and as clean as possible.

The National Biscuit Company[1] has a laundry which takes care of the table linen, the towels and the various overalls and aprons which are worn by the employés. Each department has its own uniform suited to the work, and these uniforms are laundered and mended at the company's expense.

In the works of the Sherwin-Williams Company, cleanliness extends not only to the floors and machinery of the workshops, but the employés as well, and in order to insure its thorough observance, the factory is provided with a large number of lavatories, shower-baths and lockers, and a plentiful supply of clean towels is furnished from the company's own steam laundry.

Employés are encouraged in every way to use the shower-baths and to do so freely; but in the dry-color department, in order to guard against lead poisoning, the frequent use of the baths is compulsory. As a further safeguard, each man is provided with an entire change of clothing every day. The result of this caution is most strikingly shown in the facts that previously the average time a man cared to work in the dry-color department, or could do so with safety to his health, was about one month, he now stays as long as he wants to or is wanted by the management. Where in the past at least every other man was affected by the lead, there is now not more than one in 20 injured by it, and then generally only in cases where the man does not make proper use of the system.

Several bath rooms, including shower, tub and a recently added Turkish bath, are at the service of the employés at East Aurora.

A New Jersey glass manufactory provides a bath room for the special benefit of the boys, although it is open to all the workmen employed by the company.

At the Ferris Bros. factory in Newark, N. J., where they employ 400 women and girls, bath tubs are provided in the factory with hot and cold water, towels and soap. Oak finishing, nickel plated trimmings, rugs and first class sanitary ar-

[1] National Biscuit Co., New York City. Manufacturers Biscuits and Crackers. Organized 1898. Number Employés, 2000.

rangements make the rooms bright and clean. Each employé is allowed thirty minutes for a bath at the expense of the company.

Directly under the dining hall of the Weston Electrical Instrument Co. is the swimming pool, 160 feet by 35, with a 20 foot ceiling—light, bright and cheerful. The tank, cement and enameled brick, is 150 feet long, 18 feet wide, and from 4½ to 9 feet deep. The flooring is a handsome white mosaic tiling, tastefully bordered in green, with a couple of two-colored marble steps, about 75 feet long, leading up to the batteries of shower and needle baths and tubs. A filtering plant has been installed. Here, as in the lavatories, the plumbing is fine in quality and pleasing in style. Connecting on the north is a large dressing room and the arrangements are such that the men may go directly to or from bath and work. Bathers are required to take the shower before the plunge. Certain days and hours are set apart for the women.

In the basement of the big factory of the Natural Food Company are elaborate lavatories, finished in marble and mosaic and furnished with shower and needle baths and hot and cold water. These have been provided for the employés at a cost of $100,000; each employé is allowed time at the expense of the company for the use of these baths.

In 1893 J. H. Williams & Company [1] established the first baths in any manufactory in this country. Notwithstanding that they are conveniently located in the same rooms with the lockers, that the temperature of the room is comfortable at all seasons, and that they are always clean and in good order, with an abundance of hot as well as cold water, they are not used as much as could be desired. Some of the men use them regularly, some on Saturdays only, and some not at all; others who have facilities at home prefer bathing there. They are patronized mostly in the warm season, even then not as generally as would be expected. This can be accounted for from a desire on the part of the employés to leave the premises as quickly as possible at the termination of the day's work, and also from the fact that, not having acquired the habit in early life, they are generally slow in adopting a custom of daily or

[1] J. H. Williams & Co., Brooklyn, N. Y. Manufacturers Drop Forgings and Drop Forge Specialties. Established July 1, 1884. Number Employés, 400.

frequent bathing. In addition to the shower baths, each wash trough is provided with a spray, so that the workman can thoroughly clean his head from dust and dirt. The original baths, however, are not a failure, for since then more have been erected, but, on a smaller plan, in other departments than the forging shop. In the new buildings it is the intention to include shower baths in the toilet rooms and lavatories, which they expect to make more attractive with individual wash-basins, hoping to still further encourage their use.

If this firm would follow the practice of certain others, giving the men the privilege of a bath on the company's time, it might have the desired effect of a greater use of the baths.

The Hygienic Chemical Company[1] of Elizabethport, N. J., has furnished a bath room with hot and cold water, also soap and clean towels, free. Every employé is allowed twenty minutes once a week during working hours for bathing purposes without deduction of wages. The only formality required is application to the foreman for a bath ticket. There is no restriction as to the use of the bath after working hours except the avoidance of conflict. Hot and cold water and all toilet accessories are furnished by the company. Each employé is permitted to take one bath each week in the winter and two baths each week during the summer season on the company's time.

The Colorado Fuel and Iron Company has provided a wash-house for the accommodation of those who work about the company's coke ovens and coal tipple at Redstone. Its equipment comprises 24 white enamel wash-basins, supplied with hot and cold water, 2 closets and an enclosed shower bath located at one end of the room, and lockers for those who desire to change their soiled working clothes for other attire. The floor is of cement and so laid as to permit daily flushing.

In a factory of 4000 employés, an employer has provided 120 shower baths for the men and 14 tub baths for the young women. These are located on the various floors and conveniently accessible from any department in the plant.

The Weston Electrical Instrument Company has put in sanitary drinking fountains and has found them such a success in the new building, that they were also installed in the old forge

[1] Hygienic Chemical Co., Elizabethport, N. J. Manufacturers Chemicals. Organized 1893. Number Employés, 30,

departments. In maintaining these drinking fountains in the forge departments, a valve was put in so that each workman can control the spray of water, and underneath the fountain are coils of pipe on which is placed the ice that ordinarily was put into the drinking barrels. This keeps the water very cool, but at the same time perfectly fresh and clean.

"We believe these drinking fountains have saved us money all through our factory; both from the fact that the quantity of ice used is so much less, and water so much better for drinking purposes; we find the men take much less time at the drinking fountains than when they were obliged to use the cups."

The "delivery water tanks" have been used in the Eastman Kodak factory for a number of years. The tank has two receptacles, one to hold the drinking water and the other to receive such as is not used, and is mounted on rubber tired wheels.

The one used for wash water is similarly constructed, only larger than the others, and likewise contains two receptacles, one for fresh and the other for dirty water. Clean waste is carried with the cart with which to wipe the basins. During the warm weather, three and sometimes four men are employed on these carts and in the winter usually two. The cost of maintaining these tanks is compensated for by the men not having to leave their benches to go for drinking water.

For drinking purposes in a Massachusetts factory, the water from the city water works is used, but it is put through a filter, thence through a coil pipe on which is broken ice. From this coil the water is drawn into carboys, which are enclosed in boxes packed with cork chips, so that the water is kept cool for twenty-four hours or more. The water is delivered in the various rooms in the factory, and is used simply for drinking. For other purposes the water direct from the pipes is used.

At the Weston Electrical Instrument Company, connecting with the dressing room is a lavatory (75 by 40, with a ceiling 16 feet high) lighted and ventilated by many windows, with an individual porcelain wash-basin, individual soap, mirror and locker for each man. The plumbing and all appurtenances of this department are of the highest quality and best style so as to obtain perfect sanitary conditions.

The toilets are in every respect of equal grade with the lavatories, marble stalls, tiled floors and walls, hardwood doors and seats, in all particulars of as high quality as are to be found in any hotel in the land. The closets are ample in number, and so distributed as to be convenient of access from any part of the works—connected with each group is a lavatory. All lavatory and toilet arrangements are duplicated for the women, who constitute a third of the force.

In the same factory drinking water of excellent quality and temperature is supplied by the company's artesian well, and is distributed throughout the departments by automatic jet fountains, thus doing away with cups or glasses.

No drain pipes come into any of the main buildings or work rooms. All closets and lavatories are in wings independently ventilated, and are so divided from the main buildings that gases and odors are excluded.

Three distinct systems of drainage are employed: (1) The roof-drainage, which is carried through the main columns to independent pipes; (2) The wash-water (lavatory) drainage, which is also a separate system joining the roof-drainage about a quarter of a mile from the works, and (3) the toilet-drainage, which nowhere connects with the others, but discharges on the level some hundreds of yards away from the factory—the constituents being absorbed by nature.

The Walker & Pratt Manufacturing Company,[1] of Boston, believe that care for the comfort of their employés is dictated by sound business, as well as humanitarian considerations. They find that workmen in a comfortable well-lighted building will do more and better work. They can also secure a better class of workmen when they consider the men's comfort.

Foundry work is necessarily very dirty, but this firm decided that each one of their workmen may go home clean, hence self-respecting. In the sanitary appliances it was the design that they should be convenient, easily kept clean and repaired with the least delay and effort.

The regular set bowl of the plumber, with its wiped joints on outlet and overflow, is dispensed with entirely. Two substantial cast-iron standards have a plain rectangular slab of iron bolted to them on each side, while central posts support

[1] Walker & Pratt Manufacturing Co., Boston, Mass. Manufacturers Heating and Cooking Apparatus. Organized 1877. Number Employés, 400-450.

a wooden frame which carries mirrors and a shelf for other toilet necessaries. The wash-bowls are of cast-iron, made in the works and covered with white enamel. Lugs on the under side slip over the longitudinal bar and support the bowl without fastening. A trough of sheet copper beneath receives the discharge from the bowls and carries it to the outlet at one end, where it falls into a covered gutter in the concrete floor. Thus the whole apparatus is open to inspection and cleaning. Over each bowl is a hot and cold water faucet attached directly to the iron pipe system, so that no plumbing work was required even here. The water pipe system, moreover, is entirely independent of the frame which supports the bowls, so that there is no chance of strains and leaks in the pipe from any movement of the latter. Soap powder canisters are secured to each bowl, an element of neatness which any one who has seen a cake of soap in a factory wash room can appreciate.

At this same establishment each molder has his individual bathing compartment in a room 105 by 35 feet. The entire floor is covered with concrete, the water draining to a covered central gutter. The workman stands on a movable wooden grating. Each bathing compartment, 3 by 5 feet, contains hot and cold water faucets, a seat, a pail, and hooks for clothing, a locker fitted with a Yale lock enables the man to leave his ordinary clothing and valuables in security. Overhead incandescent lamps furnish light, and steam pipes keep the room comfortably warm; white paint has been freely used on all the fixtures. One man is in charge of bath and washrooms, so that everything is kept neat and orderly. He has some time left for odd jobs in other parts of the works.

The value of physical exercise is constantly emphasized at the Roycroft Shop. Fifteen minutes per day, on the company's time, are devoted to exercise, either gymnastics indoors, under the guidance of a physical director employed by the company, or to walks for those outside who prefer, participation in the gymnastics being entirely voluntary. Tramps across the country are urged at other times, and are frequently led by Mr. Hubbard or the physical director. A ball nine and an annual field day of the employés further encourages physical development, as well as a croquet ground and hand-ball court on the grounds.

The Ayars Machine Company [1] has provided a wash room with concrete floor, hot and cold water and other facilities for washing; the employés have separate lockers, which are in the wash room and all arranged conveniently so that the men may keep themselves and their belongings clean and in good order.

The women's rest room is a large apartment, fitted with couches, easy chairs and writing desks at James R. Keiser's New York work rooms. Conveniences have also been provided for employés who may be taken ill. One end of the rest room is given up to individual lockers for street garments.

Another most unique and commendable movement is that practiced at the dry goods house of A. T. Lewis & Son,[2] of Denver, Colo., where two days in each month are allowed women in their employ, with pay, at the time when nature demands rest and quiet. This two days' vacation is given only at these times and for the purpose implied. It is the testimony of this firm that the general health of the women is very greatly benefited; and although the cost to them during the year amounts to several thousands of dollars, the additional efficiency of the workers and their appreciation of the particular privilege fully offsets the cost. It may be stated that this measure was adopted at the suggestion of Mrs. A. T. Lewis.

The history of the lunch room and restaurant at the Cleveland Hardware Company is so valuable from a daily contact with actual conditions of space limitations and other adverse circumstances that I shall use the report of Mr. E. C. Adams in full.

In studying the Cleveland Hardware Company's plant, I found the employés of a very mixed class, a few machinists of the better class, down to the commonest Poles in the rolling mill yard. Mr. Adams said: "This matter of starting a restaurant was delayed some six months or a year from the fact that we were so badly cramped for room that we had no place in which to put a kitchen, to say nothing of a dining room. When we finally came to start this kitchen, the greatest obstacle to overcome was found to be the washing of the dishes.

[1] Ayars Machine Co., Salem, N. J. Manufacturing Machinists. Organized November 1, 1893. Number Employés, 78.

[2] The A. T. Lewis & Son Dry Goods Co., Denver, Colo. Organized January 14, 1902. Employés, 500 to 700.

However, after pondering over it for some time, we hit on the plan of serving all the food on paper plates, and having each man furnish his own knife and fork. In this way we had nothing but the cooking utensils to wash, so were able to put a roof over one of the light wells, between the rolling mill and the factory, and turn this into a kitchen. We could not, however, give the men a dining room, and overcame this by making a number of folding tables and arranging the men in different groups, giving each set of eight or ten a folding table which they took care of themselves. We also furnished to each man a pint porcelain pail and put up small cupboards at convenient places, similar to those in a barber shop. In these the men kept their coffee pails, together with knife, fork and spoon, and the table was folded up and hung on the wall in whatever section of the factory that particular group happened to be working.

"We then bought a number of tin boxes with shelves, and one man from each group would take the order in the morning for the meal, and place it in the kitchen before ten o'clock; the cook would then get the dinner ready and pack in these cans. The cans were then put on steam radiators, and some man who was not running a machine was allowed to quit work five minutes before the whistle blew, and get the cans belonging to his set from the kitchen. Our plan was to furnish the men a pint of coffee for a penny, and other goods at practically cost, although where we lost money on the coffee, we sold pies and other things that might be termed luxuries at a slight advance, and in this way made up the amount.

"The plan of paying for the meals was to have tickets printed in strips the same as street car tickets, in denominations 1, 2, 5 and 10 cents; these were handled by the timekeeper and the amount deducted from the man's pay; in this way we overcame the handling of any money in connection with the kitchen.

"The restaurant was undoubtedly the feature that attracted more attention and praise from outsiders than anything else. But after running it for three years, we came to the conclusion that as far as we were concerned it was not practical. We found that at the prices we were charging, we could give a man a good meal for from ten to twelve cents, but there was a deficit of from fifty to sixty dollars at the end of the month. However, even at this price, we found that out of about seven hundred men employed, we were feeding only one hundred to one hundred and fifty, and as far as we could see, it was very little appreciated. Some of the men even went so far as to express themselves that it was only another money making scheme on the part of the company. About this time, the cook whom we had employed for the entire three years and who practically had taken the entire responsibility off our hands, decided to leave, and we thought best to close the restaurant.

"After the restaurant had been closed some ten days or two weeks, the men seemed to appreciate it more than they ever had, and some sixty of them signed a petition asking the company if they would be willing to give them the use of the kitchen and outfit, provided they would make arrangements with somebody to furnish the meals. This we were perfectly willing to do, and the men then formed themselves into a club, and made a contract with a woman whereby she furnished a regular dinner for 15 cents. Outside of furnishing the equipment and light and heat for the room, the company had absolutely nothing to do with this venture. Although sixty men signed this petition, the number taking meals under this plan never exceeded thirty-five. We think this could be taken as just about the proportion of the seven hundred employés that really appreciated the restaurant when it was run by the company. This seemed too small a proportion to spend fifty or sixty dollars a month on, besides a great deal of detail work that is not taken into consideration at a money value. After running under this plan for about nine months, the woman in charge gave it up, and since that nothing has been done with it as far as the factory employés are concerned.

"This has been our experience with the restaurant as far as the workmen in the factory are concerned. However, we would not want to discourage the starting of a restaurant entirely by our experience. The Cleveland Twist Drill Company is still running a restaurant for its employés, and the writer understands that to a certain extent it is considered a success; they have room enough to have a general dining room, and in this room they have a library, piano, etc., which makes it practically a general recreation room for the employés.

"This is something which we could not do because of lack of space. I understand also that in connection with this they run a cigar and tobacco stand, and the profit on these articles to some extent helps out in the deficit on foods.

"Our men, too, are of a very mixed class. I found in talking with a good many of them about the restaurant that they were living in boarding houses, and would get no reduction whatever from these places on account of not carrying their lunches, so no matter what they paid for the dinner at the factory, it was entirely an extra expense. The keepers of the boarding house would tell them that they made preparations for lunches anyway, and could not make any reduction on account of their not using them."

Shortly after starting the restaurant for the men, the firm found that a great many of the office people were getting their lunches from this kitchen. On account of using the desks for tables, it was absolutely necessary to have a dining room for the office force. This was done by building it originally on top of the bins in the warehouse. Even in the new building they could not find space enough for a room for the men, but they did manage to partition off part of the top floor for a dining and general recreation room for the office employés. This is still maintained, and is considered a success in every way. Before giving up the shop kitchen, all the food was prepared in that department and then brought over to the office dining room. Now the office dining room has a kitchen in connection with it, and the meals are cooked by the woman who takes care of the general offices. She has a young girl who comes in for five or six hours a day and helps with the kitchen work and serving at noon.

In this dining and recreation room there is an employés' library, also a large and small pool table and piano, and a Cecilian piano player. The room is used considerably during the noon hour for dancing. It is also used at times for dances held in the evening, as well as being given to the employés for holding meetings of their Mutual Benefit Association, banquets and smokers.

"Ain't it nice," said a little girl, who was cuddled down on a heap of gay sofa pillows, "we sing every noon now. It's such fun," and even at her distance she joined in the chorus, keeping time with her foot. "It's all lovely," said her neighbor. "I guess we girls who never had such things before know that." This colloquy was overheard at the noon hour at the Patton Paint Co., in Milwaukee, where a most attractive girls' room has been installed. One end of it is fitted up with polished oak tables and chairs, and there the girls eat their luncheons, supplementing their sandwiches and bread and butter with coffee made by one of their number, who is allowed to take the time for this work and for arranging the table and taking care of the dishes afterward.

Divided from this by a row of gay Japanese screens is the rest room, with its comfortable many-cushioned couches, capacious rocking-chairs, its tables heaped up with the newest magazines and a stationary washstand with a mirror long enough for a girl to see herself from head to foot. There is a lavatory adjoining and off the corridor leading to the room are the lockers where the girls keep their street clothes, the cupboard which they are stocking with dishes and cooking utensils, and the little kitchen with its gas stove.

Every table was decorated with a pot of ferns and each was surrounded by a chattering group, which sipped its coffee and ate the luncheon in a cheerfulness that was good to see. Luncheon over, some of the girls slipped into the rest room, where they dropped down on the wide couches or rocked in the big chairs, happy as factory girls not always are. Then presently from the lunch room came a song, a merry popular air, carried clear and strong by one or two voices, with a dozen others joining in the refrain.

The men's room is not so dainty in appearance, but it is larger and its reading table is stocked with the magazines a workman cares most to read, while in one corner is a "crokinole" board, on which some exciting games are played every noon. Those who do not care to play this game smoke or read, and since smoking is forbidden everywhere else in the factory, the air gets blue in the men's lunch room before the signal for beginning the afternoon's work is heard.

The men have taken to the new departure more quietly than the girls, who are outspokenly enthusiastic. Many of the men have worked in other factories where the only place to eat was at their machines, and their delight in their pretty lunch rooms and the zeal which they show in keeping them attractive is sufficient proof of what they think of them.

On the upper floor, a large room commanding a view of Niagara is set aside for a dining room, where the employés of the Natural Food Company may gather for their noonday meal, as guests of their employers. Regularly employed cooks prepare a complete meal each day, and the young ladies follow in turn in waiting upon the tables, each corps serving a week, the selection being made alphabetically from the entire number. The wholesome noonday meal is served absolutely free of cost to the young ladies in the office of the operative departments of the factory, while a nominal fee of ten cents is charged the male employés for their luncheon, which is served in a separate apartment.

With a large number of employés it becomes necessary to formulate certain regulations for efficiency. At the Curtis Publishing Company I find the following:

"No money will be received in the lunch room, payment being made entirely by lunch-checks.

The hour for luncheon in each department will be assigned by the bureau manager and is subject to change according as the number of employés in the department decreases or increases.

Owing to the limited space in the lunch room employés must not loiter at the tables after they have finished eating.

Employés must stand in line when waiting for orders at the window. It will facilitate the service and save time if each employé will decide upon her order before reaching the window.

It is very necessary that each employé see that her place at the table is left in neat condition, that soiled dishes are taken to the proper window, and that waste paper and paper napkins are placed within the refuse receptacle. Throwing paper, remains of lunches or anything whatever around the room is positively forbidden.

Employés are requested to guard against the indiscriminate taking of paper napkins, two being all that is considered necessary for each person.

A box for suggestions and complaints has been placed below the bulletin board in the lunch room, and it is desired that this box shall be freely used. Suggestions and complaints need not be signed.

Employés remaining in the building during the noon hour either in the rest room or their own department, must conduct themselves quietly, and are not expected at that time to make use of the benches or the main hall in front of the building."

The dining room is an important feature at the Iron Clad Factory.[1] It is artistic, beautiful and comfortable. The ceiling is hidden under a mass of grapevines laden with green leaves and luscious purple grapes, through which the electric lamps shine like stars. It is a large room with many windows, each having its window box filled with growing plants and fragrant blossoms. Instead of long tables common to cheap boarding houses, there are numerous small ones arranged in the same manner as seen in all high-class hotels. Waiters in white suits serve a substantial dinner, consisting of soup, roast, two vegetables, dessert and coffee. Smoking is allowed after dinner.

The Atchison, Topeka and Santa Fé Railroad provides for reduced rates at all of its restaurants, which are very numerous, so that a man may get as good a meal for twenty-five cents as is served to passengers.

Recent additions in the factory have enabled the Waltham Watch Company to carry out a long cherished plan for establishing an attractive dining or lunch room for the use of such of their young women as are unable by reason of inconvenient distance to take their midday meal at their homes. This room is cosily provided with small tables at which congenial groups of young women may eat. Conveniences for the heating of coffee or food are provided, and a lunch counter for the sale at cost of simple forms of food.

The ordinary accommodations are for 300 at a time. The number varies from 50 to 150, but in case of sudden or severe storms the number sometimes reaches as many as 800, so that an unusual number of young women, who would ordinarily go to their homes for their midday meal, will avoid the incon-

[1] Iron Clad Manufacturing Co., Brooklyn, N. Y. Manufacturers Steel Barrels and Galvanized and Enameled Ware. Organized 1859. Number Employés, 1500.

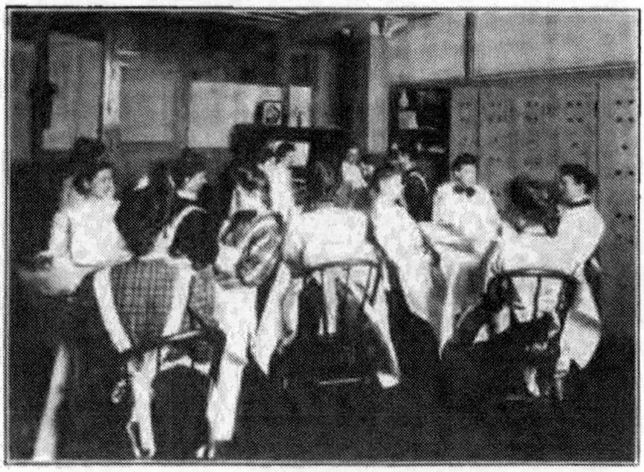

A Corner in the Young Women's Rest and Lunch Room at the Lowe Brothers Company.

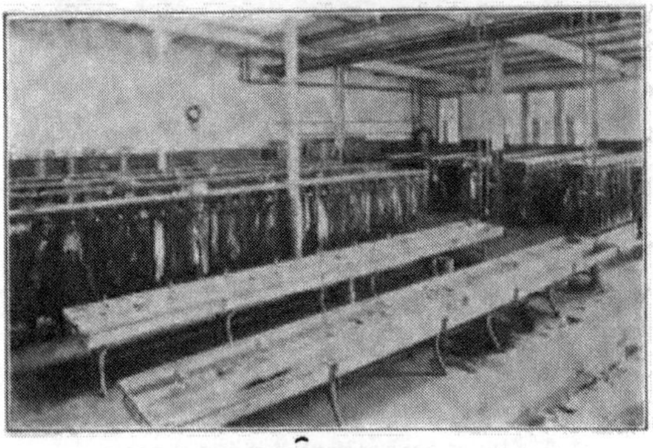

Individual Lockers and Lavatories at the Works of the General Electric Company.

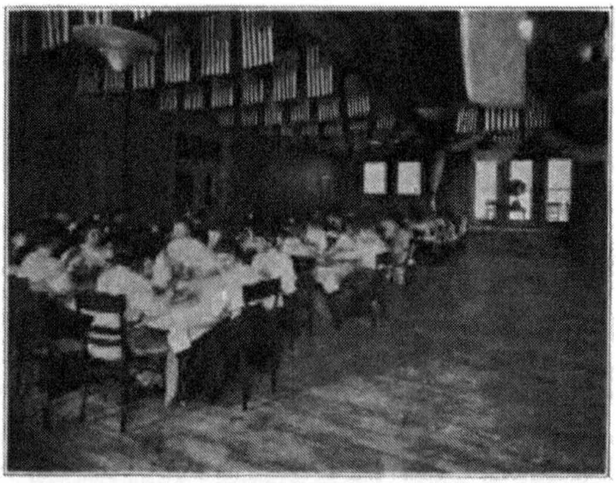

Employés at Luncheon in the Convention Hall of the Acme White Lead and Color Works.

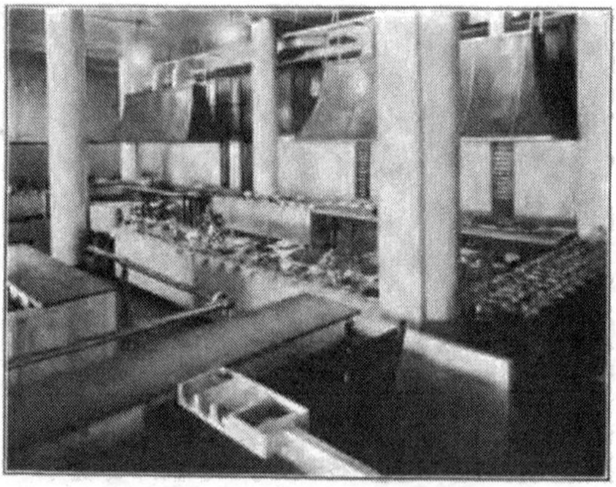

The Dining Room at Marshall Field & Company.

venience and possible danger of exposure to the storm and be sure of a nourishing luncheon.

This room is also free to those who furnish their own food. Food is furnished practically at cost, but conveniences for transportation to the homes of their people are so good that a comparatively small number of them avail themselves of the opportunities afforded them by the lunch room. The lunch room is managed by the matron of the large boarding house, so that food can be furnished to the operatives at a cost much less than would otherwise be possible. The matron is always accessible to all the young women for advice and help and in every way strives to give an atmosphere of home to the place. A large airy recreation room has been fitted up with easy chairs and settees, and also tables furnished with papers and magazines. A grand piano gives opportunity for the enjoyment of music.

Mutuality was the philosophy at the Wayne Knitting Mills[1] before any definite industrial betterment work was undertaken. This received its permanent impetus five years ago when the present office building was completed. The entire upper floor was thrown into one large room or assembly hall and set aside for various purposes in the interests of the mills' employés, and is used for meetings and lectures, but principally as a dining room. A kitchen was equipped with all necessary apparatus, and thirty small tables, seating four persons each, were placed around the room. Several girl employés act as waitresses, receiving their lunch free in payment. Three women are constantly employed cooking and washing dishes, even working evenings when it is necessary for the mill operatives to work overtime.

In 1905 the National Cash Register Company decided to build a large dining room and auditorium to take the place of the former dining room in the factory, where the space was needed for commercial purposes. It was the plan of the company to place the management in the hands of the Men's League; if, in addition, they would hire the help, purchase the supplies and serve the meals, the company would provide the building, dishes and furniture. There was the further condition that luncheon

[1] Wayne Knitting Mills, Fort Wayne, Ind. Manufacturers Hosiery. Organized 1891. Number Employés, 1500.

was to be served six days a week, at a daily cost of 15 cents for each person, or 90 cents a week. In a formal communication the company stated that they would erect the necessary kitchen, bakery, cold storage rooms, and in addition equip the dining hall with the necessary cooking utensils, cutlery and table ware. They would also furnish it with an orchestrion, piano, stage, steropticon outfit with two screens, sufficient lanterns and men to operate them.

"We will hold the Men's Welfare Work League responsible for making out in a general way the menus, which we will furnish at the cost of the raw material, the cooking and the serving of the same. We will make no charge to your organization for rent, for breakage, for heat, light, the services of the steward and the services of the purchasing agent.

The service is a question involving considerable expense, and we will leave that entirely to your league, whether you will hire people to do that, or whether your people will take turns in doing it. Your organization is not only to be responsible for the success of the dining room, but it is to have charge of the amusements, consisting of lectures, vocal and instrumental music and other entertainments. You are to charge admission for all these entertainments or part of them as you see fit.

This will also provide your organization with a suitable meeting place, which the officers of your organization have told us they have wanted for some time so that you could have more meetings of the entire league. The desire of the company to provide you with a suitable meeting place has also assisted us in making up our minds to appropriate this warehouse for a lunch room and amusement hall for the benefit of the league."

Welfare Hall is a huge permanent building, accommodating 2500 at table or 7500 when used as an auditorium. Kitchen, bakery and cold storage plant adjoin the big dining room.

The charge for noonday lunches is based on the flat cost of raw materials, the company doing the cooking and serving free. Six hundred women who lunch at Welfare Hall pay twenty-five cents a week.

In the men's dining room the charge is ninety cents a week.

Each table has a representative who reports to the proper official of the league on Friday the number of "six-meal-ticket" holders at the respective tables. This gives the steward an accurate estimate on the number of meals he needs to provide for Saturday and prevent waste.

To employés who are not regular attendants of Welfare Hall single meal tickets are sold for any day in the week at 25 cents.

Men having a "five meal ticket" who may wish to take luncheon on Saturday also, may secure a ticket for this day for 15 cents.

Table representatives are urged to make their reports promptly and correctly. These reports become valuable when made by all. The reports are prepared in the following manner:

1. Number of table and date.
2. Name of head of table.
3. Number of people without tickets, from whom a "sign up" should be taken.
4. Number of permanent vacancies at the table.
5. Punch out number of vacancies at the table.

By adding the number of persons without tickets the number of "sign ups" will be obtained. The number of permanent vacancies will show where new people can be placed. Number of punches from the form will give number of meals served, which should tally with waiters' count and auditor's record of meal tickets sold. It is absolutely necessary that this report be given daily.

If for any reason the table representative is absent he either has another man punch the ticket or notifies the president or secretary of the league.

Many a factory is so congested that there does not seem to be a single square inch of room that is not needed imperatively for the business. This was true at the plant of the Acme White Lead and Color Works, Detroit, where there was no space for a dining room. This difficulty was obviated by folding tables, 12 inches by 3 feet, hinged lengthwise, and placed on three supports. Folding chairs were stacked up in racks. At the noon hour these tables were set up in the passageway or wherever there might be temporary room, but when not in use were stored wherever most convenient.

As building after building was added to the works the restrictive features of the past due to want of space were overcome, and advantage taken of the increased facilities to further improve the environment of the worker. In the new Administration Building opened recently, for instance, every feature that could possibly conduce to the personal comfort of employés has been utilized. This is particularly to be seen in the arrangement for work, sanitary, up-to-date toilet rooms, and for recreation. The large convention hall on the second floor, with a seating capacity of one thousand, is used not only for lectures, banquets, reunions, and as a general assembly hall, but every day as the girls' lunch room. The tables, linen and chairs, besides hot coffee, are provided by the firm. It may be stated also that this provision is extended to all employés of the various departments. In addition, there is a capacious and well-appointed dining room in the new café, where lunch is served to the clerical force and to heads of departments, and a private dining room for the officers. A recent new feature is the smoking room, where men can enjoy their pipe or cigar in cold and inclement weather. Tobacco, cigars and pipes are purchased by the firm and supplied at cost.

In studying the conditions of the life and labor of their employés, the firm ascertained that it sometimes happened that some of the workers left home without breakfast or at the noon hour did not feel the usual appetite. The accidental circumstances which may have deprived them of breakfast, or the lack of appetite at noon, do not operate against their loss of vitality and energy during the day, because the privileges of the restaurant are extended to the girls, who may obtain a bite to eat even during working hours. For a cent a cup, a good cup of coffee or tea, with milk and sugar, is furnished; three cents buys a plate of soup; eight cents a portion of hot meat and vegetables; all the desserts are three cents.

At the Milford Shoe Company[1] a lunch room is furnished free by the firm, who sell food at a small margin above its actual cost, not for the purpose of making any profit, but for the purpose of accumulating gradually a fund from which the employés may draw in case of sickness or death. On the request

[1] Milford Shoe Co., Milford, Mass. Manufacturers Men's Shoes. Organized March, 1889. Number Employés, 385.

of two fellow employés in the same department, and approved by the foreman or overseer of the department in which the employé works, in case of sickness or death, a sum of money necessary to render practical aid is withdrawn from the lunch benefit fund which accumulates over the cost of operating.

In the dining hall, as in every department of the establishment, attention is promptly arrested by the spaciousness, light and cheerfulness; but a new feature attracts the eye, for in every one of the sixteen south windows is a box of flowering plants, vigorous and flourishing, which give the place a particularly homelike and refined character.

The hall of the dining room at the Weston Electrical Instrument Company is handsomely furnished; the color scheme is pleasing—white walls, buff shades, furniture of a cherry effect, and many pictures. The crockery is a good quality of porcelain, tastefully decorated and bearing the company's monogram, as does the silver and cutlery. Paper napkins are provided. When the room is set for luncheon its appearance compares favorably with a high-class hotel or restaurant.

Lunch is either table d'hôte or à la carte. The table d'hôte costs twenty cents, and the patron is entitled to as much of any or all the dishes as he may desire.

The table d'hôte lunch is served by volunteers from among the force who are compensated by being permitted to lunch at the expense of the club, and to whom the company allows enough extra time at noon to insure their having the full forty minutes' recess. They usually serve a month at a time.

For the convenience of those who do not care to take the table d'hôte, there is a lunch counter where members may buy what they choose, and wait on themselves.

When the club was started there was considerable hesitancy about permitting the sale of beer. The members who had been in the habit of having beer with their luncheon protested that it would be unfair to impose such a restriction, whereupon the club decided to make this concession, but, it was clearly understood, only as an experiment. Beer is sold whenever the club is open—at luncheon and on entertainment evenings. There has not been a solitary instance of the slightest abuse of the privilege. To the lodge-keeper has been given the right to sell tobacco.

The kitchen, 35 by 25 by 16, is off the dining room, directly over the refrigerators and ice-making plant, and connected therewith by a stairway. It is furnished with ranges, grills, copper-jacketed kettles for soups and stews, a steam heated serving table, dish-washing machinery and all the various utensils—in fact it is a complete hotel or restaurant kitchen. The kitchen help is employed by the club, and has no connection with the regular force.

The ice-making plant and the ample refrigerator—one for meats and one for vegetables—form a large element in the financial success of the restaurant. Meats, vegetables, butter, groceries and other supplies are bought in quantities. Not only does this effect a considerable saving in cost, but it permits many otherwise impossible economies. The initiation fee is but 25 cents, and the monthly dues the same—about a cent per work day. A lunch of six courses, excellent in quality and unlimited in quantity, is served for 20 cents, while for 15 cents the frugal man or woman may fare sumptuously. The more economical may bring their lunch from home and eat in the restaurant, supplementing from the lunch counter bill of fare, or not, as they choose.

In view of these facts, it is gratifying to be able to report that the club has arrived at a point where, after all expenses, including renewals and repairs, have been met, a little surplus is earned. Of course the club pays no rent; this, and the original plant and working capital, being the company's contribution.

Harris Hall, a memorial to James Harris, a director and treasurer of the Plymouth Cordage Company, is the center of the commissary department. Several years ago there was a call for hot coffee and tea among the men, and the company opened a small room for a dining room, with the necessary tea and coffee urns. After a while there came a call for sandwiches, but it was impossible in these quarters. However, a suitable place was soon found in Harris Hall, where it is the main idea to give a good, cheap, substantial dinner for 10 to 12 cents, with tea, coffee, pies and cake extra for those who wish.

The men are obliged to wait upon themselves. They buy their coffee at one place, move on to the next, buy their dinner, and then take it to their table. On the first floor is a serving room, a large dining room for men, that will hold about 200, and leading off the main room is a smaller room for the office help. The men's toilet rooms are also situated on this floor. The lower part of the building is given up to a dining room for the girls, with rest rooms and toilet. The kitchen, cold-storage cellar and manager's room are also situated on this floor. The material is the best of its character that can be procured. Everything is made in their own kitchen, so they are perfectly sure of the material that goes into the food.

A room comfortably furnished is provided for those who lunch in the building of the Ferris Brothers Company. Every day tea with milk and sugar is provided free by the firm. In comparison with the overworked, round-shouldered anxious-faced girls of the ordinary factory, these employés are trim, tidy, cheerful looking, with bright eyes and rosy cheeks.

Conditions at the Westinghouse Companies, Pittsburg, will not permit the use of any particular scheme for furnishing luncheon at the noon hour; consequently there are five different methods.

The Casino is an institution established by the company to meet certain sociological needs of the immediate vicinity and is managed by nine directors appointed by the company. These men are selected with great care from among the employés so that the board will be thoroughly representative of the different classes of employés. The income from the bowling alleys, pool and billiard tables assists in defraying a portion of the expenses incurred in connection with the Casino Technical Schools and the lunch room. On this account food is served at a very nominal charge. A substantial meal consisting of meat, two vegetables, bread and butter, coffee and dessert is served for 20 cents. The quick lunch plan where each individual waits on himself enables them to feed 1000 persons in one hour. The tables are of the folding type and can be closed up and stored away in a very few minutes, permitting the dining room to be used as a lecture hall on short notice. This plan has been in operation for three years and has proven all that could be desired.

The East Pittsburg Club is frequented by the office force, a very substantial meal being served for 35 cents. The service compares very favorably with that rendered in connection with the dining room of a first class hotel. Soup, two vegetables, choice of four different meats, salad, choice of four different desserts cover the bill of fare. The club is managed by officials of the company, and the food is furnished at cost. The women shop employés have a large dining room where coffee, sugar and milk, and table appurtenances are furnished free —other food being brought from their homes. The dining and rest rooms for female office employés are situated in the main office building, where food is supplied at cost. The officers and principal heads of departments assemble in a dining room located in the office building, thus bringing them together once each day.

A large dining hall, 40 by 100, with all modern conveniences, is to be provided for the comfort of its 300 employés by the Eastern and Western Lumber Company,[1] a short distance from its yards in North Portland. Soup and coffee will be served free of charge.

The mills are in operation day and night, and as most of the men bring their lunches, they have been in the habit of taking the midday or midnight meal wherever they could conveniently seat themselves. The new arrangement will enable them to enjoy a rest after they have partaken of a warm meal, without extra cost to themselves.

Between the village of homes and the big mill, of the Lynchburg Cotton Mill,[2] is a large two-story brick building, 52 by 70 feet.

On the first floor is a dining hall where the operatives, instead of sitting by their machines or at the end of a plank or "any other old place," may enjoy their midday meal in comfort. Adjoining this is a smoking room and lavatories, with shower baths and bath tubs, supplied with hot and cold water. On the second floor is a large assembly room, furnished with tables and chairs, magazines and periodicals and writing material. It is also the purpose of the company to have this room so arranged that at night it can be used for entertainments and for lectures, with the object of inculcating lessons of thrift,

[1] Eastern and Western Lumber Co., Portland, Ore. Lumber Manufacturers and Logging. Organized 1902. Number Employés, 700.

[2] Lynchburg Cotton Mill, Lynchburg, Va. Cotton Manufacturers. Organized 1888. Number Employés, 550.

and encouraging the operatives in a desire to improve their surroundings.

The building, costing $10,000, is lighted with electricity and in winter heated by steam. Every arrangement for the comfort of the operatives is to be brought into service. The president of the company has other plans in contemplation for making life happier and better for those in his employ, and in keeping with the present love of athletics has allotted a level piece of ground for a baseball field.

The lunch room which is managed for the employés of the Maddock pottery company[1] is one operated by a very homelike German and his wife. It is across the street from the pottery, and is maintained by the employés. It is so arranged that if any of them should carry a cold dinner, and should want five cents' worth of warm soup, he can get it, or anything else he may wish. In fact, a good warm dinner is served for fifteen cents. The firm themselves are in the habit of dining there.

The Metropolitan Life Insurance Company provides a lunch room for the use of the women clerks, equipped by the company, but managed by a committee of the young women themselves, who engage the steward, and he employs the subordinates, cooks, waitresses and purchases the supplies. The cost of running the lunch room is met by the small weekly subscription for membership in the club, and a charge for whatever is ordered from the daily bill of fare.

There is a large lunch counter for the factory help of the Solvay Process Co., which is kept open 24 hours every day excepting Sunday, when it is closed from 3 P.M. to 6 P.M. Luncheon, consisting of griddle cakes, cookies or fried cakes, with coffee, is served from 6 A.M. to 10 A.M. for five cents. For dinner, from 11 A.M. to 1 P.M., and for supper from 5 P.M. to 7 P.M., the charge is 10 cents, the fare comprising meat and potatoes, one helping of vegetable, bread and butter, two cups of coffee or a glass of milk. Many take their luncheons between the hours set apart for regular meals, when they may obtain cold sandwiches, bread and butter, baked beans and hot coffee at a moderate price. At the lunch counter each day 250 workmen take their meals.

[1] John Maddock & Sons, Trenton, N. J. Manufacturing Potters. Organized 1895. Number Employés, 250.

At the club house, dining room and lunch counter there are served about 3000 meals a month.

The George B. Peck Dry Goods Company,[1] at Kansas City, maintains a lunch room for employés in charge of a competent man and woman, with a force of assistants. An abundance of wholesome food is served at the lowest possible cost.

Factory and office lunch rooms are maintained at a dozen different works of the International Harvester Company, and employés can get good food at a low price, the purpose being to have each one self-sustaining, no charge being made for floor space or equipment expense. Nearly all the women patronize the lunch rooms, and the number of men patrons is increasing. The lunch rooms are conveniently situated for the women workers.

The importance of a well-appointed lunch room is evidenced by James R. Keiser, who has set aside space representing a rental value of $1500 for large noonday rest rooms and lunch rooms for employés. The women's lunch room has a table seating capacity for nearly 200 persons. A gas range permits of warming food, a water heater provides abundant hot water for tea and coffee and a refrigerator preserves cream and any perishable delicacy that employés may bring from their homes. No further culinary appliances are necessary, as each employé brings his or her own luncheon. The men have a dining room adjoining.

Because of the value of gold on the work-benches, employés of Carter, Howe & Company are not allowed to remain in the factory during the noon hour; so for the convenience of those who cannot go home for dinner, the first floor of a building which adjoins the factory has been leased and fitted up comfortably for the men's use. For the women employés of the same firm there are two rooms, beside the toilet and kitchen, the latter having a cook stove with fire and tea kettle of hot water ready for them, so that they can make tea or coffee or cook any simple article of food, if they care to do so. The women's lunch room is provided with shelved closets and other conveniences for putting away dishes and cooking utensils, and for meeting other requirements of the purposes of its use.

[1] George B. Peck Dry Goods Co., Kansas City, Mo. Department Store. Organized May, 1889. Number Employés, 900.

All the rooms are heated by steam and kept clean and comfortable at the expense of the company.

In a large department store[1] in San Francisco a small room was set aside where the girls could eat the luncheon which they brought from their homes. They responded to this so eagerly that the firm added a gas range and a woman in charge, who began furnishing such food as could be prepared easily.

For adult workers at John Wanamaker's there is perhaps not as great, certainly not the same scope for personal care; at least not so large a proportion of them are in circumstances to require it. Some things are done, however, and much remains to be developed. In the lunch room ten cents buys a satisfying lunch and thereby helps to preserve health of stomach and poise of temper. There are separate lunch rooms for the men and women, and temporary outdoor porches where rest can be taken in the open air. On their porch men can smoke if they choose. In connection with the lunch room is a rest room containing a circulating library of 4600 volumes.

What is known as a "lunch club" is run in connection with the Tide Water Oil Works. The company furnishes room, utensils, fuel, cook and waiters. The members of the club pay for provisions, wear and tear of linen and other supplies. The club membership is open to all employés. Some fifty men have availed themselves of the privileges.

The National Biscuit Company has a large and well-equipped restaurant, where good food is supplied at reasonable prices to an average of 1500 people a day. The plan is to make the restaurant support itself, but not have it make any profit. In this way the employés who patronize it may know that they are getting their full money's worth.

The Gorham Company,[2] Providence, R. I., opened a casino which was to be a social center for their 1900 employés. The plan was a success from the start, in fact so successful that the company decided to double its capacity. October, 1907, it was re-dedicated with appropriate remarks and social

[1] Hale Brothers, San Francisco, Cal. Dealers in Dry Goods, etc. Organized 1903. Number Employés, 800.

[2] Gorham Co., Providence, R. I. Silversmiths and Goldsmiths. Established 1831. Number Employés, 1900

festivities. The purpose of the casino is to afford the employés comfortable and agreeable surroundings for eating their midday meals, instead of staying in the shops. A restaurant is in charge of a competent chef, where food is sold to the employés at the lowest possible rates, with no gain for the company. Off the main room is a dining room where a three-course dinner may be bought for 25 cents. There is also a dining room for the women, where the feminine employés of the company may have all the advantages of a meal at home.

On the upper floor are the rooms occupied by the caretakers of the building, besides various sleeping apartments. Commercial men or buyers who do not wish to go downtown over night will find in this building sleeping apartments such as any hotel would do well to duplicate. On the upper floor also is a large dining room, used once a year for the dinner of the heads of the departments, and used all the year round by the directors of the company and their guests. It is one of the largest in the building. The kitchen also is on the upper floor, and the food is sent down by means of two dumb-waiters.

The lower floor is devoted to the use of the employés, and is fully as well appointed as the rooms above. There are reading and sitting rooms for women, which from their appearance will attract many of the women employés to them, while the library, reading rooms and smoking rooms for the men are equally comfortably appointed.

Intimately connected with the preparation of good food, is the ability to purchase the purest foodstuffs at the right price. At the corporation stores of the Vermont Marble Co.[1] the purchase of pure food is an important matter. This company has at its quarries and works in Vermont 3300 employés. Its business is scattered over a considerable district in Rutland County, Vermont, and requires some fifteen miles of railroad to connect its different quarries, mills and shops.

The company has always believed and still believes that from the nature of the case it ought to maintain in that village a first class store for the accommodation of its employés, and that, situated as the village is, its people would not be provided

[1] Vermont Marble Co., Proctor, Vt. Quarrying Marble. Monument Builders. Organized 1902. Number Employés, 3300.

with the variety and quality of goods which they ought to have nor at economical prices except through the instrumentality of a store such as the company with its capital and facilities is able to maintain.

For many years stores have been run at as low a margin of profit as safe business would warrant. In 1902 on a business almost as large as they had ever done until then the per cent. of profit to the company on their entire sales for the year was only 3.6 per cent. They endeavored to make a specialty of staple goods and necessities and in some cases, through the facilities of the company, were able to make marked reduction from the regular price. For example, for years the employés of the company have had coal delivered at their houses by these stores at from 50 to 75 cents per ton cheaper than it was sold in the neighboring city of Rutland or could be bought anywhere in the vicinity. This was accomplished by the company buying the supply in connection with its coal for commercial uses and being able to forego the profit upon it.

May 1, 1903, the company announced that it proposed to divide among its employés according to their trade at each store the entire profits of that store. The management of the store was continued in the hands of the company. A representative committee, however, of five employés was appointed for each of the stores to take a consultative part in its management and particularly to supervise and audit the settlement of its business and the distribution of its profits at the end of the year. These committees are from time to time consulted and suggestions are sought from them as to changes or improvements which would help the service, but the real responsibility for the management of the store has continued as before in the company, which advances all the money required for their business and through its executive officers directs their general policy. The purpose has been to continue to keep the prices of the stores as low as possible and assure a reasonable margin of profit.

The total sales for the first eight months, that is, from May 1, 1903, to January 1, 1904, were $251,620.11, of which $179,716.38 were sales to employés of the company, and the balance, $71,903.73 were sales to non-employés. The profits from the business of the three stores, including both its sales to employés and non-employés, were for the same period $16,296, or 6.4 per cent. of their entire sales. That gave the employés trading at the Proctor store a dividend of ten per cent. upon their purchases, those trading at the West Rutland store a dividend of nine per cent., and those at the Center Rutland store a dividend of six per cent. These dividends were paid to the employés in January, 1904, by bank check.

The R. D. Wood Company[1] has always maintained a store in the village in which its works are situated for the sale of goods to its operatives, leaving entirely to their option the question of purchasing goods there. Their store has never been profitable, owing to the prices being placed on the lowest possible basis consistent with the policy of paying the cost of running. They have, however, continued to run it, so that the cost of living in the village should not be influenced by those who might otherwise charge unfairly high prices for goods.

The advisability of starting a corporation store had been discussed several times by the Ludlow Manufacturing Associates, but no action was taken, until recently the corporation started a restaurant, in connection with which they sell bread, pastry and cooked foods. Believing that the credit system is a curse to manufacturing villages, they have run this store on a cash basis. The result has been that the operatives generally confine their purchases to stores which give them less for their money but allow them credit and deliver at their doors.

A coöperative purchasing committee is appointed by the Seattle Electric Company,[2] whose business it is to make arrangements with such merchants as may be selected, by which the members of the association are enabled to secure the lowest possible prices for clothing, groceries and all immediate supplies, and this same committee endeavors in other ways to promote the economic and business welfare of the members. The dues of each member of the association are 75 cents a month.

As the Plymouth Cordage Company is situated some distance from the town, many small groceries sprang up to supply the employés with their staples of food. The company, not satis-

[1] R. D. Wood & Co., Florence, Millville and Camden, N. J. Iron Founders. Organized 1803. Number Employés, 558.

[2] The Seattle Electric Co., Seattle, Wash. Street Railway and Electric Lighting. Organized January, 1900. Number Employés, 1500.

fied with existing conditions, bought out some of the stores and started a large one under the head of the Employés Coöperative Store. The company furnished sufficient capital to start it along the following lines: That the company would not receive any interest on the money invested; that it should be a coöperative business entirely for the employés' benefit, they to receive their share of the profits pro rata as their accounts showed on the books.

In 1895 the head of a large firm noticing that the employés were in the habit of using lead pencils, matches or sticks in removing foreign bodies from the eyes, arranged to have a number of workers in the different departments equipped with emergency outfits and trained to do the first aid work. Later the work was turned over to a foreman, who made a special study of first aid treatment. With the large increase in the number of employés a permanent relief station became necessary. A room has been set aside for the care of injured eyes. This emergency room contains an equipment for first aid treatment equal to that of almost any practicing oculist. It is under the charge of a student of ophthalmology, who has had several years' experience in this work. The daily average is 12 cases in winter and 20 in summer, when the windows are open and the dust blows. Few of these cases are serious and none is due to dangerous processes of manufacture.

When the injury is one of a grave nature, the patient is sent to a specialist, only first aid measures being taken at the factory. In the last five months 15 cases have required expert treatment.

During certain hours of the day an optician is on duty at the factory, and consultation and treatment may be had by employés without cost. Lectures on health are also given to the factory employés. Requiring all employés to pass a physical examination when they enter the factory, in order to protect the other workers, the company spares no effort to keep them healthy and make their work safe and pleasant. The employer is repaid many times for any expense incurred in promoting ideal health conditions.

At the Cleveland Hardware Company the work is quite hazardous, and there are necessarily many accidents. A small room about eight by eight, which had formerly been used as a serving room, connected with the kitchen, was fitted up as a hospital. The firm consider it a great success, and practically a necessity in a factory of their kind, and a good thing to have in any place where there are a large number of employés.

The room is located practically in the center of the plant; in fitting it up it was painted with white enamel, an enamel wash-basin put in with hot and cold water, small glass-top surgeon's table, two chairs, a rattan couch, two blue army blankets and towels and other accessories. In this room are kept liniments, salves and other things for use in emergency cases. First of all the injured employé is taken direct to the hospital, where the wound is thoroughly cleansed and washed. The first dressing is given at the hospital, and if a man feels sick or faint from the injury, he stays in this room until he feels strong enough to go to his own doctor or to a hospital located in the vicinity of the factory. The firm state that this is an excellent thing from a humanitarian standpoint, and in addition they have found that very often an employé getting a slight wound will not in the first place wash it thoroughly, and then perhaps will wrap a piece of dirty cloth around it, and in three or four days the wound has begun to fester, and while it probably would not have been much if attended to properly, it has become a serious matter, and may keep him from work for some time. This is a loss to the company, not only on account of the absence of a good employé for some time, but also on account of the employé sometimes making a claim for damages. In this way all accidents are reported immediately to the office. On the bottom of a special report is a detachable order; if in the opinion of the person attending the injured employé he should need medical attention, this is filled out immediately, and the company pursues the plan of paying for the first attention which is necessary. The amount that is paid by the company later on account of such injury of course depends upon circumstances.

One can easily see also the benefit of having a complete record of every accident that happens in the factory, no matter how slight, from the fact that if later on there is any claim for damages made by the employé, it is very easy to refer back to the original report and get intelligent information in regard to the accident.

It is to the company's advantage to give out such remedies as cholera cure and headache medicine, for very often an employé may be cured from one of these ailments in a few minutes, that will allow him to continue his work during the day, and in this way increase the output of a manufacturing plant, which of course is one of the things that all manufacturers are working for.

Employés who are slightly indisposed understand that they can make application at any time and go into this private room, and get a good thorough rest during the noon hour.

In connection with the factory hospital of this same company arrangements have been made with the Cleveland Visiting Nurses Association for the entire time of one nurse to be given to the employés of this factory. She is a trained nurse of the very highest quality, and this arrangement was made through the Visiting Nurses Association, so as to have the benefit of their supervision. The nurse has regular hours at the factory hospital, to give consultations and dressings. She also makes visits to the homes of sick employés, and will also make calls to give advice in case of sickness in the employés' families. She furnishes a daily report.

Case reported July 25, 1907.
Case investigated July 26, 1907.
Name: T. H.
Address: St. Clair Avenue.
Nationality: Slav.
Married or Single: Single.
Home or Boarding: Boarding.
Medical Attention: Dr. S.
Ailment: Gastritis.
Probable period of disability: Able to return immediately.

Resident Conditions: Boards with family living over a saloon. Rooms clean and light.

Statement of Patient: Man said the Doctor had told him that he must stop drinking beer before his stomach would be much better. Said he was going to work Monday, July 29th.

Statement of Nurse: Called to see man July 25th; was not

at home; called again July 26th, not at home. People where he boarded said he was at the Doctor's. They went for him. I waited about one and a half hours before he came home. Doctor said he was not there July 26th, had not been to see him for one week. From every appearance the man had been drinking. This young man's case indicates saloon boarding house environment bad.

A hospital and medical department has been organized with a large central institution at Pueblo, known as the Minnequa Hospital, with branches or emergency hospitals at all of the leading camps of the Colorado Fuel and Iron Company. These are in charge of skilled physicians and surgeons, whose duty it is to care for the sick and injured employés, and to exercise general supervision over sanitary conditions at their respective stations.

The Minnequa Hospital at Pueblo was completed in 1902 at a cost approximating a quarter of a million dollars. The entire hospital plant, including grounds and buildings, covers 13 acres and comprises a central or administrative building, three ward and operating buildings, a hospital for communicable diseases, a physician's residence, a recreation hall for convalescents, a kitchen and a dining room, a laundry, a light and power plant, a well and pumping station, and a stable and ambulance barn. The hospital now accommodates 240 patients, and it is planned to add other wards as they are needed.

This same company places a local doctor at each of the mines to care for the sick and slightly injured. Great stress is placed upon preventive measures, and the doctors are required to deliver monthly lectures of a popular nature on various health topics, not only to the children in the schools, but to adults in evening courses. Further, a monthly bulletin treating of sanitary subjects is circulated free to all employés.

It may not be generally known that the railroads maintain at an enormous expense well-equipped hospitals, with all necessary surgeons, physicians, nurses and attendants, for the sole purpose of relieving as far as possible the pains of those unfortunates who have been injured in one of those wrecks, the cause of which is sometimes due to negligence, and again because of some unforeseen, some well-nigh inexplicable, happenings which come to all roads.

A feature of the betterment work of the Southern Pacific Railway[1] is the hospital car service by means of a car which is in every particular a model hospital with all the necessary equipment, and which was constructed at a cost of $18,000.

It is the intention of the railroad company to place these cars at certain stations on their line, when in the event of serious accidents they can be attached to special engines and hurried to the scene of the accident, carrying surgeons, nurses and all the emergency appliances with which all well-regulated hospitals are equipped.

The car is not only a model in so far as the hospital appointments are concerned, but a device permits the berths to be automatically lowered when not in use to spaces prepared under the floor of the car. By this it will be seen that the usual overhead berth is done away with, and that space affording more ventilation is gained in the car. The floor space gained by the lowering of the berth affords room for chairs and tables and makes a delightful dining or reading room. The remainder of the car can be occupied as a sleeper.

One remarkable feature in connection with the operating room on the car is that it is provided with double swinging doors on each side of the car, and so arranged that injured passengers may be brought to the operating room and placed on the operating table or in the beds without having to be lifted from the stretcher. The beds, too, are unique. They are so arranged as to permit the stretchers being placed in the space usually occupied by the mattresses, thus being designed to avoid the additional suffering which might result as the patient was being transferred from stretcher to bed. The construction of the car provides for making the operating room an absolutely private ward during an operation or the dressing of a wound; after which the sliding doors are thrown open and the operating room becomes a part of the principal division of the car.

In building the car the company has not overlooked the com-

[1] Southern Pacific Co., Chicago, Ill. Railroad. Organized 1884. Number Employés, 80,304.

fort of the surgeons, nurses and other attendants. They have provided a private room, with stationary bed, toilet and shower bath, lavatory and lockers for the surgeons; kitchen quarters for the nurses and servants, where every needed convenience for surgical apparatus, medicines and supplies are kept, and an observation room, with stationary revolving chairs.

The Erie Railroad Company maintains a special hospital car 60 feet long, divided into two compartments; the operating room, 15 feet 10 inches by 8 feet 8 inches, is equipped with an operating table having a movable head and foot extension. This is located in the center of the room. An instrument sterilizer is on the right and a surgeon basin on the left of the operating table. This room also has three lockers fully equipped with surgical instruments, and is fully stocked with bandages, plasters, sponges and all anesthetics, antiseptics, astringents and other medical and surgical necessities. Sliding doors on each side of room, four feet wide with portable steps, permit an easy entrance for a stretcher to the operating room, which has six windows, three on each side, as well as those in the side and end doors.

Two chandeliers equipped with four mantle lamps each as well as one portable lamp, furnish the necessary light at night in the operating room. A gravity water system furnishes both hot and cold water from tanks just under the roof of the car. The flow of water can be regulated by a surgeon with his foot, thereby avoiding the necessity of handling any of the equipment. The head lining and interior of the car is very plain, thoroughly enameled in white. The floor is covered with white rubber tiling.

The ward room is 43 feet 4 inches in length, equipped with 11 iron beds enameled in white, and a lavatory. It has white rubber tiling on the floor and composite board sides enameled in white. There are white rubber curtains around and between each bed, which makes the space enclosed equal to a private room, giving to each patient the necessary privacy required.

Equipment boxes underneath the car are provided with crutches, splints, army stretchers, surgical implements, wrecking tools and other accessories. Six-wheel trucks insure the utmost freedom from vibration.

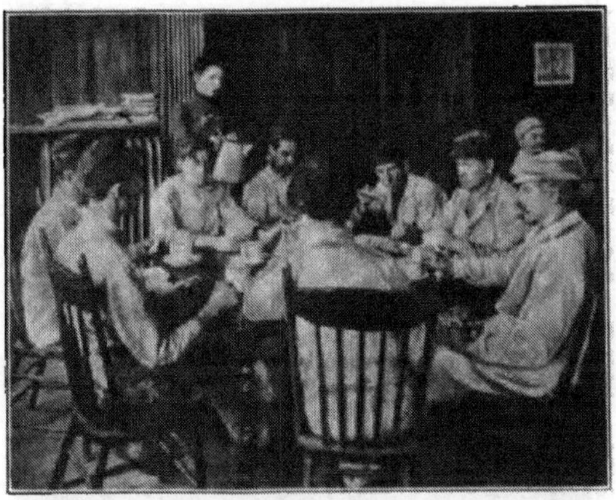

A Corner of the Men's Dining Room at the Patton Paint Company, Milwaukee, Wisconsin.

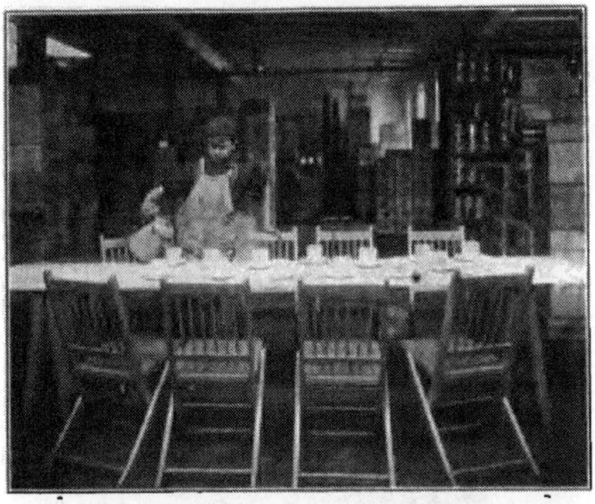

Where There's a Will, There's a Way. Folding Tables and Seats Set up for Dinner at a Crowded Factory Where Every Inch of Space is at a Premium.

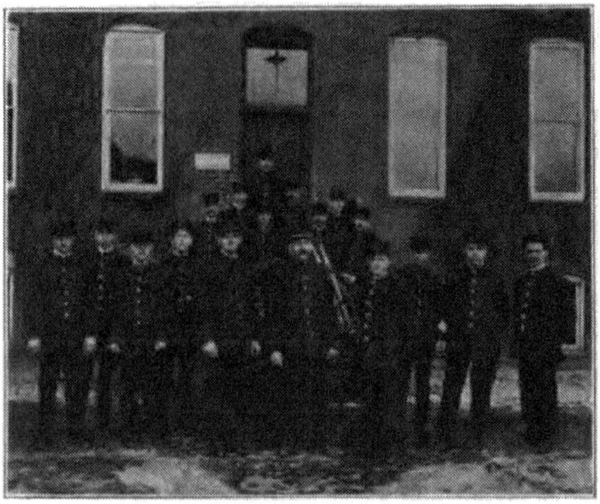

Fire Fighters at the Remington Typewriter Works.

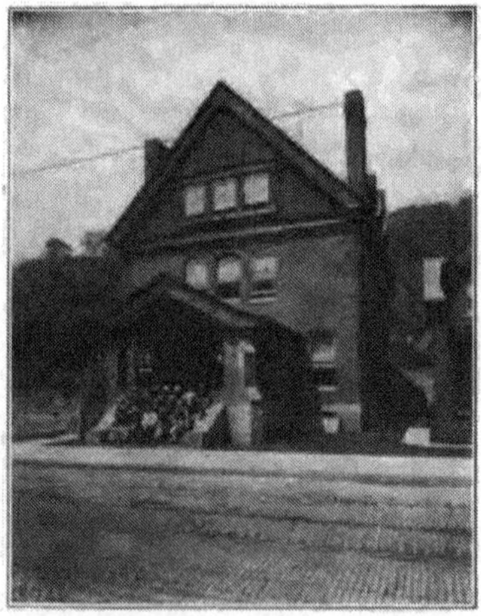

Where the Fire Fighters Live at the Westinghouse Electric and Manufacturing Company. Dormitory Equipped with Reading Room, Pool Room, Piano and Shower Baths for Thirty-two Men.

An annual subscription to the Paterson General Hospital is paid by the Ludlum Steel and Spring Company,[1] for which employés who need treatment through accident or sickness are taken in free of cost.

Liberal contributions are made by the New York Switch and Crossing Company[2] to a local hospital, which is a charitable institution, so that employés in case of accident or sickness may have a place to go where they will receive proper medical treatment.

Another company provides no hospital of its own but furnishes four free beds in the city hospital.

A Brooklyn drop forge company encourages during the holiday season a collection among its employés for the benefit of one of the city hospitals. This annual fund has increased in twelve years from $40 to over $200. This custom has good influence in promoting self-respect in the men, and especially when they become beneficiaries of the hospital.

The American Steel and Wire Company has 20 emergency hospitals, operated at, and in connection with, its various manufacturing plants, all of these hospitals being fully equipped with surgical instruments and dressings. Every hospital is in charge of a competent surgeon, who is paid by the company. Very serious cases are sent to public hospitals at the company's expense, and all injured men, irrespective of the manner in which they get hurt, are nursed back to health entirely at the expense of the company. Upon the recovery of the injured men financial assistance is given them if they have been off duty upwards of from three to four weeks, provided there has been no misbehavior on their part in the meantime. The amount of personal injury gratuity is not arbitrarily fixed, but determined on consideration of the character of the injury and the actual needs of the man, based on his age, his family relations and his record as to term of service and faithfulness.

The Standard Bleachery Company[3] supports hospital beds

[1] Ludlum Steel and Spring Co., Pompton, N. J. Manufacturers Steel and Springs. Organized March 12, 1898. Number Employés, 75.

[2] New York Switch and Crossing Co., Hoboken, N. J. Manufacturers Railroad Frogs and Switches. Number Employés, 110. Organized May 13, 1896.

[3] Standard Bleachery Co., Carleton Hill, N. J. Bleaching Cotton Goods. Organized 1855. Employés, 1100.

and contributes liberally to the support of libraries and other institutions in surrounding towns for the benefit of its employés, who appear to be satisfied and to appreciate the advantages thus provided for them.

The Baldwin Locomotive Works carries its own insurance against accident to employés, and deals personally with its men who become injured, or whose families are in need from any cause. The men are perfectly free to consult with the superintendent when in difficulty, and cases warranting investigation are met by sending a competent representative to their homes, who is authorized to furnish the relief which the case requires.

For those employés who are in poor health and convalescent Strawbridge & Clothier make arrangements with private parties in the country and at the seashore where such employés, when not otherwise provided for, are sent by them. This service will be extended as the necessity for it may increase.

Systematic hospital collection was started by John Maddock's Sons, who take from the envelopes of the employés the last pay in each month ten cents; the total contribution so received is divided equally between the hospitals of their city. A receipt for the contribution, like the following, "Monthly contribution of 10 cents for the support of William McKinley Memorial Hospital and St. Francis Hospital," is placed in the envelopes. This method of collection has proven entirely satisfactory to the men, and the hospitals are trying to introduce the same system throughout the plants of the city. It is an interesting proposition both to the employé and employer. It avoids all factory collections, which are at the least annoying and expensive from both sides, and it is believed that the reports of the hospitals will prove that by this system they receive more during the year than by the old method of collection made individually through the shops two or three times a year.

The health of her employés is of great importance to Mrs. Seaman, head of the Iron Clad Company. A doctor is in constant attendance to help the sick to get well, and to help the well to keep so. Lectures are given every month on "How to Keep Good Health." A small hospital ward is maintained in the factory to give immediate relief to the injured and sick. The Mutual Aid Committee visits the sick and cares for them and in the event of death does all in its power to console the bereaved.

In 1896, W. L. Douglas,[1] Brockton, Mass., placed a doctor at the disposal of his employés, who consulted him during the noon hour for any ailments. They were at liberty to call at his office at any time, or if confined to the house the doctor called upon them, the service being entirely free to the employés.

In 1906 a special surgical and medical department was established, with a trained nurse in charge daily from 8 o'clock until 5 o'clock; and a physician in attendance from 8 A.M. to 10 P.M., and from 3 P.M. till 5 P.M. daily. This department includes nurses' rooms and rest room, where employés desiring to rest, but not sick enough to go home, lie down for an hour or two at a time, a doctor's consulting room, from which he also dispenses medicines used, and a most complete surgical room, with practically every appliance known to modern surgery.

There are also emergency sets in the different parts of the factories, with men who are competent to handle them in case of sudden injury, previous to the arrival of a doctor. In the new plant there will be an emergency room and surgical department, with a physician in attendance at all times, so that any case can be handled promptly and effectively.

At the United States Shoe Company's plant is located an emergency hospital with modern appliances and in charge of a competent attendant, free to all employés.

[1] W. L. Douglas Shoe Co., Brockton, Mass. Manufacturers Leather Shoes. Incorporated 1902. Number Employés, 3200.

CHAPTER IV

SAFETY FOR LIFE, LIMB AND HEALTH

CHIEF among the perils to social and industrial life, night and day, is fire. While the insurance companies and the state laws insist on certain rules and regulations, there is a large field which can be occupied by volunteer effort; the greater the measure of coöperation or good feeling in the plant, the prompter and more efficient will be the response to fire fighting, the success of which means safety for life and property. A case in point: A Detroit factory has its own private fire department of ten men living close to the plant, who stand ready at any moment, day or night, to respond to any alarm indicating that the buildings are in peril. The chief of this department is the engineer who lives next door to the factory. He and his comrades (as well as the night men on duty) recently late at night, when a fire was discovered which threatened the lumber yard, turned out so promptly and worked so intelligently that the fire was under control when the city department arrived.

Parke, Davis & Company afford adequate fire protection by numerous fire escapes; a well-drilled fire department of their own with an excellent equipment of pumps, hose and other appliances; a complete sprinkler system covering the entire plant; private connection with the city fire department and, finally, the location of one of the city's powerful fire boats at the wharf in front of the new science laboratory.

The Curtis Publishing Company issues a special book of instructions on fire protection to each one of its 1000 employés.

"The subject of fire protection has received careful attention by the company, and its extreme importance is fully recognized.

The buildings are supplied with readily accessible and serviceable outside fire escapes and there are sufficient stairways and exits, so that in case of fire the opportunity for a prompt and safe escape is at hand. The drills in the publication building have shown that all the employés can leave that building comfortably and quietly in from two to three minutes if there is no confusion or panic.

There are plenty of fire hose, fire apparatus, fire extinguishers, water buckets and axes in every department, and a fire marshal is in constant attendance, who makes daily inspection of the buildings and frequent examinations and test of all the fire-fighting apparatus and signals.

It is well known, however, that all mechanical means of fighting fire may be useless at the critical moment unless some one has been instructed in their use in advance and the duty of using them in an emergency has been assigned to him. It is also a fact that something more is necessary than the mere provision of facilities for escape from fire, for more accidents occur from panic following the alarm of fire—when there is little or no fire—than occur from fire itself, showing that in excitement people cannot be depended upon to reason correctly, and that, if they have not been taught the thing to do in an emergency, they are likely to wait for some one else to do something and then all follow. This may lead to many going to the same exit and there getting jammed and panic-stricken and perhaps hurt.

With this in view and wishing to avoid casualties of any kind, the company has established a complete fire-drill organisation among the occupants of the buildings, together with a fire-alarm system so devised that in case of a fire a general alarm will be sounded in time to give ample opportunity to all employés to leave their building while the fire is being extinguished or held in check by the fire brigade.

For the purpose of accustoming employés to prompt and orderly action in case of fire, general fire drills are held in the publication building at intervals during the year. In the mechanical building no general drills are held, but special instruction is given regularly to the members of the fire brigade. No advance notice of the drills in the publication building is given, but the fire alarm gongs are sounded exactly as if there were a real fire, and the light signals show the floor on which it is located. Part of the special duty of the fire brigade is to direct and assist the other employés in making their exit from the building as quietly and quickly as possible and by the proper routes.

Whenever the fire alarm sounds all valuable books and papers must be instantly returned to the safes and vaults where they are kept, the safes and vaults closed and all employés who are not in the brigade must leave the building as expeditiously as possible. After the sounding of the alarm employés should first always look at the signal boxes, where the floor on which the fire starts is indicated, and then be guided by these signals in determining what exits to use.

All those who are working on floors above the fire should go upstairs and over the bridge to the Mechanical Building. Those working on the same floor as, and on floors below the fire, should go downstairs and out to the street. Always keep to the right in passing, to avoid congestion, and do not return to work until the recall bell is sounded.

It is confidently hoped that all employés will appreciate the importance of these drills and coöperate cheerfully and earnestly in making them effective. With this coöperation there cannot be at any time any great danger to the employés from fire in the buildings, for the fire should be put out before it obtains headway, while everybody is being quickly removed from the building and beyond its reach.

GENERAL RULES AND REGULATIONS

1. Fire escapes and all windows, hallways, aisles and approaches leading to them must be kept clear. Open aisles must always be kept throughout all floors, allowing free access to fire escapes and apparatus.

2. All fire equipment, extinguishers, buckets, lanterns, and so forth, are for use in case of fire only, and must not be disturbed or used for any other purpose.

3. There must be no tying of electric drop lights by strings or wires. No paper shades are allowed on electric lights.

4. At the closing hour all windows are to be shut and all electric lights turned off except in the hallways and stairs.

5. No smoking is allowed in the publication building before or after business hours, nor in the mechanical buildings at any time.

6. No inflammable material (paper, cardboard, cloth, wood and so forth) must ever be placed on or close to steam pipes.

7. Candles are not allowed to be used in any part of the building. Movable electric lamps must be used instead, and portable cord for this purpose will be furnished either by the electrician or the fire marshal.

8. Safety matches only are allowed. No fuse or wind matches must be brought into any of the buildings.

9. No waste paper or other refuse material must be thrown from the windows of any of the buildings.

10. The doors over switch and panel boards must always be kept closed.

11. All oily waste, floor sweepings and other refuse must be placed in covered cans provided for the purpose, the covers kept closed and the cans removed at the close of each day.

12. Anything that in the judgment of any employé appears to be out of order should be reported at once to the bureau manager and by him to the fire marshal.

13. In case of the discovery of a fire it is most important that there be no shouting or cries of "Fire!" which would unnecessarily alarm people and might lead to a panic. The proper method of giving notice of any fire that may be discovered is stated below.

PUBLICATION BUILDING

1. Fire-alarm boxes, painted red, are located on the wall near the front stairs on each floor, also in the machine shop and lunch room in the basement, in the rest room on the first floor, beside the rear elevator on the second and third floors, in the daily mail bureau on the fourth floor, in the manuscript room on the fifth floor, and inside the rear hall door on the sixth floor.

If a fire is discovered anywhere in the building go at once to the nearest fire-alarm box, break the glass and turn the button, and remain there until the fire brigade arrives. This signal will notify the fire marshal, who will at once summon the fire brigade.

2. Indicators which will show at once by a red light the floor on which a fire starts will be located on the north and south ends of the light-well at the fourth floor, on the first floor beside

the front elevator, and in the fire marshal's office, and in the lunch room in the basement.

In case of a fire during working hours, an alarm will be sounded for employés on the gong which is located at the south end of the light-well on the fourth floor, and also on the fire bells on the first floor and in the basement. Upon any sounding of this alarm employés should first look at once at the fire indicators to ascertain the location of the fire and then be guided by these signals and the directions of the fire brigade in determining which exits to use. All valuable papers and books should be immediately returned in the manner arranged by the bureau managers to the safes and vaults where they are ordinarily kept at night, and the safes and vaults locked and all employés excepting those in the fire brigade must leave the building speedily and quietly, and not return until the recall bell has been rung.

A simple regulation for the prevention of congestion, provides that all the employés at work on floors above the fire, should go upstairs, using the bridges to the other buildings; all those working on the same floor as the fire, should go downstairs and out into the street. Particular emphasis is laid on the direction to always keep to the right in passing.

MECHANICAL BUILDINGS

If a fire is discovered anywhere in the buildings report it instantly to the manager of the bureau or notify the superintendent's office."

In conclusion a list of fire escapes and exits, which are always marked by red lights, is given.

The Acme fire department of the Acme Lead and Color Works of Detroit, Mich., was organized early in the year 1900. Mr. Thomas Neal, Secretary and General Manager, thought it would be a good thing to have such an organization as an adjunct to other precautionary measures against fire. The employés thought so too and took hold with a vim, turning out with alacrity to practice drills, individually and collectively evincing such an interest and willingness to coöperate as to make the plan a success.

The fire department is officered by a chief and assistant chief. They assume the responsibility of maintaining a fire company that is prepared to fight fire anywhere in the Acme Works at an instant's warning—night or day. What the chief and his assistant say about fire protection "goes." They make precautionary rules and regulations, and by these all employés are guided. In the plan of organization there is a force of "regulars" and "auxiliary" fire fighters. They are prepared to do the fighting at whatever point may be indicated by the fire alarm signal—and do it quick. The auxiliaries are a reserve force in constant training, ready to take the place of absent "regulars," and assist night watchmen in case of emergency.

In addition to the "fire fighters," employés in all departments are organized to take prompt precautionary measures regarding escape from the buildings and the protection of property. In order to keep the employés in practice they are liable to be started at any moment by the signal "fire drill," when all work is instantly dropped, and the alert and quick way in which the machinery is shut down, windows closed, fire extinguishers, hose, sand pails and axes are ready for business with the employés lined up for a quick and orderly exit, is astonishing. In forty-five seconds from the time the alarm is sounded the "regulars" have two streams playing on different buildings. To do this the men must quit their work and get into their "harness" of rubber coats, hats and belts before reporting at the fire station, indicated by the alarm. These fire stations are located at different places on the ground and in the works, and each station is supplied with from 100 to 200 feet of hose.

It is also the duty of the "regulars," who are selected from all the various departments of the factories, to examine weekly the condition of all fire apparatus in every department, and make a written report to the chief. The hose, fire extinguishers, sand pails, pike poles, fire axes, ladders, lanterns, coats, belts, hats, spanners, hose and ladder straps must all be in place and ready to do service at a second's notice.

Everything from electric signal to the huge steam force pump which is capable of forcing 1800 gallons of water per minute through the arteries of the automatic sprinkler system, must be kept in perfect "trim." It consists of an automatic sprinkler to about every eight square feet of area. The sprinklers are sealed with soft solder that will melt at 155 degrees, so that a fire in the vicinity of one or more of the sprinklers immediately starts them working.

The fire pump, with a capacity of 1800 gallons per minute, supplies the sprinkler system automatically in accordance with the volume of water used. The supply is drawn from an underground tank or cistern with a capacity of 40,000 gallons, which is filled and replenished by the city water works. The fire pump is reinforced by a tank containing 15,000 gallons, located at the top of a tall water tower, which automatically assists the pump, should the demand be beyond its capacity.

Night watchmen are employed, under the control of the Acme fire department, whose duty it is to make regular rounds through the factories, visiting the stations which are located throughout the building, and send in electric signals, which are recorded on a time detector. As an extra precaution one of the "regulars" is detailed to visit the factory at some hour at night unknown to the night watchmen.

The night watchmen are provided with blank forms, which must be turned in every morning upon which a complete report must be made of anything out of order which they discover during the night. Auxiliary fire alarm boxes are located in the different departments, from which an alarm can be sent to the city fire department.

An alarm, entirely unexpected by the men, was turned in. It took 28 seconds to man the first line of hose and get the water on; the second line was longer, because the men had to set up ladders and carry the hose on the roof; it was done in 58 seconds. In a paint shop, a few seconds gained mean safety instead of loss.

The fire signal at J. H. Williams & Company, of Brooklyn, is a continuous blast of both steam whistles. One man with an assistant is in charge of each room; under them are men for detailed duties, giving the city alarm, placing fire pails on the platform, closing the windows and doors, arranging the monitor nozzle and the various lines of hose. Each man has one duty and is held responsible for its accurate and intelligent performance. The fire extinguishing and protective apparatus is inspected every week. Each workman has a complete description of the general scheme, with details, so that he may know his individual relation to it. The following are the general instructions:

"Each foreman will see that all apparatus in his department is in perfect working order. If a member of the fire department is absent, appoint one *promptly* to take his place. Do not let the fire department be crippled by the absence of its members.

The best way to prevent fire loss is to prevent fire starting. Cleanliness is necessary everywhere; fires do not start in clean places. Let no rubbish accumulate. Use no sawdust. Keep clean waste in the iron cans or tin cabinets provided for it, and burn all oily waste daily. Keep shaft bearings free from accumulations of oily dust.

Men in charge of hose lines will see that hose is properly oiled, ready for instant use; that extra spanners and washers are at hand; that nozzles are screwed tight and *everything* always ready for service.

In case of fire each department will act under its own head. Each man will take his own place and do his own work, not another's. Use care with water; it often does more damage than fire. At night leave elevator level with first floor."

The fire department at the Westinghouse Electric and Manufacturing Company consisting of 8 companies of 10 men each, affords ample protection against fire. The works are equipped with a complete automatic sprinkler system, fire walls, doors of fire resisting material, slow burning construction for floors, and wired glass. Underwriters consider the fire protection very superior.

The companies are quartered in a well-appointed dormitory immediately adjacent to the works. Two companies are always instantly available when the works are closed. The building is equipped with a reading room, pool room, shower baths and sleeping quarters. These men are drilled bi-weekly, all watchmen taking part in the drill. Time and one-half is paid for drilling. The whole force is in charge of an experienced fire fighter.

The Walthan Watch Company maintains a Fire Department in connection with its factory, the members of which are employés in the machine department. They are liable to be called out for drill at any moment, and are paid for their time while so engaged. The chief of the fire department was formerly one of the engineers of the city fire department, and is now foreman of the machine department.

A recent report of an insurance inspector comments on the fire drill at Strawbridge & Clothier's, Philadelphia, where 4000 people are employed.

A fire drill of the employés was given on the fourth floor at 8 A.M. The first alarm brought 14 men from the fourth floor in twenty seconds; a second alarm brought 112 men from all parts of the building in eighty-five seconds. In that time four lines of hose were out and ready for action. Another general alarm was given on the second floor with like results. Similar drills were made in the factory and at the Race street warehouse, all being characterized by very prompt response to signals. The drills were highly satisfactory. The men with their captains and chief deserve commendation for the fireman-like way of carrying out the purpose of the brigade.

On the hill near the Lynchburg Cotton Mills are two reservoirs, one in case of fire with a capacity of a million gallons, and the other fed from a spring, giving to each house its own supply of clear pure water. On the occasion of a recent fire in the mill, so excellently trained are the employés, and so fine is the supply of water, that what at first threatened to be a big blaze was extinguished in a few brief minutes. Insurance men have repeatedly stated that the mill has excellent fire protection.

At the Baldwin Locomotive Works the fire insurance is carried in the Factory Mutual Fire Insurance Company, and the protective apparatus is laid out in accordance with its rules. There are seven fire pumps, six of which are located in the main part of the works. These draw their suction supply from the city mains, and discharge into an underground feed system.

Each building is equipped with automatic sprinklers and storage capacity provided in each block by tanks situated on the top of stair towers and elevator towers. Each block contains two controlling stations, situated in most cases in the fireproof stairways. These control stations consist of an underground header which is connected to the feeder system and to the overhead storage tanks sprinkler supply. Tower standpipe and inside hose lines are laid out from these controlling stations.

This system makes it possible in case of fire to control the apparatus for any block from the controlling stations, and at the same time makes it possible to have an immediate water supply from all of the overhead storage tanks in the system applied directly in the building where the fire may occur. It also allows all of the fire pumps to be brought to bear through the underground feeder system. The sprinklers on each floor are controlled by a valve which always remains open except when the system on the floor is under repair. The foreman of each shop must make a daily report on blanks of the condition of all the sprinkler valves. These are countersigned by the inspector and the chief of highway.

At the Broadway Department Store,[1] Los Angeles, the proprietor installed an intricate electric alarm system. From a switchboard one man commands 76 volunteer fire-fighters, equipped with extinguishers and axes, and divided into squads of ten or twelve each. It is possible for the operator to assemble them in any one place, or direct them to many different points. They are called from their work by the sound of gongs which ring on each floor, when an alarm is turned in from one of many boxes distributed about the building. The employés on their own initiative organized themselves into a private fire service. Still other employés have been trained to act under direction of lieutenants. Special provision is made for the safety of patrons who may be in the store. At a demonstration drill the chief of the city fire department praised the efficiency and rapidity of the service. The proprietor of the store stated that he would rather see his entire establishment in ashes than have a fire in the building cause the loss of a single human life.

During the last two years, a special committee of experts of the U. S. Steel Corporation[2] has been investigating the question of preventable accidents in their various works, and as

[1] The Broadway Department Store, Los Angeles, Cal. Organized 1896. Number Employés, 823.

[2] United States Steel Corporation. 210,180 employés.

n the machine department.
drill at any moment, and
aged. The chief of the fire
engineers of the city fire
of the machine department.
recent report of an insura
drill at Strawbridge & Clotl
ople are employed.
A fire drill of the employés w
.M. The first alarm brought
twenty seconds; a second al
parts of the building in eight
lines of hose were out and re
alarm was given on the seco
drills were made in the fac
house, all being characteriz
nals. The drills were highl
captains and chief deserve
way of carrying out the pu
On the hill near the Ly
voirs, one in case of fire
and the other fed from
supply of clear pure w
in the mill, so excellent
is the supply of wate
big blaze was extingu
men have repeatedly
tection.

At the Baldwin L
ried in the Factor
protective appara
There are seven f
part of the wor
city mains, an
Each build
storage capa
the top of
tains two
fireproof
ground

Sling chains, chain hoists, small runways, trucks, trestles, buildings are inspected on the second week of each month and reported. The number of pieces inspected, kind, size and condition must be mentioned.

All cables must be Roebling's Plow Steel "Baldwin Special," 5-8" and under shall be six strands of 19 wires per strand. 3-4" and over shall be six strands of 37 wires per strand. A cable must be scrapped when 5 wires become broken in 24 inches. Tiller rope must be Roebling make.

All crane and elevator chains shall be Bradlee make. These chains shall be taken out of service when they show a certain amount of wear, measured on a single link.

The inspector must be sure that one link is not worn more than the one bearing against it. All defective crane and elevator chains are to be returned for repairs. All crane and elevator chains must be annealed and repaired at least once a year. Care must be exercised in the use of sling chains not to twist or knot them. Chains with links bolted together are not allowed. All sling chains must be laid out in center aisle of each shop on one Saturday night of each month, according to a prescribed schedule.

Side pulling on cranes is forbidden under penalty of discharge; the overloading of cranes, elevators or shop floors is forbidden. If there is any doubt, the chief of highway department must be consulted.

All line shafting, countershafting, footing pieces for runs, and any other millwright work must be put up by the highway department only. The shop tool room men must keep the bolts and lag screws in the footing pieces, hangers or runways tightened up in good shape and report anything dangerous to highway department. All moving of machinery and heavy tools must be done by the highway department only.

No alterations to buildings, locations of tools, fixtures or pipe, are to be made except under the supervision of the highway department. The cutting of joints or drilling of ironwork is forbidden.

When it is necessary to do any work on a crane or crane runway, the crane runner must be notified before commencing the work and when finished. When from any cause the crane runner is not on the crane which is to be repaired, the foreman of the shop must be notified and asked to appoint a watchman for the protection of the men doing the work.

For crane runway work, one of the following methods of protecting workmen must be employed:

Remove the fuses from the crane switch and hang a sign over it, "Men working on the line."

Put track stops on the rails between the workmen and the cranes, notifying crane operators of their location.

Put the watchman in the cage with the crane operator.

Any tools, machinery, chains, or slings, not in first class order, must not be used and should be reported at once so they can be repaired.

In every case before putting belts on pulleys, the engine or motor should be stopped or reduced to not more than half speed.

Ladders must not be used unless they are fitted with iron spikes on ends, nor must they be pieced out in order to increase their length.

Before doing any work on line shafting, the engineer must be notified at the time of commencing the work and when finished. In case of shafting driven by motor, remove fuses and hang a sign over the switch, "Men working on the line."

"

It takes a workman some days to familiarize himself with a new factory or workshop, especially if there are large numbers of employés. It is therefore essential that the new worker should be promptly informed of the conditions and requirements of his new work. For that object, the Baldwin Locomotive Works posts this notice:

"Owing to the gradual increase of the Works and the number of men who are continually being taken on, it is of the utmost importance that every precaution should be taken to prevent accidents.

The contractors should see that their men keep from standing under heavy weights which are being lifted or carried along by cranes.

Slings, chains, etc., must be carefully examined, and only those that are amply strong and in good order are to be used for the work.

Lifting chains must not be twisted as it considerably reduces their strength.

Notices are posted on all floors giving safe loads they will carry, and workmen are cautioned not to exceed the prescribed limit.

In your effort to get out the most work in the least possible time, every precaution should be taken against having an accident or injury to any one. I particularly caution you all to use the utmost care, and have everything done in the safest possible manner."

At the Westinghouse Works in East Pittsburg, every dangerous piece of apparatus, elevators, crane tracks, pulleys, band saws, etc., is provided with a safety device in the nature of a screen or guard. There have been cases of indifference on the part of the employés to make full use of protective devices, although this is not general. These devices are rendered as nearly "fool proof" as possible.

One regular resident physician is employed, while there are others available for emergency calls. This physician delivers an occasional lecture on "First Aid to the Injured" to which all employés are invited. This lecture was published in *The Electric Journal*—edited by The Electric Club.

MUSEUM OF SAFETY AND SANITATION

It is generally conceded that America is the greatest manufacturing country in the world; we are constantly striving for higher speed and increased efficiency in the machine or tool. The whole wealth of inventive genius was lavished on the machine with little or no thought for the protection of the workman running it. No country can be in the front rank of industrial civilization until as much care is taken for the workman as in the perfection of the machine. However, the public is beginning to take cognizance of the enormous number of accidents of which it is the opinion of the engineering and technical profession that many are preventable.

This thought took concrete expression in the city of Amsterdam in 1893, when a Museum of Safety Devices was opened for the express purpose of showing how machines and processes may be so safeguarded as to prevent accidents to labor and the general public.

It was an exhibit of this Dutch Museum in the Section of Social Economy at the Paris Exposition of 1900 which profoundly impressed me that a little country like Holland should have the forethought to assemble for her industrialists methods and devices for protecting life and limb.

Amsterdam's Museum of Safety has served as a model for Germany, France, Russia, Switzerland, Italy, Austria, and lastly, the United States; the idea having been brought over by the author at the close of the Exposition of 1900.

After a campaign of education lasting several years, in which two expositions were held, the Museum of Safety and Sanitation was incorporated in 1909, the first of its kind on the Western Continent. The Chairman is Charles Kirchhoff; Vice-Chairman, T. C. Martin; Secretary, Albert Spies; Treasurer, Frank A. Vanderlip; Director, William H. Tolman. A committee under the chairmanship of Prof. F. H. Hutton includes Dr. Thomas Darlington, *Commissioner of the Health Department;* Philip T. Dodge, *President Engineers' Club;* William J. Moran, *Attorney-at-Law;* Henry D. Whitfield, *Architect.* The executive offices of the museum are at the United Engineering Societies Building, 25 West 39th Street, New York City. At the museum will be gathered the best methods and devices for protecting the workers in mining, transportation, textiles, building trades, agriculture, chemical and varied industries, and for the sake of stimulating the need for the wider use of safety devices in dangerous trades and occupations. The department of sanitation will include military hygiene, foods, water, ventilation, lighting, infectious diseases, tuberculosis, disinfection, offensive trades, and alcoholism.

The idea of a Museum of Safety was so novel in this country that it was decided early in 1907 to hold an exposition of two weeks in New York, for the sake of showing the community the practicability of the movement. The exposition, which closed in February, was successful in attracting a number of exhibits from the United States, and also from Belgium, France, Germany, Austria and Italy, sufficient to justify the fact that this was an international exposition. After its close the educational work was continued by the organization of a committee

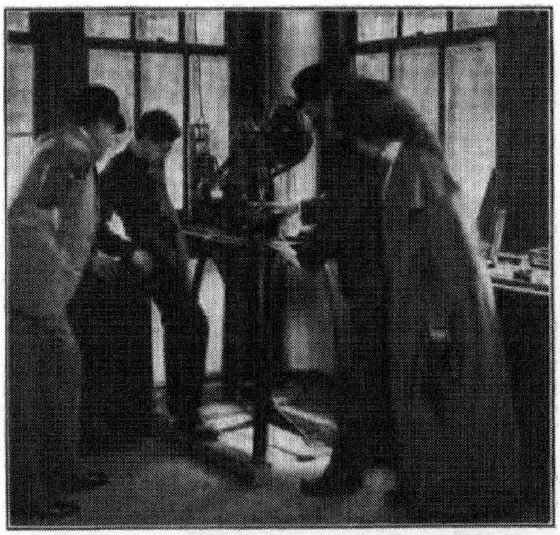

A Punch Protected so as to Guard the Workers' Hands and at the Same Time Increase the Output. Exhibited by the Travelers Insurance Company.

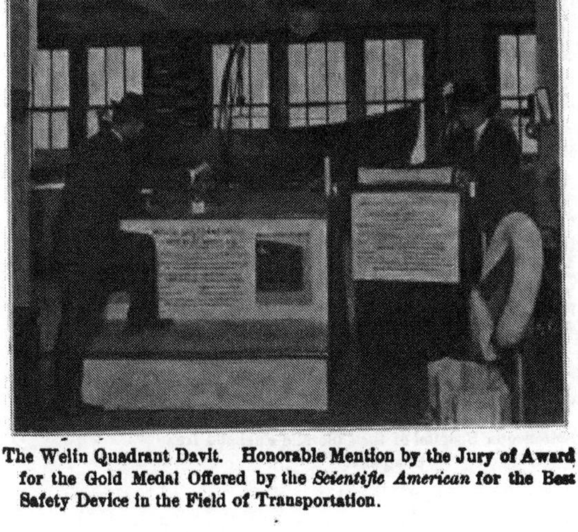

The Welin Quadrant Davit. Honorable Mention by the Jury of Award for the Gold Medal Offered by the *Scientific American* for the Best Safety Device in the Field of Transportation.

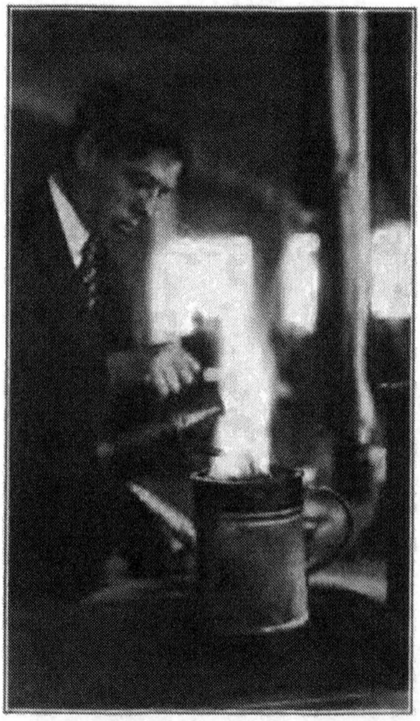

Pouring Lighted Gasolene at the Exposition of Safety Devices and Industrial Hygiene (The Safety Device Worked, McNutt Patent, Awarded the Richards Gold Medal).

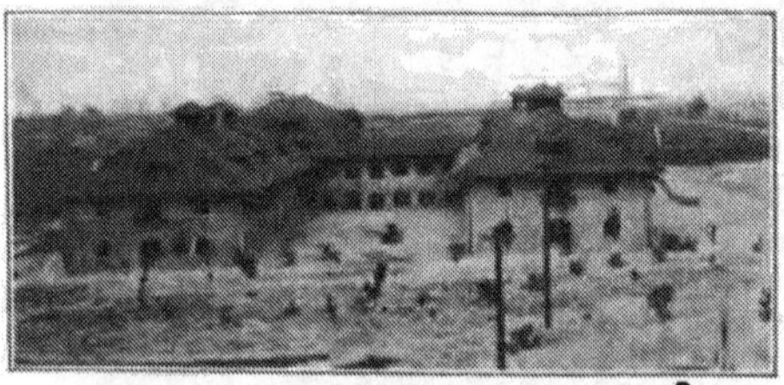

The Minnequa Hospital of the Colorado Fuel and Iron Company.

of direction, consisting of Charles Kirchhoff, of the *Iron Age*, chairman, T. Commerford Martin, of the *Electrical World*, vice-chairman, Albert Spies, *Electrical Record*, Secretary; F. S. Halsey, *American Machinist;* H. W. Desmond, *Architectural Record;* J. R. Dunlap, *The Engineering Magazine;* W. R. Ingalls, *Engineering & Mining Journal;* Chas. Whiting Baker, *Engineering News;* E. F. Roeber, *Electrochemical and Metallurgical Industry;* G. Gilmour, Chief Engineer Travelers Insurance Co.; J. M. Goodell, *Engineering Record;* Chas. W. Price, *Electrical Review;* F. Webster, *Insurance Engineering;* F. E. Rogers, *Machinery;* Professor F. R. Hutton; S. S. McClure; F. R. Low, *Power;* W. H. Boardman, *Railroad Gazette;* A. Sinclair, *Railway and Locomotive Engineering;* A. A. Hopkins, *Scientific American;* H. W. Blake, *Street Railway Journal;* James H. McGraw, President McGraw Publishing Co.; Charles T. Root, President Textile Publishing Co.; Dr. Louis L. Seaman, with Dr. W. H. Tolman as Director.

The Committee authorized the holding of a second exposition of safety devices for six weeks, from the middle of April to June 1, 1908. It was decided that there should be no charge for space, and to guard against the admission of "fake" or unreliable exhibits, a jury of admission, with Prof. F. R. Hutton, chairman, George Gilmour, Chief Engineer of the Travelers Insurance Co., and A. A. Hopkins of the *Scientific American*, were appointed.

In view of the fact that a very large percentage of accidents is absolutely preventable, the editors of the *Scientific American* offered a gold medal annually for the best device for the protection of life and limb during the year; this award to be given by the American Museum of Safety after a board of experts of the highest professional standing have passed upon the devices submitted.

For 1908 the field of the award was limited to transportation. Every device to be in competition must have been exhibited at the museum. The members of this jury were Stuyvesant Fish, George Gilmour, F. R. Hutton, John Hays Hammond, Samuel Sheldon, H. H. Westinghouse, Cornelius Vanderbilt.

A second gold medal was offered by Francis H. Richards, limiting the field to safety devices in connection with auto boats and auto vehicles, S. S. Wheeler, Caspar Whitney and A. G. Batchelder constituting this jury. For the best safety device in mines and mining, the Travelers Insurance Co. offered a gold medal, the jury of award including W. R. Ingalls, Charles Kirchhoff and Prof. Henry S. Munroe.

The exposition opened April 13th, and included 112 entries, some of which were live exhibits; others were models, actual or reduced size, photographs and diagrams. Among the exhibitors were the United States Steel Corporation, Westinghouse Air Brake, Travelers Insurance Co., Brown and Sharpe Mfg. Co., Carnegie Steel Co., Draper Mfg. Co., Holophane Glass Co., International Sprinkling Co., Johnson & Johnson, Henry Maurer & Son, McArthur Portable Fire Escape, Niles-Bement-Pond Co., Pennsylvania Railroad, Rich Marine Fire Indicating and Extinguishing System, Rutherford Pneumatic Wheel Co., Non-Explosive Safety Naphtha Container Co. (McNutt Patents), The Welin Quadrant Davit, the Lane & Degroot Life Boats, Simmen Automatic Railway Signal Co., Emil Greiner Co., H. B. Smith Machine Co., Ætna Life Insurance Co., Coston Signal Co., Automatic Signal Gate Co., American Suspension Railway Co., Montauk Fire Detecting Wire Co., Buchanan Safety Rail Joint, the Quern Fender, Quincey-Manchester-Sargent Co., Thatcher Car Step, the Dubè Railroad Spike, the Brandau Emergency Brake, Pay-As-You-Enter Car Co., U. S. Engineering Co., Automatic Door and Gate Co., Standard Safety Window Guard & Exit Lock Door Co., Standard Plunger Elevator Co., Jones Safety Device Co., Security Elevator Co., Dellock Mfg. Co., Stillman Safety Lamps, Kaplan Automatic Water Gage, Safety Fire Extinguisher Co., National Safety Gas Cock, the Sherwin-Williams Co., the Ideal Ventilator Co., and the Malsin Safety Clothes Line.

On entering the exposition the visitor saw in front of him a miniature mountain, the model of a mine gallery, to show scientifically how the construction of steel instead of wood is being used to make the galleries of the mines safe and strong, for it is already coming to pass that steel is becoming cheaper than wood. Then, too, in the case of fire there is no fear that the steel will burn. The steel beams, the lagging and the track were all of natural size, and this mine gallery installed by the

Carnegie Steel Co. could be studied in all of its detail, without a trip underground in the midst of perilous descents and dangerous passages from below the surface of the earth. In close proximity, safety lamps, respirators, helmets, detectors of dangerous gases indicated the grave perils that necessitate methods and processes of precision for overcoming them. While the exposition did not contain flying machines or seven-leagued boots, there was one device which well might figure in the "Arabian Nights" brought down to date. The inventor of this eighth wonder in simple and convincing words told how the despatcher in the seclusion of his own office, with the train sheet in front of him, indicating the whereabouts of every train on the line, could at will at any minute talk with any engineer in his cab, at any point on the line, warning him of the peril in the block just ahead of him. If this warning to Mr. Engineer should not be heeded, the despatcher, by the simple turn of a lever, could shut off the power of the locomotive so that it would come to a full stop.

"That concerns my government," said the consular representative of one of the great European powers as he saw the model of a quadrant davit whereby two men lower a life-boat filled with people from the deck to the water inside of one minute. Continuing he came to a safety lamp, "That touches my own pocket. I must have one of those lamps for my villa."

Safety exit and fireproof doors, automatic sprinklers, fire escape ladders, the invention of a woman, and a fireproof house of hollow tile were other exhibits of safeguards from fire.

Wood-working machines, with the saws and knives revolving thousands of times a minute, seek in vain to mangle the hands and fingers of the workman, while cunningly devised guards permit the workman's hands to push the work along or to glide harmlessly over knives or cutters; at the same time there being no interference with the speed or limitation of the output.

Safety elevators, emergency brakes, rail joints, automatic gate crossings and signals, life buoys and collapsible life-boats, safety hatches, life guns, safety clothes lines; and methods for safeguarding the milk and food supply of New York City, were among some of the other exhibits in this exposition for saving life and limb.

An exhibit of unseen perils, which are disclosed only by the examination of expert inspectors, was made by the Travelers Insurance Co. of Hartford. It was in a class all by itself, and was frequently referred to as the "Chamber of Industrial Horrors." On entering their section, the visitor could study a series of photographs illustrating the havoc and ruin caused by explosions of all kinds, whether in the buildings or in the street; unguarded stairs, wells and elevator shafts; machinery before and after protecting devices had been applied, and other industrial perils. Continuing the study, there was a whole series of defective chains and cables used on elevators and other hoisting machinery, illustrating excessive strains, twists and other defects that had caused the accidents, in some cases fatal. Broken cogs, gears, wheels, sheaves and bolts showed other causes of accidents; boiler plates, flanges, tubes and rivets, and other accessories illustrated causes of boiler explosions. Those in charge of the exhibit explained how the accident could have been avoided.

Leaving these exhibits, the clank, clank, clank of a press in a corner arrested attention, because it is well known that the presses and punches are prolific sources of perils in cutting off fingers. This model press exhibited by the Travelers Insurance Company has an arm or small bar which operates at right angles to the descending press, knocking away the operator's hand so that it is impossible for the fingers to be crushed. At the same time the return stroke of the bar pushes off the work, thereby increasing the output. Simple and cheap, hence the American industrialist can afford to use it.

The closing exercises of the exposition were held at the Engineers' Club May 18, 1908, when the exhibitors gathered for a luncheon conference under the chairmanship of Charles Kirchhoff. The director of the museum presented the following report from the Jury of Award for the *Scientific American* gold medal:

"The Jury of Award to select from the safety devices exhibited at the Exposition of 1908 the most meritorious invention in the field of transportation among those there brought together, present the following report as their recommendation and award:

After extended conference and consideration upon the

rules which should govern the procedure of the jury, it was agreed:

1. That the term 'field of transportation' covered by the deed of gift of the *Scientific American* Medal included the devices and apparatus having to do with the safety of transfer of the public and of the operatives in control on the railways, by elevators and on the water.

2. That by the terms of another provision for a jury of award for devices and meritorious inventions in the field of transportation by motor vehicle, this section of transportation was specifically excluded.

3. That devices usable in transportation in which safety was a secondary although necessary element, and hence subordinated to a primary purpose other than safety, were not to be considered in competition. Safety must be the primary and perhaps the only object to be sought by the device.

4. That devices exhibited which were meritorious inventions were not necessarily entitled to award if there existed other devices not exhibited seeking the same object and having equal or greater claims for consideration.

Within these limitations the jury decided that any devices to claim consideration must possess the following elements or attributes; and that the device exhibiting these qualities to the highest degree should receive the award, viz.:

1. Applicability, wide or narrow. Does the device procure safety for a large number of persons, or in a great variety of conditions?

2. Practicability. It must be capable of being used successfully. It must not be too cumbrous or intricate to apply or to operate.

3. Simplicity. It must not be so complicated that experts are required to handle it or to keep it in repair and operation.

4. Reliability. It must not be liable to derangement, causing failure to work in emergency.

5. Durability. It must not be so delicate, or require such fine adjustment that when installed it will not last in service.

6. Commercial availability. It must not be too expensive in first cost to install, or in operation to maintain.

In applying their rules and requirements to the exhibits shown in the exposition of 1908, the jury awarded the medal tendered by the *Scientific American* to the Rich marine fire indicating and extinguishing system. They are glad to make honorable mention of The Welin Quadrant Davit Co., and The Simmen Automatic Railway Signal Co."

The Rich marine fire detecting and extinguishing device may be stationed in any convenient part of the ship, preferably in the chart room or wheel house. Galvanized iron pipes are drawn from each hold or bunker, or other inaccessible compartment where fire protection is deemed necessary, into this station case, the lower end of each pipe being provided with an end-bonnet-shaped smoke receiver of about 8 inches in diameter. A clock located in front of the upper section of the station case is set to keep regular time, so that every 15, 30 or 60 minutes, in accordance with the time desired, electric contact will be made and a current operate a motor driven fan placed in the upper part of the station case. This fan draws air through the pipes from the several holds and bunkers. If there should happen to be a fire in any one of these holds or compartments smoke will issue from that particular pipe. A flexible steam hose attached to a standpipe, and being part of the extinguishing apparatus, can be coupled on to the smoking pipe, and steam turned on at a valve on the standpipe.

Models of metallic life-boats, rafts and collapsible unsinkable self-bailing life-boats were exhibited by the Lane & Degroot Co. Those for general use are constructed of No. 18 B. W. gage galvanized iron, in sizes up to 20 feet in length, and of proportionally thicker material in boats from 22 feet in length up. Countersunk tinned rivets, staggered, are used in the construction of the hull, all seams being calked with cotton. These life-boats as well as the metallic cylinder life-rafts are built of heavy galvanized iron cylinders, divided into air-tight compartments by iron bulkheads, and are designed in various sizes from a capacity of 28 persons down to 7. The Engelhardt collapsible life-boat is designed to enable a passenger steamer to carry life-boats sufficient to accommodate all on board without crowding, three of these lift-boats, nested, occupying the same space as one ordinary life-boat, under one set of davits. This company also had an interesting display of life preservers, the exhibit including life-buoys, belts and a chair-buoy.

This chair-buoy resembles certain types of life-buoys used aboard ship, but has in addition a network chair wherein the person is seated.

The exhibit of the Welin [1] quadrant davit consisted of a section of the deck, rail and cabin of a yacht or other vessel, on which is installed a tender operated by a single davit. The tender, which is of goodly proportions and strongly built, can be swung clear of the vessel without any effort simply by the operation, single-handed, of a crank handle on a threaded spindle. The movement inboard and over the rail is performed by the demonstrator with equal ease. The davit used in this exhibit has been especially designed for use on good-sized power boats and yachts, where it is the practice to carry the tender or other boat on the top of the trunk cabin. Ordinary davits are in such circumstances more or less unsatisfactory, as it is impracticable to give them a sufficient amount of overhang to lift the boat outward, from its position in the chocks, to clear the side of the vessel. It is claimed that the heaviest life-boat equipped with the Welin quadrant davit can be swung clear by two men in the remarkably short space of 20 seconds.

The Francis H. Richards gold medal was awarded to the McNutt [2] Non-Explosive Manufacturing Company (McNutt patents), with honorable mention to the Rutherford Pneumatic Wheel Company.

"If that man's going to light up some gasoline, he'd better build an iron cage, or else I'll have to get out," remarked an exhibitor at the exposition, as he saw a demonstration of pouring lighted gasoline from one container into another lighted receptacle. But the safety device worked and the speaker soon felt that he was perfectly safe. It was this device of the Non-Explosive Safety Naphtha Container Co. that was awarded the F. H. Richards gold medal for the most meritorious device for safeguarding auto boats and auto vehicles, using gasoline. The device consists of a double fold of thin brass plate punctured

[1] Welin Quadrant Davit, 17 Battery Place, New York City. Constructors of davits for ships and life-boats. Organized 1906. Number Employés, 60.

[2] The McNutt Non-Explosive Mfg. Co. Manufacturers non-explosive devices, 509 West 56th St., New York. Organized 1908. Number Employés, 25.

with a mesh of fine holes. The volatile liquid burns at the vent, but the flame can not reach the substance in the container; the can is fitted with a fusible plug, which melts at 300 degrees F., thus allowing the liquid to burn at the vent and preventing an explosion.

The Rutherford wheel is constructed on the principle of a wheel within a wheel, the inner one consisting of a hub connected to a rim or tire by means of steel plates or spokes. The outer wheel is a rim or tread which runs upon the ground, connected to an inner rim by means of a flat circular steel plate or ring. The inner rim of the outer wheel is of smaller diameter than the outer rim of the inner wheel and travels inside of it with the pneumatic tube between, the wheels moving in an upward or downward direction independently of each other, while spokes and plates prevent any lateral motion.

Thus the weight of the vehicle is suspended upon the upper half of the circumference of the pneumatic tube, instead of resting upon a few inches of bearing surface on the ground. This distributes the weight of the vehicle over more than ten times the pneumatic surface afforded by the use of the ordinary pneumatic wheel, greatly increasing its carrying capacity and resiliency.

The outer rim, to which is attached a solid tread of wood, metal, or rubber composition, is of a fixed circumference which cannot change. Should the tube become deflated while the vehicle is in motion, the wheel will continue in the same direction as before, and accidents from swerving and loss of control are impossible. In addition, the vehicle can continue the trip on the deflated tube without danger or discomfort, and it need not be refilled with air until the destination is reached.

The Exposition of Safety Devices of 1908 was a working model of what a permanent museum of safety should be, and showed the necessity of its immediate organization.

Museums of safety are no longer experimental, but the world movement has come to stay, as has been demonstrated by their establishment in Berlin, Paris, Vienna, Milan, Budapest, Stockholm, Zurich, Moscow and Munich. In Germany they are supported entirely by the government, which says, "We regard the saving of life of paramount importance. Every life saved is a national asset." Recently the director of the Berlin Museum requested 83,000 marks for the enlargement of the building already overcrowded; his request was instantly granted and it was intimated that he could have all the money he needed, as the government was only too glad to maintain this life-saving station at its highest point of efficiency. The other European nations are not slow in realizing the importance of museums of safety, which have received their great impetus during the last decade.

America, the greatest of industrial nations, needs a museum of safety devices more than any other. The object of such an institution is not coercive but suggestive. The law says the dangerous parts of machines must be protected. The museum through its jury of experts places on view every known device, so that the industrialist may select the one best adapted to his particular needs; in other words, the museum becomes the experimental laboratory for every industrialist in the country.

It is therefore to the best interest of every American employer that he should keep himself informed regarding the movement already under way for the Museum of Safety and Sanitation. Such interest will be an evidence of good faith in his desire to protect his workers by making use of the necessary devices drawn from the museum and will be a strong argument against hasty and undigested legislation.

This movement for the promotion of an American Museum of Safety is not commercial but humanitarian, and as such must depend on the generosity of the public. The high standard and the technical experience of the Committee of Direction is a guarantee for the wisest administration.

The philosophy of the scope and object of this movement for safety and security for life and labor in America was admirably expressed by Professor Charles E. Lucke of Columbia University at the formal opening of the Exposition:

"There is ample proof that the number of personal injuries and deaths from accidents in this country is unusually large. Any movement that has for its object the protection of the person, whether directed toward those engaged in their daily occupations or toward the general public, should receive the support of every good citizen. In order, however, to justify such support the remedies proposed should be sane, reasonable and free from mere sentimental impulse. It must be shown that some accidents are avoidable and that the preventive measures are not oppressive. This broad problem is not by any means a simple one, and its solution involves a divisional classification. One of these groups of cases in which I am more particularly interested is concerned with the protection of workmen engaged in producing and operating machinery. All work with tools or machinery or that involves the moving of heavy weights, the inhalation of harmful dusts or gases, is by its very nature essentially dangerous. The source and nature of the danger, are, moreover, best known to the interested parties; that is, to employer and employé, and need no demonstration by statistics or by kind-hearted philanthropists.

"It appears, therefore, that a reduction of accidents to workmen of these classes may be brought about most easily by common consent of both parties to adopt preventive measures, and one strong contributing factor to this coöperative action is the existence of such a museum of possible devices as is here in course of establishment. It may be, and probably will be true, that in many cases employer and employé cannot agree. The workman may refuse to use a device that would protect him, because it may be annoying to him in his work, and he prefers to take the chance of injury rather than be bothered, or it may be, on the other hand, that means for rendering the occupation of his men more safe will involve a prohibitive cost on the part of the employer. He is in business distinctively to make money, and if he cannot make money or should his profits be reduced by prohibitive appliances or methods he will close his works. Between these two extremes of refusal to accept a remedy on the part of the workman, and the refusal to adopt the remedy on the part of the employer, I believe there is a very large middle ground, involving perhaps a forcing of one or the other party, perhaps by gentle educational means, perhaps by legal enactment. This museum contributes to the former, employers' liability laws to the latter, but perhaps better than either of these alone, but involving both of them, is the means offered by liability and accident insurance.

"If the insurance companies can be induced to grant to the employer lower liability rates and to the workman lower accident rates for the use of this or that device, it will appeal most decidedly to the employer, as it touches his earnings, on the one hand protecting him from damage suits and on the other hand giving him his protection for lower rates, to permit the purchase and maintenance of the safety appliance, and it will appeal to the man carrying accident insurance in an equally obvious way. Before any safety device is adopted its true nature—that is to say, the precise extent of the protection it affords—must be determined. Safety appliances may be more harmful than useful when by lulling into a false security by promises of protection, there results a relaxation of vigilance that is the surest protection, with perhaps a failure of the appliance at a critical time. A safety appliance is not a safety appliance because its inventor asserts it to be such, but becomes a safety element only when it has been proved and tested and when it has by use proved to be absolutely reliable. To accomplish this a series of tests must be made by a thoroughly reliable and disinterested party, such as are made, for example, on fire protection appliances in the laboratories of the Fire Underwriters and at the laboratories of various technical schools, but whatever tests are made the results must be widely published for the general information of the entire public. To sum up the problem as it appears to me as a mechanical engineer, there is no necessity for the proving of the danger of the occupation to either the man engaged in it or to his employer. Every sort of appliance for removing danger must be invented, tried, tested, results made public and the successful appliance placed on exhibition, together with the results of the test to assist in bringing about common consent for its use between employer and employé. Without common consent, one or the other may be forced, and in this forcing process educational policies, employers' liability laws and accident or employers' liability insurance practice are, I think, the most potent factors."

Richard Watson Gilder in a *Century* editorial, entitled "The Passion for Saving and Risking Life," wrote, "When one reads the accounts constantly appearing in the newspapers of instances of the heroic saving of human life, especially in fire and mine disasters, one is impressed by the value put by all men upon life. The rescues of miners, continuing sometimes from day to day, have the whole country, sometimes the whole world, for sympathetic audience. The city of New York was thrilled lately by the story of the rescue of a fireman, after twenty-four hours of exertion on the part of his comrades, the first hours of which were with the hope of finding his dead body only. Incidents like these awaken a passion of tenderness, of heroic struggle, of widespread sympathy. As for firemen, they are proverbial for reckless courage in saving endangered lives, and when it comes to the rescue of one of their own number, they will actually fight for the privilege of flinging themselves into positions of deadly peril in order to save a threatened comrade. There never was a time, moreover, when such good care was taken of the sick and afflicted; or when so much time, money, equipment, and individual devotion were given to the discovery and application of remedies for disease, and of means for the prolongation of human existence.

"Reading of such things from day to day, and nothing else, one might, as we have said, come to the conclusion that in America the sacredness of life is keenly felt throughout the community. But, as a matter of fact, the newspapers that give us minute details, in column upon column, of these heroic rescues, on the same page chronicle events which bring the observer to the very opposite conclusion.

"Here we read of scores of men working day and night, without thought of self, to save a single life: and then we read, for instance, of automobile tragedies where the speed craze leads to the loss not only of the life of the speed-crazy, but of the innocent passer-by. We read of railroad accidents where many lives are lost through some phase of recklessness. We are given the appalling statistics of railroad fatalities and of often easily preventable accidents in the various trades, and we find that America is far behind Europe in the use of safety devices in the various occupations.

"Such exhibitions of safety-appliances as that held in New York, under the auspices of the American Museum of Safety inform the public usefully of specific means of saving life and limb. But perhaps the most useful function of such a demonstration is the awakening of public opinion. It is an aroused public opinion that we need—a sort of national conversion. There is need to spread abroad a new respect for the human frame; a conviction that it is unneighborly, that it is wrong, that it is wicked, that it is unendurable, that people should amuse themselves in a way that endangers the bodies and the very existence of their fellow-citizens. Railroad trains, electric trolleys, and automobiles are constantly put to speed that implies an outrageous spirit of recklessness.

"A man has no business to take reckless chances with his own life, much less with that of his fellow citizen, who has an equal right to the safe use of the public highway. This should seem to be a truism, but too many people act with total disregard of so elemental a principle as this. There are so many delinquents, there is such a lack of persistent defense on the part of the public, that perhaps those are wise who think that a counter-movement should be started, and that the scattered and ineffectual indignation of the community should find effective expression in a special organization."

One very valuable feature of a permanent museum is the prevention of wasted effort and time. Quoting from one of the exhibitors, "A permanent exposition of safety devices should be a clearing house for new ideas, where an inventor can quickly prove the success of his invention or be made to see the uselessness of further efforts along the line he is working. Such a clearing house of new ideas would save many a waste of honest effort.

"As it is to-day, an inventor often devotes the best years of his life to bringing his invention into practical use, without success, although he may have a very good device.

"A striking example of such a case is our friend and co-exhibitor, Mr. George Brandau. Here is a man 66 years old. For 14 years he has devoted practically all his efforts to bring his invention into public use. The efforts he expended in this task would put many a man, who is noted for hard work, to shame. As yet he has not succeeded. He has a practical device.

"Therefore, let me say again, give the inventors a clearing house for their ideas, and above all give them all the assistance possible to bring their devices into use. As a rule, nine-tenths of an inventor's ambition is to see his device in practical use, seldom more than one-tenth is commercial gain."

A commentary on this letter was instanced by the visit of a poor inventor, who came to the exposition. One device already patented instantly arrested his attention, because he saw in it the visualization of ideas which he had been trying to realize during the last four years. A museum will prevent this economic waste to society.

A conservative estimate of the number of annual accidents resulting fatally or in partial or total incapacity for work is 500,000. Reckoning the wage earning capacity of the average workman at $500 a year (this makes no allowance for the professional men, railroad presidents, industrialists and other high salaried officials who are injured or killed by railways, mines, building trades, or other occupations) we have a social and economic loss of $250,000,000 annually. What we are losing in work efficiency, Germany is saving.

"One billion marks annually we conserve for Germany through our sanatoria, museums of safety, convalescent homes and other forms of social insurance, by which we safeguard the lives and limbs of our workmen and prevent the causes and effects of diseases that would lessen the workmen's economic efficiency," said Dr. Zacher, Director of the Imperial Bureau of Statistics, in reply to my inquiry how much Germany saved every year.

The chairman of the museum's committee of direction, at the 1907 annual dinner of the U. S. Steel Corporation, made a general plea for the more adequate provision of safety appliances, particularly in reference to the steel industry. At the dinner for 1908, Judge Gary announced that Mr. Kirchhoff's remarks had been applied by the Steel Corporation. Twenty-five hundred suggestions had been received from the various plants, resulting in the adoption of the greater part of them, at an expense of some $55,000. Furthermore, the cost of their installation was not a charge against the individual plant.

Two years ago Governor Hughes was the guest of honor at a banquet in New York inaugurating the first International Exposition of Safety. Early in January, 1909, Dr. Darlington, Commissioner of the Health Department, paid a visit to one of the large city breweries. He was much interested in their new methods for casking beer in steel barrels lined with glass. While making his rounds he noted everywhere the thorough

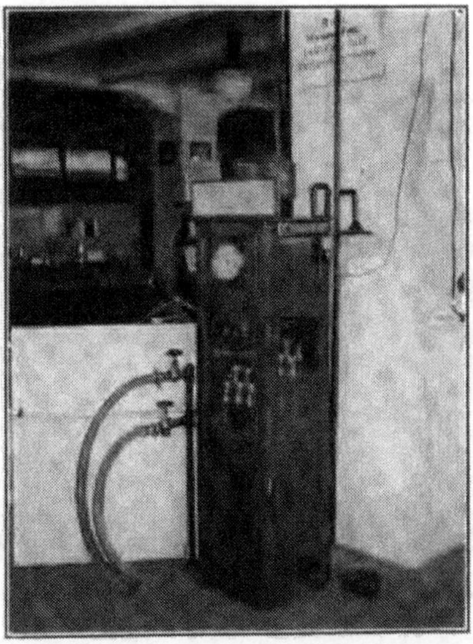

The Rich Marine Fire Indicating and Extinguishing System, Awarded the Gold Medal of the *Scientific American* at the Exposition of Safety Devices.

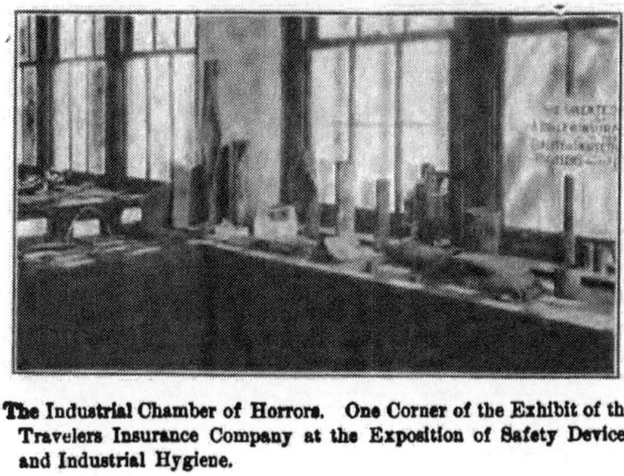

The Industrial Chamber of Horrors. One Corner of the Exhibit of the Travelers Insurance Company at the Exposition of Safety Devices and Industrial Hygiene.

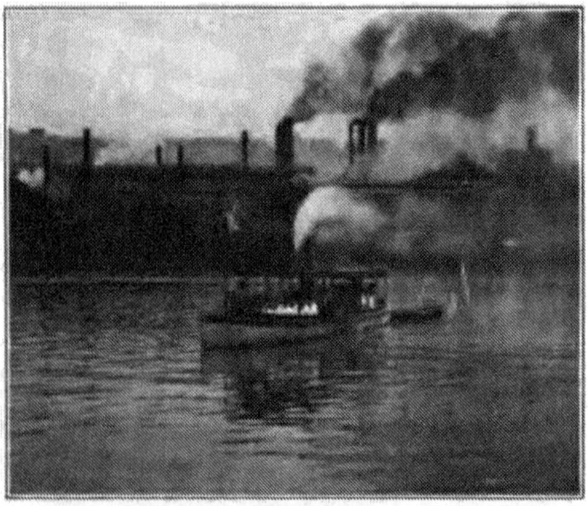

Recreation for the Convalescents at H. J. Heinz Company.

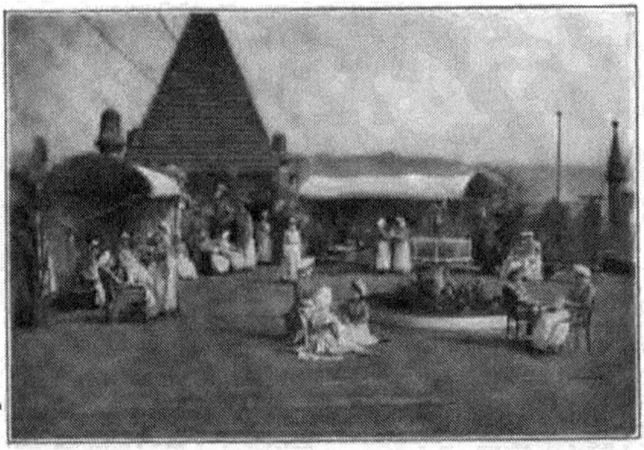

The Roof Garden for the Women and Girls of the H. J. Heinz Company.

installation of safety devices; he felt this to be so unusual, that he inquired how they came to be so well equipped. The superintendent replied, "We attended the safety inaugural banquet; we were impressed by the lantern slide presentation, and at once determined to put our own house in order."

CHAPTER V

MUTUALITY

This chapter will include the various organizations which have for their object the provision of weekly payments in case of sickness or accidents, payments towards the burial expenses, or death benefits to the beneficiary or the nearest relative of the member. In the majority of cases the form of organization is mutual, the active members concerning themselves with the administration, the firm acting as the custodian of the funds and making annual or special contributions to the treasury. In some cases the beneficial society combines social and educational features.

For the social and financial benefit of the employés of the company, what is known as the Seattle Electric Employés' Beneficial Association was organized and incorporated, having for its object the relief of the members in case of sickness, death or disability; the promotion of social relations and good fellowship, and also the education of its members in the best methods of conducting the business of the Seattle Electric Company. Membership in this association is entirely voluntary, and it is governed by a president and a board of trustees, duly elected from the members. This board represents as nearly as may be each of the six departments of the company, and there are also two members-at-large.

The membership of this association includes the motormen and conductors, artisans employed in the repair and care of cars, electrical workers of all descriptions, mechanics and other employés, and, as well, officers of the company, clerks and members of the administrative department. The assistant treasurer of the company is the treasurer of the association and has charge of the funds under the direction of an executive committee. All officers and regular employés of the company who have been in the employ of the company not less than four consecutive weeks, are eligible to membership except employés on temporary duty and those whose monthly compensation is less than $25, or those afflicted with chronic diseases.

When this association was instituted some years ago, to provide immediate funds for sick benefits, the Seattle Electric Company contributed a very considerable sum each year, but at present, as the association embraces a membership of nearly the entire working force of the company, the regular dues provide sufficient funds to meet all claims, and the association now has a substantial surplus in its treasury.

The association employs a doctor, and also arranges for medicines at a less rate than would ordinarily be charged to an individual. Each member unable to attend to his or her duties from sickness or disability, upon proper notification and report by the association's physician, is entitled to receive from the association, after the first week of illness, no more than $10 a week for a period of 26 weeks for any one illness or disability. On the death of a member in good standing, a death benefit is paid to his or her legal representatives, consisting of not more than $250, within 15 days after due notice has been given to the secretary and proof of death filed.

Membership in the benefit association at the Farr & Bailey Company,[1] Camden, N. J., is limited to those at present in its employment, but members who leave the company to work elsewhere are allowed to retain their standing and interest in the benefit association for one year after the severance of their relations with the firm.

No admission fee is charged; the dues are 50 cents per month, which must be paid in semi-monthly sums of twenty-five cents.

The benefits paid by the association are $5 per week in case of inability to work, not caused by immoral conduct. No benefit is paid for less than one week's illness, nor for any longer period than twelve weeks in any one year, the year to begin with date of first week's benefit.

[1] Farr & Bailey Co., Camden, N. J. Manufacturers Oil Cloth, Linoleum and Cork Carpets. Incorporated 1889. 500 Employés.

Upon the death of a member, a death benefit of $150 is paid to the person who has been designated by him to receive it. In case no one is selected as beneficiary by the member, the money is paid to his wife or to his nearest surviving relative.

The board of managers of the benefit association has entered into a contract with the employing firm, under which the latter pays all the expenses of maintaining the association except the sick and death benefit. The paymaster of the company, or his representative, deducts assessments due by members from their weekly wages and pays the same over to the treasurer of the benefit association. The company also pays all assessments due from members who are temporarily laid off but not discharged, and continues to do so until they are reinstated in employment. It also guarantees to make good any deficiency that may be found to exist in the funds of the association at the time of the annual meeting, after twenty-four assessments have been paid during the year, and to advance all moneys necessary to pay benefits at any time the funds in the treasury may be exhausted.

In the case of a member who has been ten or more years in the employ of the company becoming disabled and remaining so for a longer period than twelve months, he is carried for an additional twelve months at the same rate per week, the funds for that purpose being furnished by the company. There is also a provision in the contract which allows an additional twelve weeks' benefit to members whose disability is the result of injuries received while on duty in the factory, the total amount of which is paid by the company.

The mutual benefit association among the employés of the Cleveland Hardware Company was suggested to the men by the company, but is run entirely by the employés. The company in promoting this work made a donation of one hundred dollars in cash to give it all the encouragement possible. When the association was first started all the men were urged very strongly to join it; of course none of them were forced to do so. Now each employé is asked whether he is willing to join the mutual benefit association; if he says no, the company has reserved the right to hire a man who is willing to join it, and in this way has kept up the membership. This does not necessarily mean that every one that is hired becomes a member of the association, because after hiring the man, his name is handed to the officers of that association, telling them that this man has been hired and has made application to join. Then they have the privilege of accepting or rejecting him. It very often happens that the men know more about the people hired than the firm themselves; sometimes on inquiry why the man was rejected by the mutual benefit association, it has been found that it has been for such a good reason that the firm did not care to employ him.

One member of the firm takes more than a special interest in this society and for a year has been associated with the visiting committee, thus going into the homes of a number of employés. Aside from giving him a very good idea of the home life of the workingman, in which he is very much interested, he thinks that it has been a benefit in a business way. The officers who have been on the visiting committee for the last year are two assistant foremen in different parts of the factory and an old German, who is to some extent the banker of the employés, advancing them money on their salaries. The member of the firm has found very often after spending a Sunday morning in company with these men on a visit to some homes, that he has found out more about the different employés and the inside working of the factory than he could learn the entire week in his regular position. One of the firm says this knowledge very often is used to good advantage in dealing with problems that are brought up during the week.

While the Solvay Process Company has done much toward advancing the interests of the children of its employés, it likewise has adopted and successfully executed important plans for the direct welfare of the workmen. On November 12, 1888, the Solvay Mutual Benefit Society was formed among the wage earners to render them financial relief in case of sickness, accident or death. None but employés of the company are eligible to membership in this society. They are obliged to pass a medical examination and to pay an initiation fee of ninety cents. For members who receive at least $5 per week in wages the dues are thirty cents a month, and those whose compensation is less than $5 weekly are charged one-half of the regular initiation fee and dues. For every thirty cents paid in dues by its employés the company contributes fifteen. The corporation's paymaster is authorized in writing by members to retain initiation fees and dues from their wages. These sums are collected by the treasurer of the society, who deposits them with the company's treasurer, to whom are addressed all orders for the requirements of the benefit association, the latter's treasurer keeping accounts of its financial condition and making a monthly statement of the same; together with a full report at the end of his term of office. Ninety days after joining the organization members are entitled to sick, accident or death benefits. An employé disabled from work by illness or injury receives $6 per week for not more than six months if his earnings be $5 weekly or over. One-half benefit is paid to those receiving less than $5 a week. Provision is also made for the payment of a funeral benefit of $100 and a half benefit of $50, and upon the death of the wife of a member he receives $50. In addition the company defrays all expenses incurred in the treatment of injured workmen who are taken to hospitals, and it also engages and compensates medical specialists when occasion demands their services.

Skilled physicians and surgeons are appointed by the company to attend the sick and injured. Their remuneration is fixed by the board of trustees. The physicians notify the society's secretary of all sick and accident cases and make a weekly report of the condition of disabled members, always holding themselves in readiness to immediately respond to calls in the event of necessity. Members on the sick list must be at home by sundown to entitle them to benefit. Those who meet with accidents are required to be in their residences at the setting of the sun unless the society physicians or a majority of the trustees grant them written permission to be out. In the way of penalties, any member whose disability is occasioned by the use of intoxicating liquors, or who becomes intoxicated while on the sick list, is liable to suspension from the society for a period determined by the trustees.

The last annual report for 1906 shows receipts $21,638.25; disbursements $17,336.94. Receipts since organization November 12, 1888, $243,203.25. Disbursements since organization $238,901.31.

Before the Mutual Benefit Association of the Celluloid Club[1] was organized, difficulties were frequently encountered in determining the real merits of cases wherein applications for help were made by employés, who, from sickness or through accidental injury, were unable to work. The situation in this respect and the thought given to the question of how to deal with it, so as to take care of deserving cases of want and guard against fraud at the same time, finally resulted in the establishment of the mutual benefit association, which now provides both the machinery for investigating claims and the money to assist those found to be entitled to relief.

The suggestion which led to this action came from the officers of the company and was eagerly adopted by the employés, who saw in the plan a certain means of changing their dependence for help, when sick and in need, from a charitable to a business basis. In other words the insurance principle pure and simple was adopted, and every employé was thereby at once placed in a position to make such provision for his family in the event of his own sickness or disability, as he felt able or disposed to pay for out of his weekly wages. The officers of the company made a very liberal donation of money to the association at the commencement, which placed it in an independent financial position and fully able to meet all demands.

A full set of officers consisting of a president, vice-president, secretary, financial secretary and treasurer is provided by the constitution of the mutual benefit association for conducting its business. These officers are elected at the regular annual meeting for a term of one year. There is also a board of trustees, seven in number, the members of which serve one year and are so elected that the terms of three and four of them respectively terminate alternately every six months.

Any male employé of the Celluloid Company under 50 years of age, of good habits, and moral character, may become a member by passing a medical examination; but to qualify for holding an office it is necessary to be 21 years of age, a member of the association and also of the Celluloid Club, and to be in good standing in both organizations.

[1] The Celluloid Co., Newark, N. J. Manufacturers Compounds of Pyroxyline and articles made therefrom. Organized November 28, 1890. Number Employés, 1500.

The board of officers and trustees acting together are required to consider and pass on all applications for membership, and decide on the qualifications of members for holding office, and also all other questions connected with the regular business of the association, such as auditing accounts and deciding on applications for benefits.

The board of trustees and officers hold at least one meeting each week to consider applications and to hear reports from the sick visiting committees. Two classes of insurance are provided; one against sickness and the other against death. Members are required to insure themselves in both classes. The maximum amount of insurance against sickness allowed to a member is ten dollars per week, and the minimum three dollars per week. The rate charged is two cents for each dollar of weekly benefits desired. The death benefits allowed are fifty dollars and one hundred dollars; for which amounts the weekly payments are, respectively, two cents and four cents per week. Members are not allowed to insure themselves against sickness for more than the amount of their weekly wages.

Sick benefits do not begin until a member has been connected with the association for three months, and unable to perform his regular duties at the factory for at least one week. Death benefits are paid only after the deceased member has been in good standing in the association for a period of three months. Claims on account of sickness or disability originating in intemperance or other vicious or immoral conduct are not allowed.

Before sick benefits are allowed, a doctor's certificate stating the nature and probable cause of the sickness must be sent to the board of trustees by the applicant, and the same must be done every two weeks thereafter while benefits are being paid. The amount of money paid as sick benefits to any one member is graded into four classes according to the duration of the case of sickness or disability. Full benefits, that is to say, the exact weekly sum for which the beneficiary is insured, are paid for only a period of thirteen weeks in any twelve consecutive months from the date on which the sickness or disability began; if the disability continues beyond that time, benefits are reduced to three-quarters; if it extends past six months, only one-half is paid; if more than nine months, the benefits are reduced to one-quarter of the full amount, which sum is paid until the completion of one full year of disability, when all payments cease.

The greatest possible care is taken in handling applications for disability benefits to protect the association against fraudulent claims. All requests for benefits are made to the president, who turns them over to a visiting committee. This committee is required to visit the applicant at least three times each week for the purpose of satisfying themselves in regard to the genuineness of the disability on account of which relief is claimed or is being paid. Their reports are made regularly to the board of officers and trustees, who have power to order that the payment of benefits be discontinued whenever in their judgment the reports of the sick committee would seem to warrant the adoption of such a course. Claimants for benefits are required to furnish a physician's certificate of disability not only with the application in the first instance, but at any time thereafter during the payment of benefits if required to do so by the board of officers and trustees. If a claim is found on investigation to be fraudulent, charges are promptly brought against the offending member, which may, if sustained, result in his expulsion from the association, and possibly, also, from the employment of the Celluloid Company.

The constitution provides that when the surplus funds of the association have grown to an amount equal to twelve dollars for each member in good standing, payment of dues by all members who have been on the rolls for more than a year shall be suspended, and not resumed until the surplus has diminished to a sum equal to ten dollars per capita of the membership in good standing.

Of the several forms which the movement toward organization among the employés of the Celluloid Company has assumed, the mutual benefit association may, with the possible exception of the parent organization, the Celluloid Club, be regarded as most beneficial to the company's workmen and their families. Through its assistance many have been saved from want or from running into debt because of a suspension of income, which, among wage workers, is generally the sure accompaniment of sickness or inability to work.

The 39th semi-annual statement of the Hopedale Mutual

Benefit Association,[1] December 1, 1907, showed receipts for $1764.91. The expenses were $1135.83. During nineteen and a half years of the association, the income has been $26,548.85; outgo $25,920.77. The present membership is 769.

The cost per member during the last six years was, 1907, $3.30; 1906, $2.85; 1905, $3.30; 1904, $2.70; 1903, $2.85; 1902, $2.35. The benefits are $5 per week (after the first week's sickness) for 12 weeks, with $100 death benefit. The association is a distinct organization, the only connection with the company is the privilege that the bills for monthly assessments be collected through the pay roll.

The Westinghouse Electric & Manufacturing Company's Foremen's Association was organized March, 1903, for the object of fostering social gatherings for mutual benefit in forming acquaintance with one another. Among the means to this end are the holding of meetings at which some official or officials of the company are invited to be present and address the members; the holding of smokers and an annual banquet.

The membership is composed of foremen, inspectors and chief clerks connected with the shop force of the company. An application for membership must be made through the general foreman of the section with which the applicant is identified; in case the applicant does not come under a general foreman, his application must be made in writing to the board of directors. All applications must be approved by the board of directors before applicants can be admitted to membership.

A member three months in arrears is considered suspended from all privileges and benefits of the association; and if not paid within three months from date of suspension, he is considered as expelled from the association. If the expelled member wishes to be reinstated, he must make out a regular form of application, and he will be admitted upon the approval of the board of directors and payment of all dues and assessments up to the time of his expulsion.

The dues are $3 per year, payable quarterly in advance, and an assessment of one dollar to assist in defraying the expenses of the annual banquet, the menu of which does not contain any intoxicants. At the death of a member in good standing each

[1] Draper Co., Hopedale, Mass. Organized 1896. Manufacturers Cotton Machinery. Number Employés, 3000.

member is assessed $5, to be paid to the beneficiary of the deceased.

All employés of the Westinghouse Electric Company, between the ages of 16 and 45, of good moral character, perfectly sound and not habitually subject to any bodily disease, have the privilege of joining The Westinghouse Electric Beneficial Association, subject to the rules and regulations.

Every person applying for membership must be in the employ of the Westinghouse Electric Company for two months, and be proposed in writing, through the secretary, by a member in good standing.

A relief committee consisting of three members is appointed by the secretary, to serve until relieved. It is their duty to visit the sick within 48 hours after having been notified of such sickness by the secretary, and to report to the executive committee.

It is the duty of the chairman of the relief committee to visit, or to have the sick or disabled members visited, at least once a week, and report their condition to the executive committee, who, after having been notified, attend to that duty or procure a substitute. All necessary expenses of this committee are paid by the association. A fine of one dollar is imposed on any member of this committee failing to attend to this duty, unless in case of contagious disease.

If sick or disabled for two consecutive weeks or more, he shall be entitled to $5 benefits for each week. The character of the injury or sickness is passed upon by the relief committee, and decided by the executive committee before benefits are allowed. Benefits are paid only from the date the member is reported to the president or secretary.

Every sick or disabled member reports or is reported to the secretary or president. In case of death arising from sickness or any injury by accident, the sum of $100 shall be allowed for funeral expenses.

No member, if taken sick, is entitled to benefits if over two months in arrears in dues, and if taken sick during such arrearages, he cannot, by payment of the same, claim benefits during that sickness, nor can a member while receiving benefits become in arrears so as to debar him; a sufficient amount being withheld from his benefits to prevent any arrearages, to the amount of one month's dues. Any member allowing himself to become over two months in arrears for dues is suspended from sick and funeral benefits for one month from the date of payment of such arrearages.

A member who feigns himself sick or disabled for the purpose of fraudulently obtaining benefits, or who shall be found at any time under the influence of intoxicating drinks while in receipt of benefits, shall be reported to the executive committee and dealt with according to the judgment of said committee.

The beneficial association provides for cases of sickness through the payment of $5 per week, and in case of death the sum of $100 is paid; the company adds $100 to this amount.

The object of the Curtis Mutual Benefit Society is to relieve its members in case of sickness, injury or disability which may unfit them for their daily labor, and to provide also for the payment of funeral expenses. The board of directors has general supervision over the affairs of the society, and meets regularly once each month.

Investigating committees to visit the sick, consisting of not fewer than two members, are appointed within 48 hours after notification of sickness has been received by the secretary. Such committees visit the sick at least once a week thereafter, and report the condition of the member or members visited to the secretary in writing. When in doubt as to the propriety of allowing benefits such committees may call in the society's physician to assist in reporting a case. In case of protracted illness, the secretary may accept the attending physician's certificates in lieu of reports by committees; and in all cases the president may at discretion call a paid visitor to the service of the society in place of a committee.

A relief committee composed of three members of the board of directors, including the secretary, is appointed by the president immediately after the annual election. The duty of this committee shall be to act upon all applications for relief. This committee shall meet whenever it is necessary.

The board of directors shall have power, at such times as in their judgment it is just and necessary, to levy an assessment on the members of the society to meet the contingencies of excessive sickness or accident.

When an officer of the society shall leave the employ of the Curtis Publishing Company his office shall be declared vacant, and such vacancy shall be filled by the board of directors for the unexpired term. The Board shall also have authority to fill any other vacancies.

Any person in the employ of the Curtis Publishing Company shall be eligible to membership in the society, upon application to the secretary and the payment of 25 cents for admission to Class A or C, or 50 cents to Class B or D. All applications, however, shall be subject to the approval of the board of directors. Such approval shall constitute election to membership.

Membership shall cease upon the resignation, suspension or expulsion of a member, upon his ceasing to be in the employ of the Curtis Publishing Company or upon his neglecting to pay his dues for a period of two months, and it shall be the duty of the board of directors to cause the names of all persons coming within any of the above classes to be erased from the roll of membership. Any member suspended from work for a period of less than six weeks shall not be considered as ceasing to be in the employ of the Curtis Publishing Company.

Any member leaving the society but remaining in the employ of the Curtis Publishing Company may again become a member by paying all back dues and assessments from the time he left the society and discharging any other obligations, subject to the approval of the board of directors.

The membership shall be divided into four classes: Class A shall be open to all employés in robust health; Class B shall be open only to those employés in robust health whose weekly pay is $7 or more; Class C shall be open to those employés who are otherwise eligible to Class A, but who are not in robust health; Class D shall be open to those employés who are otherwise eligible to Class B, but who are not in robust health. No employé shall be admitted to more than one class. The dues in Classes A and C shall be 5 cents per week, and in Classes B and D 10 cents per week, to be paid to the secretary in advance. Failure to pay within 24 hours of the time specified by the secretary as the regular time for making payments shall subject the member to a fine of one cent per week in Classes A and C, and two cents per week in Classes B and D, for such period as the dues may remain unpaid; all fractions of a week in such cases to be counted as a full week. No member shall be eligible for weekly dues during such period as he may be sick.

The board of directors shall have the right to transfer members by a two-thirds vote from one class to another; if the condition of health in a member in Class A or in Class B warrants a transfer to Class C or to Class D; or if a member in Class A or in Class C applies to the board to be transferred to Class B or to Class D on account of an increase in salary to $7 or more weekly; or if the salary of a member in Class B or in Class D is reduced to less than $7 a week.

When the general fund of the society shall amount to $1500 there shall be no further collections from members in Classes A and B until the funds shall have been reduced to $600; after which the regular dues shall be collected from members in these two classes until the general fund shall again amount to $1500.

Any member of the society unable to attend to his duties through sickness or disability, shall notify the secretary at once of the date of the beginning of such sickness or disability and, subject to approval by the relief committee, shall be entitled to receive from the society out of the funds then on hand, if a member of Classes A or C, $2.50 per week, and if a member of Classes B or D, $5 per week, for a period of not more than thirteen weeks in any one year, such year to be reckoned in all cases as dating from the first week for which benefits are paid. Benefit payments shall begin with the first day of absence from work, provided notification shall have been received within a week from such date; but no benefit shall be paid to a member for less than one week of sickness. When the duration of sickness shall extend to one week or more, then benefits shall be paid for the full term of sickness, including fractional parts of a week.

The relief committee shall have the right in all cases to demand the certificate of a physician in good standing in regard to the sickness or disability of any member who claims benefits.

On the death of a member in good standing—one who has been a member at least six months—payment on account of funeral expenses shall be made to his legal representative, as follows: In Class A or C, $50; in Class B or D, $100—within five days after due notice of death has been received by the secretary.

Any member detected in obtaining or attempting to obtain benefits fraudulently, either for himself or for some other member, shall be expelled from the society by the board of directors.

Any one between the ages of eighteen and fifty years of age who is employed in the works of the Keuffel & Esser Company [1] and desires to join the Employés Sick Benefit Association can do so, subject to a vote of the members. The admission fee is two dollars.

The monthly dues are fixed at forty cents, which must be paid promptly, under penalty of forfeiture of benefit during the month for which payment has not been made. Members are allowed to fall in arrears for three months' dues, after which, having been notified by the secretary, one week is allowed for paying up all arrears; failing to do this, the delinquent member is expelled at the next meeting of the association. An expelled person cannot be again admitted to membership until six months after expulsion.

The association allows its members, in case of sickness, a benefit amounting to the total sum of one hundred and seven dollars, as follows: Six dollars a week for a period of twelve weeks, and three dollars and fifty cents a week for a period of ten weeks, no matter what interruption there may be. With the drawing of this sum the membership of the recipient practically ceases. Should he desire to continue his connection with the association, he must be proposed for membership again, and present with his application a physician's certificate of the state of his health. If reported on favorably by the physician, the member may be admitted again, even if not any longer employed in the factory, or if he should have already passed the age limit of fifty years. A new admission fee in such a case is not required.

Members must be in the association for a period of three months before they are entitled to benefits, and no payments are made for sickness or disability that lasts less than three days. Benefits may be withheld from members found engaged in work for which their physical condition unfits them, and

[1] Keuffel & Esser Co., Hoboken, N. J. Manufacturers of Drawing Materials and Mathematical and Surveying Instruments. Organized 1867. Number Employés, 750.

benefits are not allowed to a member on account of an incurable disease, if it can be shown that he had already been suffering with such sickness or complaint before being admitted to membership without the same having been mentioned in his application.

Besides the weekly relief paid during sickness or disability resulting from accident, the sum of seventy-five dollars is paid on the death of the member from the funds of the society, and twenty-five dollars additional from the officers of the company.

There is thus assured to the family of a deceased member an amount of money sufficient to meet the expenses of a respectable burial which is the joint offering of his fellow workmen and his employers. On the death of the wife of a member the sum of fifty dollars is allowed by the benefit society.

A visiting committee of three members, who are appointed by the president to serve one month, are required to visit patients once a week, and must sign their names to the call book left with every member who is on the sick list.

The president and the visiting committee have power to cause an examination to be made of a patient at any time. Should the physician report the member able to work no benefit will be allowed.

A member who leaves the employ of the Keuffel & Esser Company may continue his relations with the benefit association if he lives anywhere within a radius of twenty-five miles of the factory.

The men elect their own officers, look after their own cases and make all their own investigations in connection with the sick benefit association at the Emerson Manufacturing Company. The firm attends to the clerical work, and whenever the funds get below a certain point, assists by making a subscription to bring them up again. This, however, has not been necessary more than two or three times.

The members pay in twenty-five cents per month and in case of sickness are given one dollar per day, and in case of death their family is paid $50 to assist in defraying the funeral expenses. This has been in operation three or four years and has proven of great benefit to many of the men and does away entirely with passing subscription papers when fellow workmen are sick and in distress.

All regular employés of the Fitchburg & Leominster Street Railway Relief Association [1] are eligible to membership, but they must be elected by the governing board. The dues are 50 cents per month with a payment of $5 per week for sickness or bodily injury for the first week, and $10 for each succeeding week; the entire liability must not exceed $50. In case of sudden death the family or beneficiaries of the deceased receive the sum of five weeks' benefit. A special assessment of one month's dues is made when the fund amounts to less than $100.

The Scranton Railway Beneficial Association [2] pays to members, who are totally unable to work by reason of injuries, $4 for each week, and after six months the payment is reduced to one-half and after one year the payment ceases. For sickness it pays $4 a week after the first week, provided the sickness entirely incapacitates the member for work. No member may receive benefits for more than thirteen weeks in any one year. The association further pays $100 for the death of a member and $50 for the death of the wife of a member, and $50 for the death of the mother of an unmarried member. Contributions, assessments and dues of members are paid in advance and are deducted by the Scranton Railway Company from the wages due members. The dues of members are 25 cents per month, but an assessment of 25 cents is levied on the death of each member, and one of 25 cents upon the death of the wife of a member or of the mother of an unmarried member. No assessments are made when the unexpended balance in the treasury amounts to $4 per member.

In addition the company has entered into an arrangement with one of the local hospitals whereby they have a private room always at the disposal of their members free. This includes medical attendance, nursing and any other necessities required. "We maintain this feature at an expense of $300 per year, and the investment is thoroughly satisfactory to all concerned," it reports.

[1] Fitchburg & Leominster Street Ry. Co., Fitchburg, Mass. Organized 1886. Number Employés, 125.

[2] Scranton Ry. Co., Scranton, Pa. Organized December, 1896. Number Employés, 726.

The Clifton Silk Mills,[1] Union, N. J., organized a benefit society for the assistance of its employés, which has proved very successful. The company employs about seven hundred and fifty persons, and about one-half of them are members of the association. The incidental expenses, outside of doctor's fees, are all provided for by the company, so that practically every cent contributed by the employés is returned to them in the form of benefits.

Membership in the association is divided into three classes, based on weekly earnings:

Class A, all whose earnings are ten dollars a week or over; Class B, earnings from six dollars and fifty cents to ten dollars per week, and Class C, earnings less than six dollars and fifty cents per week. The entrance fee for Class A is seventy-five cents; Class B, fifty cents, and Class C, twenty-five cents.

The dues charged and benefits paid the several classes of members are as follows: Class A, fifteen cents, due every two weeks, benefits seven dollars per week; Class B, ten cents, due every two weeks, benefits, four dollars and seventy-five cents per week; Class C, five cents, due every two weeks, benefits two dollars and thirty-five cents per week. Dues are deducted from wages by the company's paymaster and turned over to the treasurer of the association. A receipt for the amount taken from the wages of members is enclosed in their pay envelope.

To be entitled to sick benefits a member must have been connected with the society at least one month, and is not to receive anything for disability lasting less than one week, nor more than a total of eight weeks' benefit in any one year.

The society also provides death benefits arranged by classes as follows: Class A, seventy-five dollars; Class B, fifty dollars; Class C, twenty-five dollars.

Members of the society may resign at any time by giving thirty days' notice to the secretary, during which time dues must be paid as usual. A member who leaves the employment of the mills or is discharged forfeits at once all right of membership; but if discharged the two previous payments of dues are restored when the member is finally paid off.

Proper notification blanks to be used in case of sickness or

[1] The Clifton Silk Mills, Union, N. J. Silk Manufacturers. Organized 1900. Number Employés, 750.

death are supplied to members, and these must be used in bringing claims for either form of benefit before the board of directors of the society. A visiting committee investigates all cases, and advises the directors as to the facts underlying the claim.

The management of the benefit society is vested in a board of directors, four of whom are elected by the members, and one appointed by the board of directors of the mills. These serve for six months or until their successors are elected or appointed.

At the Plymouth Cordage Company the Old Colony Mutual Benefit Association was organized June 27, 1878. The dues of the association are $4 a year. This gives an accident benefit of $4 a week for twenty weeks; also includes a death benefit of $150. If the employés are not fortunate enough to belong to these societies the men are generally ready to start a paper through the mills for their benefit.

Membership in the sick and burial club of the firm of John Maddock & Sons, Trenton, N. J., is limited to male employés who earn at least seven dollars per week.

The amount paid to the family of a dead member is absolutely on the assessment plan, the rate being fifty cents for each member in good standing at the time the death occurred.

The firm has encouraged the workmen in every step taken in relation to the benefit society, and has helped financially when occasion required; the management is entirely in the hands of the workmen themselves, and much interest in its affairs is displayed by every member.

The firm writes, "The work is producing good results; we have a membership in the club of about 90 per cent. of the employés, and we would very much dislike to see the organization disbanded for any reason whatever."

The National Saw Company,[1] Newark, N. J., contributes to the funds of the employés benefit association, but not in fixed amounts nor according to any regular plan. Its contributions are given whenever needed, which is, generally speaking, when the treasury is unable to meet claims against it. The company's contributions average about fifty dollars a year.

[1] National Saw Co., Newark, N. J. Manufacturers Saws and Brick Trowels. Organized 1893. Number Employés, 325.

At the Keystone Leather Company,[1] Camden, N. J., the employés have a beneficial society formed for the purpose of aiding those who are taken sick or who may become disabled by accident, and assisting the families of members in case of death.

The dues amount to fifty cents per month. The benefits paid to sick or disabled members are five dollars per week for a period of six weeks.

On the death of a member the sum of fifty dollars is paid to his family to assist in meeting the expenses of burial.

The company contributes liberally to the funds of the association, and in all possible and necessary ways encourages the efforts of its employés in this direction.

The employés of the Adolph Raudnitz Company,[2] Hoboken, N. J., have a sick benefit association membership which is limited to men and women employed at the works. The object of the society is to relieve those of the membership who may be incapable of working through either sickness or accident.

At present it pays a weekly benefit of five dollars for a period of twenty-six consecutive weeks, after which payments are optional on the part of the society, but they are always continued in greater or less amounts according to the necessities of the member as long as disability continues.

The dues per member are ten cents per week. The firm takes an interest in the beneficial society and helps its work along financially, although the management of its affairs is entirely in the hands of employés.

February 12, 1907, the 27th Annual Meeting of the Strawbridge and Clothier Relief Association was begun at 5.30 P.M. in the store, with a luncheon, followed by the business meeting. An orchestra and a double quartette of the employés furnished the music. The annual report showed that more money was received and disbursed last year than in any previous year; $7860 were in benefits for sickness to three hundred and eighty-three members; $1600 on account of deaths, and $341.75 for expenses, leaving a credit balance of $377.97.

That these results have been accomplished at a cost of $3.75

[1] Keystone Leather Co., Camden, N. J. Tanners of Goat Skins and Horse Hides. Organized November 19, 1895. Number Employés, 400.

[2] The Adolph Raudnitz Co., Hoboken, N. J. Manufacturers Fancy Leather Goods. Organized December 29, 1906. Number Employés, 185.

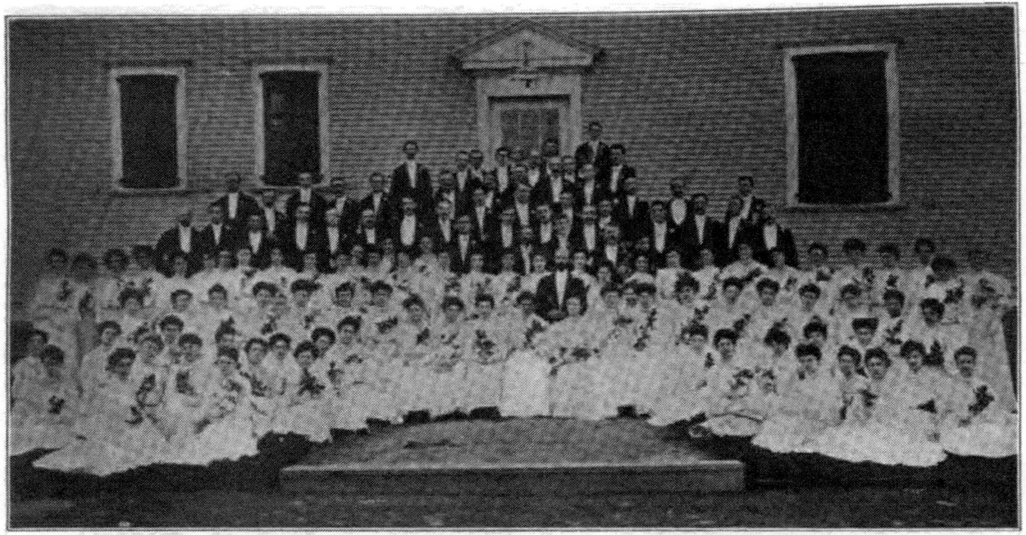

The Choral Society of the Employés at Strawbridge & Clothier's, before Singing to an Audience of Fifty Thousand People at Willow Grove, Philadelphia.

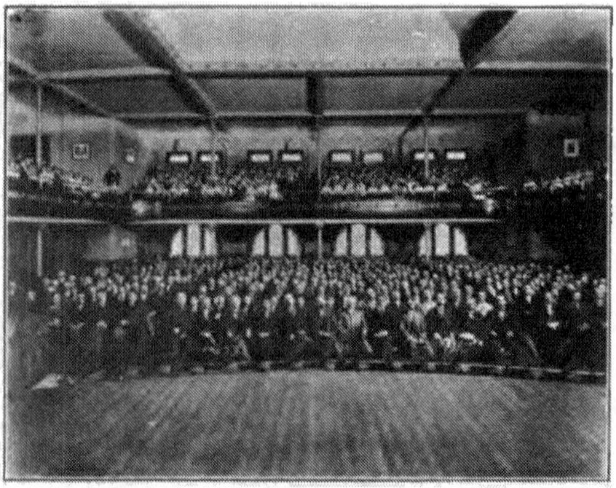

An Entertainment at the Auditorium in the Factory of the H. J. Heinz Company.

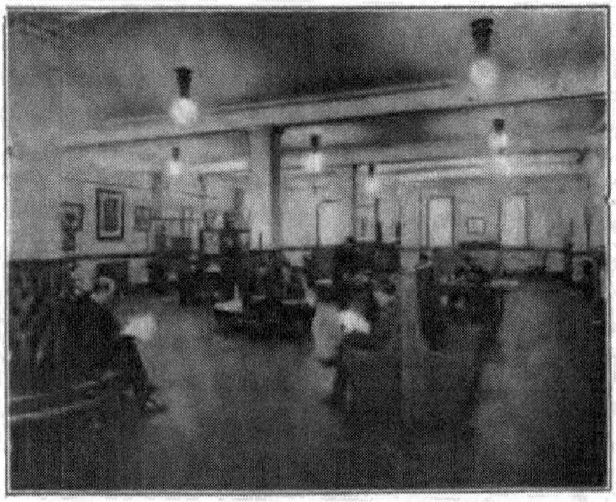

The Library and Reading Room for the Employés of the New York Edison Company.

to the individual member was due to a contribution of $4,277.40 by the firm. The membership at the beginning of the year was 1280; during the year 333 persons had joined, 4 were reinstated, 239 left the employ of the firm; 4 had withdrawn, and 16 had been removed by death, making the membership at the end of the year 1358.

This association was organized in 1880 for the relief of any member who may be detained from business on account of sickness, disability, or accident, and the raising of a benefit fund in case of the death of a member. Whenever the treasury has more than $1000, there is no assessment: otherwise it is 25 cents a month. The sick benefit is $5 per week, payable weekly, but no benefits are allowed for less than one week's illness, or fraction thereof, nor for a longer period than fifteen weeks in any one year, beginning said year with date of first week's benefits. The death benefit is $100.

Since the organization in 1880, the assessments have amounted to $69,217.75; the firm has contributed a total of $58,642.25; and new members have paid $3,295.22, the grand total amounting to $131,155.22. $107,384.72 were paid in sick benefits; $17,679.75 in death benefits; the expenses were $5,737.78, making the total disbursements $130,802.25.

An organization that combines the beneficial with the educational and recreative, is the Association of the Employés of the New York Edison Company. Organized in 1905, it provides that any one in the employ of the company for three months is eligible to membership, $2 for the entrance fee, with annual dues $2.60, payable quarterly in advance. There are the usual officers. The general business is conducted by the board of trustees.

The benficial feature consists of a mortuary fund, from which is paid at the time of the member's decease, to his family, the sum of $100, to which the company contributes an equal amount. It is always the intention to pay this amount within 24 hours after the death of a member, where possible.

The entrance fees are devoted entirely to the mortuary fund as well as $2 of the $2.60 annual dues, 60 cents being sufficient for general expense. The money derived from field days and entertainments is kept as a contingent fund, and may be used either for general expense or turned over to the mortuary fund at the discretion of the board of trustees. There are at present nearly 800 members.

Should a member leave the employ of the New York Edison Company his membership in the association ceases, unless he leaves owing to illness and dies as a result of that illness and is not employed elsewhere between the time of his leaving the company and his death. In the latter event, provided of course his dues have been paid, he is considered a member in good standing, and his family receives the benefits as though he had been actually on the pay roll of the company at the time of his decease.

Regular meetings are held monthly, and during the winter months special meetings are usually held between the regular meetings. At the regular meetings general business is transacted, after which there is usually a short entertainment given by the members. The special meetings consist of technical papers, general talks on subjects relating to the electric lighting industry, or addresses on some non-technical subject of general interest. All meetings are held in the auditorium of the New York Edison Company, the expense of the meeting place being assumed by the company.

The association also promotes athletic sports among the members. In the summer months a regular baseball league is organized and matches are played each Saturday half holiday between teams organized in the different departments or branches of the company. Annually a summer outing is given by the association, at which prizes are awarded for general field games.

During the winter a bowling league is conducted, the teams being organized in the different departments. A dramatic entertainment is given, the performers usually amateurs and members of the association. Both the outing and the entertainment net considerable sums, which are turned into the treasury.

In 1905 the company decided that it would work out its own problems of self-insurance against accidents in such a way that the full benefit of the indemnity should go to the beneficiary and that all the employés might feel that the company was personally interested in the individual. In the event of an accident, the employé is sent to the company's physician, by the foreman, with a card, which entitles him to free medical treatment and medicines during his disability; for this consideration he is asked to sign a release. If he is unwilling to sign, he is visited by a representative of the company, who explains that no liability insurance is carried, and that each case is considered on its individual merits. If the facts show that the accident was caused by the negligence of the company, a foreman, or fellow servant, the employé is put on the "Disability pay roll" and his wages in full are paid during his disability. If the accident was caused by the man's own carelessness or the violation of self-evident rules for protection, his length of service, fidelity, marital condition, and the number of others dependent on him, are factors determining whether he shall receive full or partial wages while disabled. If it is clearly shown that the accident was caused by carelessness so gross as to seriously endanger the safety of his fellows, or the working of the apparatus, he is deprived of his income. I am informed that such cases are very rare. In the case of fatal accidents, the mortuary expenses are paid in full by the company regardless of the responsibility for the fatality. The company does not consider that its duty to the man's family ceases because he is dead, but almost invariably the council votes a donation dependent on the previous record of the employé and the economic condition of his survivors and dependents. The great advantage to the company is the personal and intimate relations which it has been able to maintain with its staff, most of whom appreciate the individualization. The company extends the system by free legal advice to its personnel, who may be injured by outside corporations or individuals. If it appears that the man has a just claim, a representative of the company visits the one responsible for the injury, for the sake of explaining the "Edison system," at the same time suggesting that the case in question should be managed in a similar manner. Of all the accidents to its own employés, only five men have sued the company.

The B. G. Volger Manufacturing Company,[1] Passaic, N. J., in cases of idleness caused by accident or sickness, makes no

[1] B. G. Volger Manufacturing Co., Passaic, N. J. Manufacturers Self-Inking Stamp-Pads and Stamp Books. Organized May 17, 1902. Number Employés, 15.

deduction of wages, if the sick or injured person has been five years or more in its employment. In all other cases, one-half of the regular wage is allowed. Married men are required to carry $1000 of life insurance, the company paying in full the first year's premium, and assisting such as may find after payments a hardship on account of any unusual drain on their earnings.

Benefit features in the works of the Samuel L. Moore & Sons Corporation,[1] Elizabeth, N. J., are limited to an arrangement with the general hospital, under which employés injured in the actual performance of duty are received into that institution and treated without expense to themselves. For this privilege each employé contributes ten cents per month. The general hospital will treat any injured person who may apply for admission, but the workmen prefer paying this small sum monthly so as to assist the institution and also that if, through accident or sickness, they become inmates, they may not be regarded as charity patients.

Relief and aid or accident funds are in operation at some of the works of the International Harvester Company, and a plan is under consideration which shall afford benefits in case of sickness, as well as accident and death benefits, and its scope is as liberal as any known scheme for aged and disabled employés. A pension plan is also contemplated. No permanent outside hospitals are maintained, but the company contributes to the regular hospitals and dispensaries, and resident physicians at three plants afford much relief, while medical service on emergency call is available for a regular portion of each day at other plants.

W. W. Herrick, manager of the accident and pension department of the American Steel and Wire Company,[2] sent a circular concerning this pension system to its employés in 1902. June 1st there were one hundred of the old employés on the

[1] Samuel L. Moore & Sons Corporation, Elizabeth, N. J. Engineers, Machinists and Founders. Organized January 9, 1905. Number Employés, 275.

[2] American Steel and Wire Co. Manufacturers Steel and Wire Products. Organized January 13, 1899. Number Employés, 28,443.

pension list. Each workman will receive from $5.00 to $20.00 each month as long as he lives. One of the pensioners, Samuel Overend, has been with the company 51 years, practically since its establishment. Two others have served more than 50 years, six over 40, nine over 35, twelve over 30, seventeen over 25, and twenty-two over 20. The circular follows:

Pension Department of the American Steel and Wire Company of New Jersey:

REGULATIONS

1. The Pension Department is a department created for the purpose of enforcing the action of the officers of the American Steel and Wire Company, requiring that all employés who have attained the age of 65 years shall be retired, and such of them as have served ten years, either with the present company or its predecessors, may be pensioned. However, an employé 65 years of age can obtain permission, through recommendation of the manager, to continue for a longer period in the employ of the company. Persons more than 55 years of age, who have been in the employ of the company for ten years, may make application for retirement, and if full examination shows they are unable to continue their vocation, they may be recommended to the board of administration, whose decision to pension or not shall rule. Persons not in continuous service for a period of ten years shall not be entitled to a pension.

Neither the action of the board of administration nor the board of directors, in establishing a pension system, nor any other action now or hereafter taken by them, or by others in charge or connected with this pension fund in the inauguration and operation of the department, shall be construed as giving any officer, agent or employé of the company, a right to be retained in its service, or any right or claim to any pension allowance, and the company expressly reserves the right and privilege to discharge at any time any one employed by the company when the interests of the company in its judgment may so require, without liability for any claim for pension or other allowance than salary or wages due and unpaid.

2. A board of trustees has been appointed to care for and invest a sum set aside by the company to carry out the provisions.

A board of administration has been appointed who shall have power:

To make and enforce rules and regulations for the care and operation of the department;

To determine the eligibility of employés to receive pension allowances;

To fix the amount of such allowances; and

To prescribe the conditions under which such allowances may be made.

The powers and duties of the board of administration shall also embrace the consideration of all applications for employment in the service of inexperienced persons over thirty-five years of age, and experienced persons over forty-five years of age, who are included in the first and second paragraphs of the exceptions to the age limit established in connection with the creation of the pension fund.

They shall make rules for the government of the pension department.

In order to carry out the work properly under the ideas of the management, it is considered necessary to appoint in each mill a committee to be known as "The Mill Committee," which shall consist of the superintendent as chairman, the chief clerk, master mechanic, chief timekeeper, and superintendents or foremen of departments. This mill committee to furnish to the board of administration the necessary data from which the board of administration is to decide as to the eligibility of employés for pension; also this committee to take up further the matter of assistance to faithful employés in the service, who may become sick or destitute, and make recommendations to the board of administration for prompt assistance in such cases. The mill committee is to be appointed by the superintendent subject to approval of district manager.

3. Of the employés who are required by the organization to give their entire time to the service of the company, there shall be two classes who shall be retired from the service, as follows:

(a) All employés who shall have attained the age of sixty-five years, and who shall have served ten or more years with the company or its predecessors.

(b) All employés fifty-five to sixty-five years of age, who shall have been ten or more years in the service, and shall, in the opinion of the administration board, have become physically disqualified.

4. In the case of employés who shall have attained the age of sixty-five years, retirement shall be made effective from the first day of the calendar month following that in which they shall have attained that age; in all other cases the date of retirement shall be from the first day of a calendar month, to be determined by the board of administration.

5. In case any employé fifty-five to sixty-five years of age, ten or more years in the service, claims that he is, or should his employing officer consider him, physically disqualified for further service, he may make application or be recommended for retirement on proper blank, and the board of administration will decide whether or not he shall be retired from the service.

6. No inexperienced person over 35 years of age, and no experienced person over 45 years of age, shall hereafter be taken into the service of the company; however, persons beyond such age limit may be taken into the employ of the company temporarily, but shall have no claim to pension; provided also, with the approval of the board of administration, persons may be employed indefinitely irrespective of age limit, if the services required are professional or otherwise special in their nature.

7. In referring to the employés of the company, the expressions "service" and "in the service" will refer to employment in connection with any of the works operated by the company, and the service of any such employé shall be considered as continuous from the date from which he has been continuously employed by the American Steel and Wire Company or its predecessors. Leave of absence, suspension or dismissal, followed by reinstatement within six months, shall not be considered as a break in the continuity of service; persons who leave the service of the company relinquish all claims to pension allowance.

8. It shall be the duty of every employing officer to report at once, through the usual channels, to the board of administration, on the proper blank, all employés who have attained or who will in January, 1902, attain the age of sixty-five years, and thereafter at least a month in advance of the date of their

retirement, all employés about to attain that age, for consideration for a pension allowance.

9. The information required for pension allowance shall be sent by the immediate employing officer to his superior officer, and by him forwarded to the proper executive officer in charge of the department in which the employé may be for his information and forwarding to the district manager.

10. The pension allowances authorized by the board of administration to be paid monthly are upon the following basis:

For each year of service one per centum of the average regular monthly pay for the ten years preceding retirement; thus, by way of illustration: If an employé has been in the service of the company for forty years and has received on an average for the last ten years $50 per month regular wages, his pension allowance would be 40 per cent. of $50, or $20 per month.

Whenever at any time it shall be found that the basis of pension allowances shall create demands in excess of the amount, which has been fixed by the officers of the company in the administration of the pension department, a new basis, ratably reducing the pension allowances, may be established, bringing the expenditures within the limitations, and the decision of the board of administration in establishing such new basis shall be absolutely conclusive without appeal.

11. When pension allowances are authorized pursuant to these regulations, they shall be paid monthly during the life of the beneficiary, provided, however, that the company may withhold its allowance in case of gross misconduct on his part. The disbursing officer, with the approval of the board of administration, may adopt such a system of distribution of the monthly allowances as he may think proper.

12. In payment of pension allowances, pay rolls showing the names of those to whom allowances have been made and the amount of such allowances, shall be prepared at the close of each month by the proper officer, who shall certify to their correctness, and forward same to district manager, who shall in turn send them to the manager of the Pension Department for approval.

13. Each employing officer must keep himself advised of the whereabouts of former employés who have been retired from service and promptly advise the manager of the pension depart-

ment, through the usual channels, when any of them cease to be entitled to further pension allowances through death or misconduct. Where they do not reside within the jurisdiction of the officer of the department in which they were engaged before being retired from the service, such officer shall require affidavit to be made and forwarded to him, by such former employé, at least once a year, and oftener as may be required, that he is entitled to a pension allowance.

14. The benefits of the pension system will apply only to those persons who have been required to give their entire time to the service of the company, and will not apply to the law and surgical departments, nor will they apply to such officers and employés as may have now, or obtain hereafter, a benefit or bounty from the operative results of their departments in addition to their salaries.

15. No pension allowance shall be paid to any person for a period during which he may be receiving accident or sick benefits from the accident or benefit departments.

16. The acceptance of a pension allowance shall not debar any former employé from engaging in any other enterprise differing distinctly in character and scope from his former employment, but such person cannot re-enter the service of the company, and would lose his claim to the benefits granted, should he engage in similar employment.

17. To the end of preserving direct personal relations between the company and its retired employés, and that they may continue to enjoy the benefits of the pension system, no assignments of pensions will be permitted or recognized; such being hereby declared to be non-assignable. In case any pensioned employé should assign to any one else his claim to pension, the board of administration may stop his pension altogether.

18. Employés placed on pension roll will be expected on request of the officers of the company, to report and give to the company the benefit of their experience, and act as advisers when called upon.

Edward A. Woods, Pittsburg Manager of the Equitable Life Assurance Society,[1] has 51 clerks in his office to whom the

[1] Equitable Life Assurance Society of the United States, Pittsburg. Organized 1859. Number Employés, 205.

pension system applies. Every clerk who has been with him two years or more is assured on the 20 year endowment plan. The policies are taken and paid for entirely by Mr. Woods. They are payable to the employés, but assigned to and held by him, so that in case of any of the employés leaving the office under any delinquency or dying with such, Mr. Woods would have the proceeds of the policy, for which he himself paid, to partly offset the indebtedness. A written direction is taken from each employé as to whom he desires the money to be paid in case of death, and in such case the policy is paid to the beneficiary designated. In every case where an employé leaves, the bond is turned over to him, which he can carry or cash, as he pleases. All but one that have been turned over have been kept up, as there is great inducement to do so when several premiums have already been paid. Where the employé remains until the end of the 20 years, the endowment becomes payable, and it is the intention to give it to him as an additional reward for 20 years' faithful service, or if he is not in a condition to continue, he can retire with less hardship and strain than if this arrangement had not been systematically made over a course of years.

The advantages expected from this arrangement are as follows:

1. An appreciation on the part of the employés of some interest in his future beyond salary.

2. An inducement to a faithful employé to remain instead of making changes, hurtful both to employer and employé.

3. The avoidance of calls upon the Pittsburg office by destitute dependents of deceased employés, this provision having already been made.

4. An additional indemnity in case of the death of a delinquent employé.

5. The facilitating of the retirement upon something like a pension of an employé who after twenty years of service could be replaced with advantage by a younger and new one.

6. The encouragement of thrift on the part of the employé. Almost all of those for whom bonds have been taken ultimately take additional bonds themselves.

Looking towards a still closer knitting together of his working force, Mr. Woods has effected what he calls the "Pittsburg Veteran Legion," an organization of agents and office employés, by classes, who have been with him five, ten, fifteen, twenty, or more years. The purpose of the organization is eventually to form a basis for giving certain advantages, privileges and possibly shares of profit to old employés, thereby encouraging persistence among them.

At the first meeting in 1907, those entitled to membership in this legion were presented with certificates of membership, and with the insignia, a gold pin, the insignia of the five-year corps having no stone setting; the ten-year corps a sapphire, the fifteen-year an emerald, the twenty-year a ruby, and the twenty-five year a diamond. Hereafter as members of the agency attain five years' continuous service, or as members of a corps of a lower rank become eligible to membership in the next higher corps, they will be admitted to membership in person only at the first meeting of the lunch club that they thereafter attend.

Some of the prizes which will be distributed annually will be confined to members of the Pittsburg Veteran Legion. It is expected that this organization will ultimately make it possible for the agency to further recognize those who have long been associated with it, and contributed so largely to its success. Not only do years of experience and loyalty of service justly entitle those to credit and prestige in their profession and with the public, over the inexperienced and the beginners, but it is the desire of the management of the Pittsburg agency to show appreciation to those veterans who have year in and year out in good and evil report loyally remained faithful to the society, bearing its troubles and sharing its prosperity.

The five-year corps was composed of 26 members, of whom two were women; the ten-year corps, 12 members, with one woman; the fifteen-year corps, two members; the twenty-year, three, and the twenty-five, one member.

In March, 1901, Dr. Carnegie wrote from New York to the president and board of directors of the Carnegie Company in Pittsburg the following letter:

"Gentlemen:—Mr. Robert A. Franks, my cashier, will hand over to you, upon your acceptance of the trust, Four Million

Dollars of the Carnegie Company bonds, in trust for the following purposes:

The income of the Four Million Dollars is to be applied:

1. To provide for employés of The Carnegie Company, in all its works, mines, railways, shops, etc., injured in its service, and for those dependent upon such employés as are killed.

2. To provide small pensions or aids to such employés as after long and creditable service, through exceptional circumstances, need such help in their old age, and who make a good use of it.

3. This fund is not intended to be used as a substitute for what the company has been in the habit of doing in such cases —far from it—it is intended to go still further and give to the injured or their families, or to employés who are needy in old age through no fault of their own, some provision against want as long as needed, or until young children can become self-supporting.

4. A report is to be made at the end of each year, giving an account of the fund and its distribution, and published in two papers in Pittsburg, and copies posted freely at several works, that every employé may know what is being done. Publicity in this matter will, I am sure, have a beneficial effect.

5. I make this first use of surplus wealth upon retiring from business as an acknowledgment of the deep debt which I owe to the workmen who have contributed so greatly to my success.

(Signed) ANDREW CARNEGIE."

March 20th the board of directors of the company accepted the trust and agreed to the conditions as expressed in Dr. Carnegie's letter setting forth the terms of the gift. The board formally expressed their deep appreciation for his munificent gift for the welfare of the employés of the company, "reciprocating the kindly expressions of his personal interest in those with whom he has been so long associated, though no words can adequately express our feelings of love, loyalty, admiration, and inspiration, which have been so much a part of our service for him."

The Andrew Carnegie Relief Fund was made effective January 1, 1902, but in 1905 was changed to the Carnegie Relief Fund. The following are the constituent companies participating in the Fund: Carnegie Steel Co., Carnegie Natural Gas Co., Pittsburg Limestone Co., Ltd., H. C. Frick Coke Co., Oliver Iron Mining Co., Bessemer & Lake Erie R. R. Co., Union Railroad Co., Pittsburg Steamship Co., Pittsburg & Conneaut Dock Co., Union Supply Co., Mingo Coal Co., National Mining Co.

In the general regulations of the Carnegie Relief Fund, the administration is in charge of an advisory board appointed annually by the board of directors of the Carnegie Steel Co., serving one year from the first day of January. The usual officers are elected by the board.

A manager elected by the board has executive charge of the fund. He also acts as secretary of the board.

The advisory board, subject to the approval of the board of directors, has power:

(a) To make, amend and enforce regulations for the efficient operation of the Carnegie Relief Fund.

(b) To determine the eligibility of employés to receive accident benefits, of beneficiaries to receive death benefits, and of employés to receive pension allowances.

(c) To fix the amount of such benefits and allowances;—and

(d) To prescribe the conditions under which such benefits and allowances may inure.

All questions or controversies of whatever character arising in any manner, or between any parties or persons in connection with the Carnegie Relief Fund, or the operation thereof, whether as to the eligibility of persons to accident or death benefits, or pension allowances, or as to the construction of language or meaning of the regulations, or as to any writing, decision, instructions, or case in connection therewith, shall be submitted to the determination of the manager of the fund, whose decision shall be final and conclusive thereof, subject to the right of appeal to the advisory board within thirty days after notice to the parties interested in the decision. The action of the advisory board shall then be final and conclusive.

Accident or death benefits and pension allowances may be withheld or terminated in case of any misconduct on the part of the beneficiary, or for any cause sufficient, in the judgment of the advisory board to require such action. It shall be the duty of the manager of the fund to keep himself advised at all times of the whereabouts of beneficiaries, and to promptly advise the advisory board when any of them cease to be entitled to further benefits or allowances.

All benefits and allowances from the Carnegie Relief Fund shall be made and apply only to those employés (or their families) who have been required to give their entire time to the service of the Carnegie Steel Company or to one or more of the affiliated companies or associations. Employés who leave the service thereby relinquish all privilege of application to the benefit of the fund.

Whenever it shall be found that the basis for accident and death benefits and pension allowances, shall create a demand in excess of the annual income, a new basis reducing the accident or death benefits or pension allowances, or new bases reducing all benefits and allowances, shall be established, bringing the expenditure within the prescribed limitations. Notice of such new basis, or bases, shall be given before the beginning of the month in which it may be decided to put the same into effect.

No assignment of accident or death benefit or pension allowance will be permitted or recognized under any circumstances, nor shall any such benefit or allowance be subject to attachment or other legal process for debts of the beneficiary, nor shall death benefits be applicable to payment of debts of the deceased.

ACCIDENT BENEFITS

Payment of benefits on account of disablement by accident shall only be made upon the disablement being shown to have resulted solely from accidents or cases of sunstroke and heat exhaustion occurring to employés during and in direct and proper connection with the performance of duty in the service of the company. There must be a clear and well established history of the cause and circumstances of injury accidentally inflicted and sufficient to produce the alleged injury, with exterior or other positive evidence of such injury and satisfactory evidence that it renders the employé unable to perform his duty in the service.

Employés disabled by accident occurring otherwise than as aforesaid, including such as may arise at any time from acts or things having no proper relation to the performance of duty, or from the individual's physical condition or tendency (except in cases of sunstroke or heat exhaustion) shall not be eligible to benefits; nor shall benefits be payable for injuries arising in consequence of intoxication, or resulting from the use of stimulants or narcotics, or while engaged in any unlawful or immoral acts.

Employés shall not be eligible to receive accident benefits for time for which wages are paid by the company.

Company surgeons, or such other surgeons as may be delegated by the manager of the fund, shall ascertain and report upon the condition of injured employés and decide as to their fitness for duty, in accordance with instructions issued by the manager.

If an injured employé shall decline to permit the company surgeon (or such other surgeon as may be delegated) to ascertain his condition, or shall fail to give proper information respecting it, or shall leave the company surgeon's jurisdiction without his knowledge or permission, or shall in any manner render it impracticable for the company surgeon to ascertain his condition, he shall not be eligible to accident benefits.

In order that all employés injured and eligible to accident benefits, as prescribed in these regulations, may participate in the fund, it shall be the duty of employing officers to keep a record of such, and, when the time lost by any aggregates one year, whether in one continuous period, or in more than one period due to the one injury, to notify the manager of the fund, and the company surgeon under whose jurisdiction the injured employé is, (or such other surgeon delegated to perform such service) on proper blank; also to certify as to whether or not injured employés receive wages for time lost by disability, and to the date on which they return to duty.

When authorized by the manager, in accordance with these regulations, accident benefits, on account of continued disability shall be paid monthly, at the close of the month, and for short periods when the amounts are ascertained, to the injured employé, through the office of the employing officer.

Benefits to employés disabled by accident in service shall become payable the day after the time lost by reason of the disability aggregates one year; shall continue during the disability, and shall be governed by the following schedule of rates: 75 cents per day for unmarried men; one dollar per day for married men; provided, however, that in no event shall the accident benefits exceed the average daily wages of the employé.

DEATH BENEFITS

Payment of benefits on account of death by accident shall only be made upon the death of the employé being shown to have resulted solely from accidents or cases of sunstroke or heat exhaustion, occurring during, and in direct and proper connection with, the performance of duty in the service of the company. There must be a clear and well established history of the cause and circumstances of injury accidentally inflicted and sufficient to produce death, with exterior or other positive evidence of such injury.

The families of deceased employés who meet death from accident occurring otherwise than as aforesaid, including such as may arise at any time from acts or things having no proper relation to the performance of duty, or from the individual's physical condition or tendency (except in cases of sunstroke or heat exhaustion) shall not be eligible to benefits; nor shall benefits be payable for deaths occurring in consequence of intoxication, or resulting from the use of stimulants or narcotics, or while engaged in any unlawful or immoral acts.

In order that the families of all deceased employés, who may be eligible to death benefits, as prescribed in these rgulations, may participate in the fund, it shall be the duty of the employing officers, when such death to an employé occurs, to notify the manager of the fund on proper blank; and the company surgeon (or such other surgeon as may be delegated by the manager) shall report on the case, and certify to the cause of death.

The manager of the fund shall investigate the financial condition of the family of the deceased employé and submit the results of such investigation, together with the reports of the employing officer and surgeon, to the advisory board, and recommend in what manner death benefits shall be paid.

Death benefits when allowed by the advisory board shall be payable to the family which was dependent upon the deceased employé, as soon as possible after the required evidence of the death of the employé is obtained, and shall apply primarily to the cases of married men, and be based in such cases upon the following schedule of rates:

Five hundred dollars for the widow of deceased.

One hundred dollars additional for each child under 16 years of age, on the date of death of deceased employé; provided, however, that in no case shall the death benefits exceed $1200, including that paid to the widow.

The relative or relatives of unmarried men shall not be eligible to death benefits, unless such deceased employé shall have been the sole support of, or a regular contributor to the support of, such relative or relatives. Evidence of such support, satisfactory and conclusive to the advisory board, must be furnished, and in such cases, and in all other cases, the advisory board shall designate the person or persons who shall receive and receipt for the payment to the beneficiary or beneficiaries. Death benefits when allowed the relative or relatives of unmarried men shall be in the sum of five hundred dollars.

Payment of death benefits granted shall be made in monthly installments, depending on the financial condition of the beneficiary or beneficiaries, at the close of each month, until the whole amount be paid; such monthly amount and the date on which payment shall begin, to be fixed by the advisory board. If, however, reasons sufficient, in the judgment of the board, for payment to be made otherwise than as aforesaid shall be given, the board shall determine how payment in such cases shall be made.

PENSION ALLOWANCES

Any employé of a constituent company of the Carnegie Steel Company which has been ten years within the Carnegie interests, who shall have reached the age of 60 years and shall have been at least 15 years continuously in the service of the company, and who claims that he is, or should his employing officer consider him, incapacitated for further service, may make application to be, or his employing officer may recommend that he be retired, and the advisory board shall decide whether or not he shall be placed upon the pension list.

No employé of a constituent company of the Carnegie Steel Company, which has not been ten years within the Carnegie interests, shall be eligible to pension allowance. When such a company shall have been 10 years within the Carnegie interests, the service rendered by an employé to such company (and its predecessor or predecessors) previous to its entry into the Carnegie interests shall be included in computing length of service.

Any employé, of a company which was once, but has ceased to be, a constituent company of the Carnegie interests, shall be eligible to pension allowance, provided that at the time the company by which he is employed, left the Carnegie interests, he had reached the age of 55 years, had been 20 years in service, and his case fulfils all the other requirements of the regulations. In such cases the service rendered by the employé to such company while within the Carnegie interests only, shall be included in computing length of service.

In computing service it shall be reckoned from the date since which the employé has been continuously in the service to the date when retired, such service to have been in the Carnegie Steel Company or one of its affiliated companies or associations. Leave of absence, suspension, temporary lay-off on account of reduction in force, or disability, shall not be considered as a break in the continuity of service and time thus lost shall not be deducted in computing the length of service. Dismissal and voluntary leaving of the service, followed by re-instatement within two years, shall not be considered as a break in the continuity of service, but time thus lost shall be deducted in computing length of service.

The number of years of service shall be taken at the nearest even year, as indicated by the final result. The provisions of this regulation requiring re-instatement in two years in cases of dismissal and voluntary leaving of service shall not apply to service rendered prior to the date of establishment of the fund.

Physical examination by the company surgeon under whose jurisdiction the applicant for pension allowance is, or such other surgeon as may be satisfactory to, or delegated by, the manager, shall be made of employés in all cases, and a report of such examination shall be transmitted by the manager to the advisory board for its information.

It shall be the duty of the employing officer when recommending an employé for pension allowance to furnish, on proper blank, from his office records, the record of the employé's service, to certify thereto, and forward blank to the manager of the fund; also, at the request of the manager to approve or disapprove and to certify to, as above, the applications of employés for pension allowance.

In retiring employés from service and placing them upon the pension list, their retirement shall be made effective from the first day of a month, to be determined by the advisory board.

When pension allowances shall be authorized, pursuant to these regulations, they shall, unless and until revoked by the board, be paid monthly to the retired employé at the close of each month, and shall terminate with payment for the month in which the death of the employé occurs.

If for any reason a retired employé shall be unable to execute a proper receipt for pension allowance, the manager shall determine to whom payment shall be made for him, and the receipt of such person shall be made for him, and the receipt of such person shall be a sufficient discharge.

If an employé shall become permanently totally disabled from sickness causes or from injuries received while not on duty, before reaching the age of 60 years, he may, provided his case fulfils all the other foregoing requirements governing the granting of pension allowances, be placed upon the pension list, subject to the conditions pertaining thereto.

The pension allowance authorized shall be upon the following basis:

For each year of service one per cent. of the average regular monthly pay received for the entire term of service.

By way of illustration—An employé who had been 30 years in the service and had received an average of $70 per month, would receive a pension allowance of 30 per cent. of $70, or $21 per month.

In the calculation of a pension allowance the amount shall be taken at the nearest half-dime, as indicated by the final result.

The acceptance of a pension allowance shall not debar any former employé from engaging in other business, but such person must retire, or be retired from, and cannot reënter, the service of the company.

Summarizing the work of the last six years:

	Accident Benefits	Death Benefits	Pension Allowances	Totals
1902,—	$19,700.90	$16,316.00	$12,196.95	$48,213.85
1903,—	106,655.37	46,824.00	27,172.80	180,652.17
1904,—	128,471.57	76,948 00	36,573.75	241,983.32
1905,—	96,187.80	123,249.00	46,853.35	266,290.15
1906,—	15,023.70	101,972 50	58,212.55	175,208.75
1907,—	17,545.15	130,449 00	68,769.90	216,764.05
Grand Totals	$383,584,49	$495,758.50	$249,779.30	$1,129,117.29

The Sixth Annual Report shows the operations for the year ending December 31, 1907:

	Accident Benefits	Death Benefits	Pension Allowances	Totals
Carnegie Steel Co. (24 works and companies)	$9,267.65	$60,141.00	$44,028.75	$113,437.40
Pittsburg Limestone Co. (2 quarries)		660.00		660.00
H. C. Frick Coke Co. (60 works and companies)	4,333.25	29,418.00	18,835.50	52,586.75
Oliver Iron Mining Co. (Gogebic Range—6 mines, Marquette Range—6 mines, Menominee Range 3 mines, Missabe Range—11 mines, Vermillion Range —4 mines)	2,104.25	22,530.00	19.60	24,653.85
Bessemer & Lake Erie R. R. Co. (4 departments)	92.00	9,400.00	135.70	9,627.70
Union R. R. Co.	365.00	8,620.00		8,985.00
Pittsburg Steamship Co.		2,190.00		2,190.00
Pittsburg & Conneaut Dock Co.	883.00	650.00		1,533.00
National Mining Co.		1,840.00		1,840.00
Keystone Bridge Works			6,250.35	6,250.35

There was posted March 7, 1902, in the 26 barns, stables and power houses of the Metropolitan Street Railway Company, throughout Manhattan, a notice from President Vreeland to all employés, announcing the establishment of a pension system for the superannuated employés of the concern. This is the first pension system ever established for street railway employés, and is the final step in the system inaugurated by President Vreeland, when he took charge of the Metropolitan, for steadying and elevating the status of its 15,000 employés.

"To all Employés:

The plan I have long had in mind of establishing a pension system for the relief of the superannuated employés of this company, members of the Metropolitan Street Railway Association, whose annual maximum wages have not exceeded $1,200 per annum, has finally been perfected and will be put into effect on or before July 1st. The specific regulations are now being drafted, and will, in due course, be distributed for your further information.

This pension system provides for voluntary and involuntary retirement of all employés so included, between the ages of 65 and 70, after 25 years' service in the Metropolitan Street Railway Company, or any of its constituent companies. Employés benefited by the system will be of two classes:

1st. All employés who have attained the age of 70 years, who have been continuously in service for 25 years or more, preceding such date of maturity, and

2nd. All employés from 65 to 69 years of age, who have been 25 years or more in such service who in the opinion of the trustees of the pension have become physically disqualified. All employés of 70 years will be considered to have attained a maximum age allowed for active service, and will be retired by age limit, while those whose ages range from 65 to 69 may, upon examination, be retired under pension if found incapable.

The pension allowance to such retired employés shall be upon the following basis:

a. If service has been continuous for 35 years or more, 40 per cent. of the average annual wages for the 10 previous years.

b. If service has been continuous for 30 years, 30 per cent. of the average annual wages for the 10 previous years.

c. If service has been continuous for 25 years, 25 per cent. of the average annual wages for the 10 previous years.

The fund from which payments will be made will be appropriated each year by the company, and employés will not be required to contribute to it.

My object in establishing this department is to preserve the future welfare of aged and infirm employés and to recognize efficient and loyal service.

(Signed) H. H. Vreeland,
President and General Manager."

Again mutuality takes the form of sympathy by employé with employé. In a New England mill town where there had been a peculiarly trying strike, a sympathy sprung up between certain Italians and certain Irishmen. This arose from an appeal made by an Italian to an Irishman who had been rather prominently connected with the strike, to help him in the trouble he was having with a doctor, or rather quack, who had robbed the poor fellow of something over $150 of his hard-earned savings, pretending to be able to cure his moribund, consumptive wife. This good-hearted Irishman went to see the woman, who was a most pitiful spectacle, and found the Italian putting everything he earned into food and nursing for her, tenderly caring for her himself while out of the mill, but sticking manfully to his work to get the means to make her comfortable. It was a touch of human nature which bowled over the Irishman's sympathies, and made him at least a strong believer in the good heart and whole-souled devotion of this particular Italian. The leaven has appeared to work, and there is not much, if any evidence of friction between the two races now in this place.

One interesting feature of the Colgate & Company's[1] hundredth anniversary banquet of 1906 was the speech of the head of the firm, in which he announced the intention to give away about $40,000 to the old employés.

Toward the end of the dinner Richard M. Colgate, the senior member of the firm, asked permission to make a second speech. He was told by the toastmaster that he was out of order, but permission was finally given. He then announced that the firm had decided to give each employé, of factory or office, who had

[1] Colgate & Co., New York. Manufacturers Soap and Perfumery. Organized 1806. Number Employés, 1100.

been with the concern over one year, a five dollar gold piece for each completed calendar year of service. One hundred and fifty of the thousand employés had over ten years of service to their credit. The senior employé received nearly $250.

The employés of the Swiss Laundry of Rochester were recently given their third annual complimentary banquet by Mason Brothers, proprietors. One hundred and twenty-five persons were present.

Christmas, 1906, the Proximity Manufacturing Company gave their superintendents and overseers a banquet at the Benbow Hotel. All of the superintendents, overseers and officers of the mills met together and spent a most enjoyable evening. Between 75 and 100 people attended, and in place of set speeches, informal toasts were made, nearly everybody being called upon, and there was a great deal of fun and hilarity. The president of the company is sure that this occasion had a good effect in promoting the good will which exists between their people and themselves. This company gives annually each family a Christmas turkey, and the school a Christmas tree with a gift for each child.

At the meeting of the stockholders recently, of the Weems Steamboat Company, Baltimore, when it was decided to accept the offer made by a syndicate for the stock of the company, Mrs. Henry Williams, wife of the President of the company, and Mrs. Matilda Forbes, the chief owners of the stock, suggested that there should be some recognition of the long fidelity of the employés. The suggestion was favorably received by Mr. Williams, and it was decided to divide $25,000 in cash as a reward for their faithful service.

In April, 1907, at the Letts Department Store, Los Angeles, an organization was formed by the "Broadway Y. W. C. A. Coöperative Committee" for the purpose of coöperating with the Young Women's Christian Association, for mutual benefit, morally, mentally, physically, socially and spiritually, of women employés.

Scores of women have been visited during illness—flowers, various dainty and appetizing foods carried to them, and in many instances assistance of a substantial nature. Others have been directed to reliable physicians, dentists, surgeons, or a good church home found for them, while for many others good room and board has been found, places entirely desirable in every respect.

Employés not fitted for public work are assisted in finding other agreeable employment. Meals are carried to women who are too ill to leave their rooms and who have no one to care for them. Educational classes, as well as physical culture and Bible classes are regularly attended through the efforts of this committee.

The Good Will Association of the Strawbridge and Clothier Company was organized in 1901 for the purpose of looking after the welfare of the children employed by the firm. This society has been quietly carrying on a work of kindness and helpfulness.

In the first four years of its existence over $2000 was collected for dues and over $500 in subscriptions. These sums, under the careful administration of the officers, were expended for clothing, food, medical attention, vacations for delicate children and picnics. Members have looked after the daily well-being of the little ones, have seen that they were properly clothed, were in condition to work and on wet days that their feet were dry, and that they were provided with hot milk and wholesome food.

The present membership is more than five hundred.

A coöperative purchasing committee is appointed by the Seattle Electric Company, whose business it is to make arrangements with such merchants as may be selected, by which the members of the association are enabled to secure the lowest possible prices for clothing, groceries and all immediate supplies, and this same committee endeavors in other ways to promote the economic and business welfare of the members. The dues of each member of the association are 75 cents a month.

The purchasing committee is entirely under the direction and appointing of the beneficial association, which is entirely independent of the company, the trustees and officers of the association being elected by members who are employés of the Seattle Electric Company; the only requirement being that the treasurer of the association shall be the assistant treasurer of the company.

An association of the women of John Wanamaker's, called

The Women's League, is a stem bearing such branches as a mandolin class of 20 members; a dressmaking class of 36 members; an elocution class of 12; a physical culture class of 20; a millinery class of 22; an English class of 10; a French class of 17; a stenography class of 17; an art embroidery class of 36; a manicure and hair-dressing class of 30; a dancing class of 125. The league also provides each month, excepting December and the hot months, one evening of entertainment and social time, ending usually with a little dancing. People eminent as musicians, in reciting, reading or lecturing have most kindly given their services for these evenings. Further, this league plans, and has made some progress toward a very practical work in meeting new fellow employés who are strangers in the city, assisting them to find suitable boarding places and to gain an at-home feeling in the store and city; and also in cases of sickness or distress, by personal attentions, to supplant the work of the beneficial association. The store maintains a savings fund, with special inducements for its employés to save, and building associations, instituted and managed by the employés, are most successful means of saving.

For the seventh session of the International Railway Congress, held in Washington, D. C., May, 1905, M. Riebenack,[1] Comptroller of the Pennsylvania Railway Company, prepared a special study of railway provident institutions. This included all the features of betterment, by which the railways are enabled to get into closer and more intimate relations with their employés, and find the common ground on which both sides can meet. The various plans for betterment are integral parts of the system of many of the great lines. Although his study included all the English-speaking countries of the world, I shall use only the data which concern the United States. Out of 203 roads which were supplied with questions, 140 replied; out of the 63 who failed to reply, some had less than 200 miles of operated lines, and others were members of a large system, which had already replied. Mr. Riebenack concludes that his study embraces quite 90 per cent. of the railway mileage in America.

[1] Through the courtesy of Mr. Riebenack, the statistics are brought down to date.

Under the head of insurance and relief, there are provisions for life and accident insurance, regular or commercial, mutual insurance, endowment, railway relief department, and employés' relief association.

The Baltimore & Ohio pension feature was created in connection with the original general insurance undertaking conducted by employés of that railroad company, known as the Employés Relief Association of the Baltimore & Ohio Railroad Company. This association was established May 1, 1880, and embraced three dissimilar betterment undertakings denominated respectively "Relief Feature," "Pension Feature" and "Saving Feature." Membership in the pension feature, which went into effect October 1, 1884, is, operatively speaking, inchoate at the time of admission to relief association membership, and depends for its fruition upon a clearly promulgated contingency, namely, membership in the relief feature of the association for a period of four years. There are several points of difference between the B. & O. pension feature and the pension plan in vogue with other American railways, namely:

1. The Baltimore & Ohio pension feature is a component auxiliary of a special department of the company's service involving, in its operation, two other well-defined undertakings of relief and savings.

2. The financial arrangements comprehend three sources: (a) membership contributions to the relief feature for a period of four years before becoming eligible to provisions of the pension feature, and continued ordinary contributions to the relief feature thereafter until prescribed conditions for retirement from service, on pension allowance, come to pass, (b) use of an annual company contribution of $6000 for support of the relief feature when not needed in that relation, and (c) an annual company appropriation of a fixed minimum sum, invested with characteristics correspondent to those of other American roads, generally, conducting pension systems.

3. Pension allowances are based upon age and membership, while with most of the other railways of the country the basis is age and length of service.

At the close of the year 1907 the railways of the United

States conducting pension systems in behalf of their employés numbered 18, as follows: Atchison, Topeka & Santa Fé Ry., Atlantic Coast Line R. R., Baltimore & Ohio R. R., Bessemer & Lake Erie R. R., Buffalo, Rochester & Pittsburg Ry., Chicago & Northwestern Ry., Delaware, Lackawanna & Western R. R., Houston & Texas Central R. R., Oregon Railroad & Navigation Co., Oregon Short Line R. R., Pennsylvania System East of Pittsburg, Pennsylvania System West of Pittsburg, Philadelphia & Reading Ry., San Antonio & Aransas Pass Ry., Southern Pacific System (Pacific System), Southern Pacific System (Sunset Route), Union Pacific Railroad.

The railway pension systems of the United States, as now generally conducted, are grounded upon the fundamental principles enunciated in the provisions of "The Pennsylvania Railroad Pension Department," which was established January 1, 1900, in the interest of the employés of the lines of the Pennsylvania Railroad System East of Pittsburg and Erie, Pa. This system represents the type of an absolutely separate and distinct branch of the railroad service, possessed of a complete entity in its relation to all other departments of the service. It originated with and is exclusively financed and controlled by the railway corporation, the employés neither contributing to nor having a voice in its management.

The general object of the pension system is to provide for compulsory or involuntary retirement from service at 65 or 70 years of age, and voluntary retirement consequent upon permanent incapacitation between the ages of 61 and 69, with service ranging from ten to thirty years, on a fixed allowance, usually computed at 1 per cent. of the average monthly pay for the ten years next preceding retirement, for each year of service.

There is also provision in many of the pension regulations for arbitrary allowances for permanent incapacitation at any stage of service, such cases ranking as extraordinary, and being governed absolutely by decision of company concerned. This extraordinary provision is not called for, ordinarily, with railways conducting relief departments, for the reason that, as a rule, the regulations of these departments fully cover cases of this nature.

Some of the railroad companies, although not interested in

distinctive pension plans or organizations, pursue a purely company policy of awarding allowances, wholly from their own revenues, as pensions or gratuities, to meritorious employés upon the occasion of their retirement from the service owing to advanced age or permanent incapacitation.

Pension departments are usually created by the stockholders of the railway companies upon recommendation by the board of directors, and their administration placed in the hands of railway appointees, commonly styled either board of officers or board of pensions.

The pension allowance is purely an optional railway disbursement from railway revenue exclusively, the employé making no contribution whatever to the scheme, which is absolutely subject to company direction and control.

Financing of the undertakings is commonly based on an original contribution, supplemented by fixed annual appropriation, which, with interest returns on the original fund, are expected to meet all demands for allowances. Sometimes a fixed annual appropriation is the exclusive arrangement. Provision is usually made, under both arrangements, for ratable reductions in allowances where the company contribution does not cover fund expenditures.

The accounting system varies with the several roads, each observing a method adapted to its own convenience and requirements.

Allowances are, as a rule, based on age and service.

There is no commutation of allowance by payment of lump sum in lieu thereof or otherwise.

Allowance ceases with the death of the beneficiary.

Pension allowances are usually authorized by the board of officers at the pension departments, subject to approval by the board of directors of the companies, to be paid monthly, and are usually determined on the basis of one per centum of the average monthly pay for the ten years next preceding retirement for each year of service.

In computation of service it is reckoned from date of entry in service to date when relieved therefrom, deduction being made for actual time out of service, and eliminating in final result any fractional part of a month. Illustration: Where an employé has been in the service continuously for 41 years and

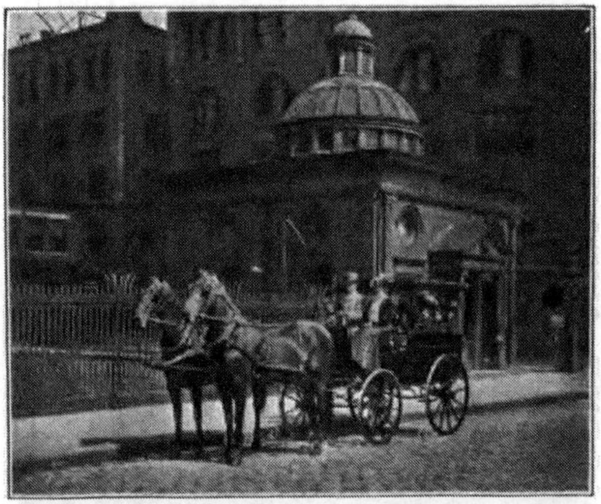

The Park Carriage of the H. J. Heinz Company Placed at the Disposal of the Convalescents for Outings in the Pittsburg Parks.

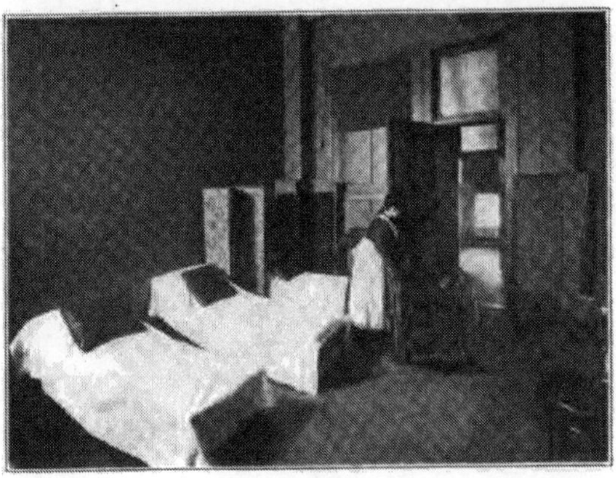

Room for Sick Girls at Siegel-Cooper's New York Store, with Maid in Attendance.

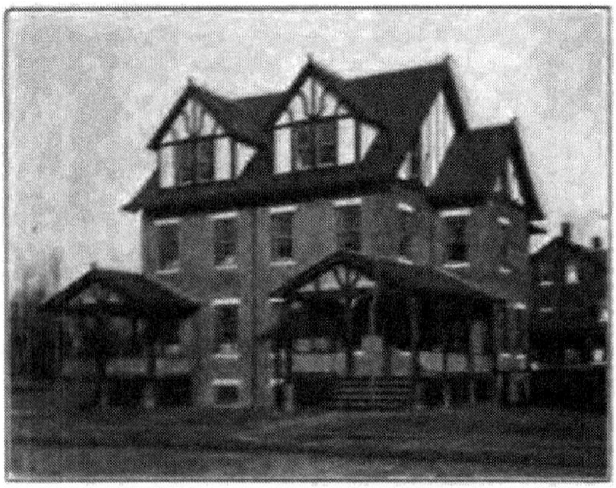

Type No. 5 of the Improved Dwellings at Kinkora.

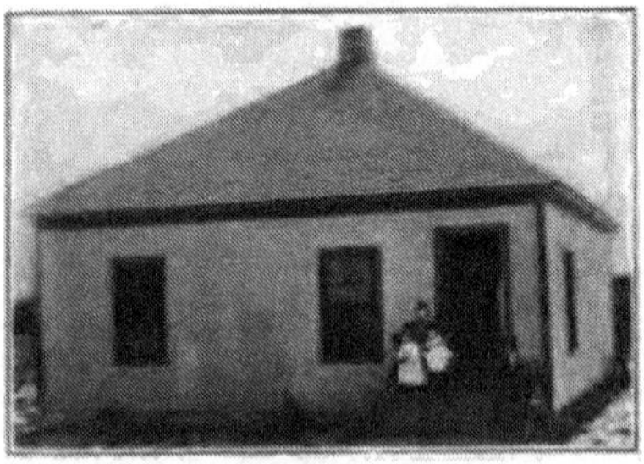

One of the Colorado Fuel and Iron Company's Houses for Miners.

during that time has been out of service for periods amounting to one year, and the average wages for the past 10 years are $40 per month, he would upon retirement, receive 40 per centum of $40, or $16 per month as a pension allowance.

The first hospital department for railway employés was organized in California in 1868 by the Southern Pacific Railway.

The hospital department differs from the various railway company insurance and relief department schemes, under which the sick and injured employé-member is insured and protected against loss of time, with accident and sickness benefits, and death benefit payments to designated representatives; a further difference existing in the fact that an employé signing an application in the company organization agrees, as a rule, to relinquish rights of litigation for injuries received, accepting in lieu thereof the benefits extended by the company scheme.

The monthly assessment is contributed for the purpose of sustaining the hospital department, and all compensations for injuries sustained are commonly settled for by the railway companies according to the legal merit of each case.

Employés suffering from chronic diseases or those arising from vicious acts are not entitled to hospital benefits.

In some instances members of the families of employés are treated in the hospitals at reduced rates.

A great many railways, particularly in the eastern section of the country, where the population is dense, and numerous independent state, municipal and private hospitals exist, do not deem the provision of distinctive hospital departments necessary, such roads having agreements with independent hospitals along their lines for the admission and treatment of their employés on liberal terms.

Other roads, while contracting with outside hospitals in this relation, have also emergency hospitals located at terminal points, which are provided with medical and surgical supplies and appliances, and are in charge of what are known as "Company Surgeons."

Again some of the roads have regularly appointed physicians, residing at various points on the lines, to give relief in cases of train accidents.

The hospital department or association usually embraces the general hospital, division hospitals, emergency stations or hospitals, contract hospitals and dispensaries.

In Cleveland, Ohio, in 1872, the first Railroad branch of the Y. M. C. A. was organized for industrial betterment among the railway men on a distinctively religious foundation. The formal opening of a room, 40 x 46 feet at a cost of $3000, was celebrated April 14, 1872. The requests for organizing effort were so numerous, from other cities, that a secretary was engaged by the International Committee to give his entire time to this work. From the small beginning in 1872, the work has grown to such an extent that to-day there are 9 executive secretaries supervising the work from the International headquarters in New York. Working with them are 471 local railroad secretaries and other paid officers; 174 railroad associations have buildings representing a cost of $3,569,200. Some phases of this Y. M. C. A. work for civic and industrial betterment are carried on on nearly every important railroad line in North America.

The following privileges and features are usually provided in connection with the branches: reading rooms, social rooms; bath rooms; rest rooms; lunch rooms; bowling alleys; classes in light gymnastics; libraries; educational classes; practical lectures on railroad topics; social receptions; entertainments; athletic fields; out-door sports; temporary hospitals; religious services.

Educational courses, conducted for the most part throughout the fall and winter months, and which are evidencing pronounced increase in the variety and usefulness of the studies comprehended, are growing in popularity and value. These courses embrace in their curriculum those commercial and railroad branches a knowledge of which is of prime importance to ambitious and progressive employés, and particularly to those who would otherwise be debarred from enjoying that encouragement and opportunity for general intellectual training and improvement which experience has shown to be essential for individual advancement in any chosen vocation.

The membership fee ranges from $3 to $5 per capita per annum.

The late Cornelius Vanderbilt, President of the New York Central & Hudson River Railroad, was among the pioneers in this work, having contributed $100,000 toward the establishment of the first branch on his road, in 1875, at New York City.

The first branch on the Pennsylvania Railroad, at Philadelphia, Pa., finally organized November 18, 1886, although originally undertaken May 1, 1876, was not fully housed until 1893, when approximately $140,000 had been raised and disbursed by the joint efforts of officers and men. The Pennsylvania Railroad Department Young Men's Christian Association of Philadelphia, Pa., is the largest on the Pennsylvania system of lines, and is also the largest railroad branch in the world in point of membership (which on December 31, 1907, numbered 1856), equipment and variety and extent of work. At the close of the same year there were 31 association branches on the lines of the system East and West of Pittsburg, with a total membership of 15,367, to which the railroad company extended financial support. Some of these branches own the buildings they occupy, but the larger number are located in structures belonging to the company. The demonstrated benefits accruing to employés enjoying membership in the association branches have enlisted the substantial and continuous support of the company and its principal officers.

Maintenance is provided by membership and railway contributions, in conjunction with nominal fees charged for special features, such as class tuition, billiards and pool, and baths.

Railway officials heartily and substantially endorse and encourage the movement, which is considered of the highest importance in developing spiritual, moral, mental and physical improvement.

Savings funds are maintained to receive small sums saved by the men and also by their families. These savings are invested and managed by the company, for the sake of encouraging prudence and thrift, thus enabling the employé to make provision against accident, sickness, old age and death. For example, on the Pennsylvania lines, at present, the savings funds conducted by the lines of their system East and West of Pittsburg, Pa., on account of their employés, had, December 31, 1907, depositors to the number of 14,093, the amount due these depositors being $5,770,641.21.

Hospitals and orphan homes are the other forms of special relief funds. The Order of Railway Conductors of America, Brotherhoods of Locomotive Firemen, Railway Trainmen, Railway Telegraphers, Railway Trackmen, Railway Carmen, Railway Bridgemen, and the Switchmen's Union of North America all have important features.

CHAPTER VI

THRIFT

The mutual benefit societies which are described in the preceding chapter are really savings societies in that they compel enough thrift to meet the regular weekly or monthly dues. There are other methods for inducing the employé to save a certain part of his earnings against a time of need; the movements that have for their object the encouragement of saving on the part of the young people are particularly commendable.

"We keep in our office a deposit ledger, which affords our employés the same facilities as a savings bank," reports R. D. Wood. When the sums to their credit accumulate to comparatively large amounts, the workmen are urged to withdraw their deposits and invest the money as may seem to them best.

The Stetson savings fund was established in 1897 for the purpose of encouraging the operatives to save their money by making deposits in small weekly amounts. These deposits are limited to such proportion of the earnings as, in the opinion of the management, the employé should retain for his future use, $10 being the maximum amount received from any one depositor in a week. The company allows 5 per cent. interest on deposits which are allowed to remain until the end of the fiscal year. If withdrawn during the year the deposit is not entitled to interest. The depositors number about 10 per cent. of the entire number of persons employed by the company.

The Baldwin Locomotive Works encourages its employés in the savings of wages, and in order that they may have opportunities for making deposits without absenting themselves from their work, they can open an account with the cashier, whereby their deposits will draw the prevailing rate of interest.

At Graniteville[1] the people have a bank of their own, where

[1] Graniteville Manufacturing Co., Graniteville, S. C. Manufacturers Cotton Sheetings, Shirtings and Drills. Organized 1845. 875 Employés.

they deposit their funds under $500, obtaining 4 per cent. interest on the same. When their savings reach $500 the company takes this amount, paying 5 per cent. interest.

John Wanamaker maintains two savings funds, one for men and women, and the other for boys and girls of the establishment. The employés themselves conduct a savings and loan association for the double purpose of encouraging saving and making it unnecessary that any one in temporary difficulties should fall into the hands of money lending sharks.

The Metropolitan Life Insurance Company [1] has agreed to establish a fund for the benefit and protection of its employés, to be known as the Metropolitan Staff Savings Fund, and to be held and administered by a board of trustees.

The fund is created from the subscriptions of the company, from the contributions of the employés and from the additions of interest.

Those who may contribute to the fund and shall be entitled to the benefits thereof are: Any superintendent, assistant superintendent, agent, supervisor, inspector, member of the clerical force (employed at the home office or at a branch office), employé of the printing and binding divison, who shall have been one year in the service of said company, and whose salary is not in excess of $3000 per annum. The word salary in the case of a superintendent and of an assistant superintendent shall mean his weekly salary. In the case of an agent it shall mean his industrial ordinary salary as computed on the amount of his weekly industrial premium collections. It shall not include in either case any commission or remuneration received from the ordinary department of the company.

The company agrees to subscribe to the fund amounts equal to one-half of the contributions of the employés. No obligation is assumed by the company to pay its subscriptions oftener than once in each calendar month.

An account shall be kept with each contributor, and shall be credited therein with all contributions made by him to the fund, and also with an amount equal to one-half of such contributions, the latter being the company's subscription. This account shall be so kept as to show the amount standing to his

[1] Metropolitan Life Insurance Co., New York City. Organized June 1867. Number Employés, 14,000.

credit as a result of his own contributions, also the amount standing to his credit by reason of the subscriptions made by the company, with the additions of interest of each.

The present amount to the credit of the fund is approximately $500,000.

Upon the death of a contributor while in the service of the company his legal representatives shall be paid the amount to which he would have been entitled.

If a contributor retires from the service of the company other than as provided, he shall, upon the termination of service, be paid the amount standing to his credit as a result of his own contributions on the preceding 31st of December, with interest at the rate of 3 per cent. per annum up to the date of retiring, together with such contributions as he has made in the year that he retires, with interest at the rate of 3 per cent. per annum, to be calculated for each complete calendar month from dates of such contributions to date of retirement, but he shall forfeit all right and title to the amount credited to him by reason of the subscriptions made by the company unless special existing conditions affecting his retirement shall be such as to induce the trustees to award him the same benefits as if he had retired on account of incapacity. The trustees shall have the power to make such exceptions to this rule.

A contributor may, at any time while in the service of the company and upon notice, withdraw from the fund the amount to which he would have been entitled had he retired for any of the reasons specified by the company, but he shall forfeit all right and title to the amount credited to him by reason of the subscriptions made by the company. A person closing an account in the fund but remaining continuously in the service of the company will not be permitted to again become a contributor except under such conditions as the board of trustees may prescribe.

Should the salary of a contributor be increased so that it exceeds the limit as hereinbefore prescribed, he may withdraw the amount of his own contribution with interest thereon, or he may allow the whole amount standing to his credit to remain in the fund and receive credit for interest; but he shall not be permitted to make any further contributions to the fund, nor shall the company make any further subscription for his benefit; nor shall he share in that part of the fund arising from the forfeitures of other contributors.

In case of the death of a contributor or the termination of his service with the company for any cause, or the withdrawal of the amount standing to his credit, his account shall be closed and no further amounts shall be credited thereto.

The rights of a contributor shall not be assignable or negotiable.

The company will pay all expenses incident to the proper administration of the fund except brokerage on the purchase or sale of investments and costs of the purchase and sale of property.

The board of directors may at any time direct that the affairs of the fund be wound up, and, in anticipation of such direction, may order the fund to be closed as to any employés not contributors at the date of such order.

Upon the closing up of the fund, all property belonging thereto shall be realized upon, and the amounts applied to the payment of amounts standing to the credit of contributors. Any surplus shall be distributed among the contributors whose accounts have not been closed, in proportion to the amounts then standing to their credit.

The powers of the directors and of the trustees to make orders and regulations shall include the power to rescind or vary such orders and regulations.

Based on the suggestion from the employés that some kind of an organization for savings and loans would be very desirable, the officials of the Mutual Benefit Association of the Celluloid Club, at the suggestion of the president of the Celluloid Company, have offered to take charge of and handle the funds and act as officers and trustees of an organization to be known as "The Celluloid Savings and Loan Association."

It must be distinctly understood that it is not the intention at present to form a separate organization, hold meetings or elect officers, and that the business of the association will be managed by the board of the mutual benefit association entirely separate from the affairs of that association, as there will be no connection whatever between the "Insurance" and the "Savings and Loan" features.

The object of the association will be to encourage savings and to furnish temporary financial assistance to those employés of the Celluloid Company who are depositors with the association, and who have been in the employ of the company for at least one year prior to their application for a loan.

It must be understood that the board does not intend to loan money indiscriminately, but will in all cases require that the applicant be recommended by some member of the finance committee, or an employé known to the committee; such recommendation will not bind the endorser in cases of default.

Any male or female employé of the Celluloid Company may become a member of the association by making weekly deposits (not necessarily a fixed amount) in sums not less than 25 cents, in amounts of 25 cents, 50 cents, 75 cents and $1.00. (No limit.)

In making deposits the week will be considered as ending on Saturday at 12 M., and any members failing to make a deposit before the end of the week shall be fined five cents for each failure, and should a member fail to make a deposit for four successive weeks, he or she will cease to be a member, and shall forfeit the right to share in any profits as hereinafter provided; the full amount deposited will be returned to them upon withdrawal less the amount of any unpaid fines and a proportionate share of the expense, which shall be first deducted.

The regular withdrawal dates shall be June 15th and December 15th of each year, when the accounts will be audited, and the amount deposited by each surviving member, after deducting unpaid fines, returned in full, and all profits accruing to the association since the last settlement, after deducting the expenses and a percentage for a sinking fund, shall be divided in proportion to their average deposits among the members of four months' membership and over.

Members desiring to leave their accumulated savings on deposit after the regular withdrawal dates, may do so. The weekly savings only in each series will participate in the profits.

Members who withdraw any part of their deposits, except as "loans," other than on the regular withdrawal dates, shall forfeit all claims to any share of the profits and shall be charged with a pro rata share of the expenses of the series.

All loans shall be for a stated period, and in no case exceed $200 to any one member, and will be divided into two classes,—"Ordinary" and "Special."

"Ordinary" loans, to be in sums from $1 to $25, will be advanced for not longer than three months; such applications will be referred to a finance committee to consist of three members of the board.

"Special" loans, to be in sums from $26 to $200, will be advanced for not longer than two months, and will be considered by the whole board.

The time limit of loans in either class may be extended provided a satisfactory reason is given for the inability to meet the payment when due. A request for an extension of the time must in all cases be made in writing to the finance committee at least three days prior to the date that payment is due.

Except in cases of emergency, applications for "Special" loans will be considered and acted upon at the Celluloid club house on Monday evenings of each week; "Ordinary" loans, and in cases of necessity applications for "Special" loans, will be, so far as practicable, acted upon on the day received; all applications will be considered confidential.

Loans may be returned in installments of not less than $2 at a time, such installments to be credited at the end of the week in an account book to be furnished to each depositor.

The premium on loans will be at low rates.

The board shall fix the salaries of the officers necessary to conduct the business of the association, also the amount and form of a bond to be given by the treasurer.

The board of the mutual benefit association is desirous of learning how many of the employés of the company really desire to have such an association as outlined above, and would support it if instituted, and to this end has furnished a copy of the proposed rules to each employé, together with a secret ballot, which they request will be returned.

When a ballot was taken on the question of instituting the savings and loan association, it was found that between six and seven hundred employés desired the "Bank." The new organization began operations September, 1906, under very favorable conditions.

This new department is now a part of the Celluloid Club; it elects its own officers from the active membership of the club, makes its own by-laws, consistent with the laws of the club; keeps its funds separate and renders a full and complete report to the club at its annual meeting. This department may receive deposits and make loans to employés of the Celluloid Company who are not members of the club, but such depositors shall have no privileges in the club house, have no vote, nor hold office.

In the first annual report of the Curtis Savings Fund Society for 1902-3, it stated that the financial report was only a cold statement of fact, and while it might be considered satisfactory in that way, it did not tell anything of the real history of the work—the troubles of collections, loans and fines, the annoyances of the backward—nor of the economies and self-denials that built the sums up week by week. It showed a return on deposits equal to 11 per cent. per annum. "Such a result, it should be remembered, could not have been obtained with an ordinary investment of the money, and has been possible only through the liberality of The Curtis Publishing Company."

The receipts from various sources were $25,152.31, of which the cash balance was $21,980.56.

The report for 1906-7 shows that there are 2794 active shares, 34 inactive; 847 shares were withdrawn. The receipts amounted to $45,641.22, of which $35,502.38 was a credit balance available at any time for distribution.

The object of the Curtis Savings Fund Society is to stimulate a desire to save money, and enable the members to lay aside a fixed sum each week.

Any employé of the Curtis Publishing Company may, on application to the secretary, become a shareholder. Shareholders leaving the employ of the company do not necessarily cease to be members of the society until the end of the fiscal year. Membership may be retained for balance of year on the same terms as apply to employés of the company.

The sum of 25 cents per week shall be paid into the association for each and every share. No person shall hold more than 20 shares; nor shall any shareholder transfer interest in the society to another shareholder. At meetings of the society shareholders shall be entitled to but one vote, irrespective of the number of shares they possess, and no voting by proxy shall in any case be allowed. All shares paid up for the year must be paid to the secretary, and not to the collector.

Any shareholder may obtain a loan for a period of not less than one month, and for a sum not exceeding nine-tenths of the amount paid in. A note to the order of the treasurer shall be given by said shareholder for the amount, with interest, payable at the time the note is issued, at the rate of 6 per cent. per annum, which being presented to the secretary, he shall issue an order on the treasurer for the amount. A charge of ten cents shall be made for each loan. Repayments of loans and interest thereon must be made directly to the secretary.

Shareholders may at any time withdraw upon giving one week's notice to the secretary. The amount paid in, less fines or charges, shall be refunded without profits to the withdrawer. To provide for emergencies, the board of directors may, if they think proper, waive the aforesaid one week's notice.

The board of directors of the society may receive from shareholders deposits of money accumulated in the savings fund to the amount of $10, or a multiple thereof, not exceeding $500, from any single shareholder, and allow such interest thereon as they may be able to obtain from reinvestment. No shareholder shall deposit more than $250 in any one year, nor shall this amount in any case be allowed to exceed the total sum accumulated by the depositor in one series of the savings fund society.

These special deposits are to be made in total within a period of not more than two weeks after the annual disbursement of savings in September of each year. Withdrawals can be made only at the expiration of a whole number of months from the date of deposit, after at least ten days' notice to the secretary, in writing.

Interest at the rate of 2 per cent. per annum will be allowed on deposits withdrawn before the end of the year. Exceptions will be made to the rule when depositors leave the employ of the Curtis Publishing Company, in which case the full rate of interest will be paid to the end of the current month, but not thereafter.

November 15, 1900, it was announced to all the employés of the Pittsburg Coal Company[1] that an association had been formed for the purpose of encouraging and assisting them to invest their savings in the preferred stock of the Pittsburg Coal Company.

Each employé is privileged to subscribe for shares of preferred stock on which he agrees to make regular monthly (or semi-monthly) payments at the rate of not less than one dollar per month per share. These subscription payments to be invested from time to time in the preferred stock of the Pittsburg Coal Company, the same to be purchased in the open market by the officers of the association, at such times, under such conditions and at such prices as in their judgment may be deemed advisable. Any unexpended balances are to be deposited currently with the treasurer of the Pittsburg Coal Company; such deposits to bear interest at the rate of five per cent. per annum.

Dividends earned by the stock thus purchased and interest allowed by the treasurer of the Pittsburg Coal Company will constitute the earnings of the association and will be added to the monthly payments of the subscribers until their monthly payments and the earnings to which they are entitled are equal to the average cost of the stock purchased and owned by the association, when each subscriber will receive the number of shares he is entitled to under his subscription.

A new series of subscriptions will be opened each month on exactly the same terms and conditions as the initial series; this to admit new subscribers and to enable old subscribers to purchase additional shares.

Subscribers who desire to pay more than the minimum amount of one dollar per month per share, with the intention to more quickly acquire shares subscribed for, shall be privileged to do so. In such cases their payments into the association will be augmented by interest on the same at the rate of five per cent. per annum, and the price of shares sold them by the association under this arrangement will be the average

[1] Pittsburg Coal Co., Pittsburg, Pa. Manufacturing Coke and Mining Coal. Organized September 1, 1899. Number Employés, 35,000.

cost of shares in the association treasury purchased during the term of such subscribers' payments.

Subscribers who fall behind in monthly payments, but who desire to keep up their payments and make formal application to the treasurer of the association for permission to pay the same at a later date, at the direction of the treasurer, may be accommodated. In such cases, however, interest at the rate of six per cent. per annum will be charged for the delayed payments during the period of delinquency.

Subscribers who leave the employ of the Pittsburg Coal Company or find for any reason they do not desire or are not able to continue regular payments and wish to withdraw from the association, may do so at any time upon thirty days' notice to the treasurer of the association, who will return to them the total amount of their payments plus five per cent. per annum, provided, however, that the association reserves the right to limit the funds to be appropriated to such payments on account of withdrawals to fifty per cent. of actual cash payments into the treasury of the association during the month in which withdrawals are made. If the said total payments with interest at the rate of five per cent. per annum are equal to the cost of one or more shares of preferred stock purchased during the term of such subscribers' payments, they will be entitled to receive stock, if they so select, at the average cost per share for shares purchased during the term of such subscribers' payments, as stated above.

Subscribers who leave the employ of the Pittsburg Coal Company may, if they desire, continue their regular payments until the closing up of the series upon which said payments are made, in which case they will receive the shares to which they are entitled under their subscriptions, the same as if they had remained in the employ of the Pittsburg Coal Company, but after leaving said employment will not be permitted to make further subscriptions.

Subscribers who find that the payment of their original subscription is burdensome, and that they cannot afford to carry as much as they have subscribed for, will be permitted to reduce their subscriptions in the following manner:

A formal notification to the effect to be addressed to the treasurer of the association on a form furnished by him upon request. Upon receipt of such notice, the treasurer will make proper entries and advise the subscriber upon what terms payments are to be made without cessation pending adjustment.

While the plan originated with the employés, it is heartily approved by the company through its executive officers, in whose name all employés, in whatsoever capacity employed, are cordially invited to avail themselves of the association's benefits, and, with its aid, take to themselves the dignity of stockholders and partners in the business in which all alike are interested.

Applications for shares of stock under the above terms and conditions may be made on the special form provided for that purpose, which may be had from any mine superintendent or head of department of the Pittsburg Coal Company, or upon application direct to the treasurer of the association. Applicants will please date and sigu the contract or application form and mail the same to the treasurer, Pittsburg Coal Company Employés' Association, Pittsburg, Pa., who will acknowledge receipt of the same and send the investor a book with rules and by-laws in which his monthly payments will be receipted for by the representative of the association who receives the same.

April 30, 1906, there were 1225 employés making monthly payments of $1.00 per share in the purchase of 10,596 shares of Pittsburg Coal Company preferred stock; the first fifteen series of purchasers having acquired 2696 shares under contracts maturing prior to the date of the report. The investment was a profitable one to the employés even at the rather low prevailing market prices for the stock. These dividends are cumulative, and hence the purchasers who have received their stock since the suspension of dividends and the purchasers whose contracts have not matured will also get the benefit of the back dividends in a ratable way when dividends shall be resumed.

The suspension of the dividends was, of course, a severe test to the employés' stock purchase scheme but, as indicated in the last report, it has been successful beyond expectations in spite of the adverse conditions of the past two years, which have very materially changed for the better during the past six months.

Mr. J. B. L. Harnberger, the controller, writes me that this department of the employés' industrial betterment has been very successful; practically all of the mine operatives are now covered although the plan is not compulsory, and when the work was started three years ago there was much indifference and even outright hostility to overcome. At April 30th there were 21,790 men purchasing the stock. At this time, being the midst of the summer business, the heaviest season of the year because of lake shipments of coal into the Northwest, there are upwards of 25,000 men enrolled in the lists of the relief department. They are now paying upwards of $100,000 per annum in relief benefits, a considerable portion of which is contributed by the company, which also joins in the pension fund. The work is coöperative in the truest sense and has done more to bring about that kindly feeling between employer and employé, that is so desirable, than could have possibly been accomplished in any other way.

The Roycroft Institution[1] was incorporated in May, 1902, under the name of the Roycrofters, when the entire capital of $300,000 was owned by the workers in shares of $25 each. No others are permitted to hold stock. Any holder quitting the employ of the company is required to sell his stock to Mr. Hubbard at the price paid for it, the latter agreeing also to pay such price. Any employé is permitted to subscribe for as many shares as he desires at par, and the stock is fully paid up, non-assessable and with no personal liability, and guaranteed to pay 12 per cent. dividends annually.

In large manufacturing establishments there is often lack of sincere enthusiasm, or discouragement, due to seeming lack of interest, by those in authority, in the individual worker. Indeed it is frequently heard said by employés, that they have never seen the president of their company, or certain other officers. An exemplification of the reverse of these conditions is to be found in the factories and offices of the L. E. Waterman Company,[2] New York, where personal touch and co-operation with all employés, heads of departments, directors and

[1] The Roycrofters, East Aurora, N. Y. Authors and Editors. Organized June 3, 1902. Number Employés, 350.

[2] L. E. Waterman Co., 173 Broadway, New York. Manufacturers Fountain Pens and Inks. Organized 1884. Number Employés, 800.

officers is so very close that the interests of the company are continually enhanced by a corps of more than 800 interested employés in both offices and workshops.

For the encouragement of saving on the part of their employés this firm credits their workers with all sums intrusted to them, and pays interest at the rate of 6 per cent., and there is no limit to the amount which may thus be placed to the credit of an individual employé.

At the Christmas season it has been the custom to present each one of the office force with a week's wages.

The company's interest in employés overcome by sickness has always been marked by appreciation. Particular attention is given to all conditions which may be of benefit to workers, in the way of properly ventilated work rooms, light, heat, and the installation of proper quarters for a comfortable rest or lunch for the female employés of the company.

The First National Bank of Chicago, under certain conditions, clearly set forth, allows any employés to buy stock, loaning them money at 4 per cent., within ten points of the market price, this loan to be repaid at $5.00 per month on each share. More than one hundred have taken advantage of this opportunity, which enables them without serious inconvenience to purchase stock that they otherwise would have been unable to obtain.

The American Swiss File and Tool Company[1] allots stock to energetic and intelligent employés. The stock is given fully paid up, and a part of the profits of the business are set aside to pay for it.

The company does all in its power to encourage its employés to become members of building and loan associations and the workmen generally show a disposition to follow the advice given them in this respect. The company also contributes liberally to the maintenance of local hospitals, to which employés have the right of admission and treatment free of charge.

The families of deserving men are looked after in case of sickness, and in many instances half the ordinary wages of

[1] American Swiss File and Tool Co., Elizabeth, N. J. Manufacturers High-Class Files. Organized July 17, 1899. Number Employés, 102.

workmen suffering through a long period of sickness has been paid to their families. In such cases the money paid has been regarded as an advance in anticipation of future earnings, and a small percentage of the wages which accrue after recovery is deducted until the money is returned. This course is followed in accordance with the known and expressed wishes of the employés who have been so assisted. They seem to feel that self-respect requires that they should not be under an obligation which they have the ability to repay.

The company looks sympathetically on the idea of sharing profits, and would adopt it if only a proper system could be devised for carrying out such a plan. Pending the time when this may be done, and also as a fixed matter of policy, the firm encourages thrift, steadiness, regular contributions to building loan societies and all other habits and practices that make men thrifty and prudent. Where the company finds a really valuable man, every endeavor is made to attach him permanently to the business by increasing his salary according to merit.

The De Witt Wire Cloth Company, Belleville, N. J., warmly expresses its interest in any movement having a tendency to improve the social and industrial condition of its employés, and as its own particular contribution to that end, has inaugurated a system of profit sharing with them. The plan of placing a certain allotment of the company's stock in the name of such employés as choose to invest in it, allowing them the privilege of paying for the same in installments, is practiced by them. The security of the investment is guaranteed by an agreement on the part of the company that stock owned by employés who may afterward leave its service shall be repurchased at par with interest, provided two weeks' notice be given of the intention to leave. The number of employés who have thus far availed themselves of the privilege is eight and semi-annual cumulative dividends of three per cent. each have been paid on the stock.

Under date of July, 1906, Robert Rogers, the president of the company, says: "I do not think that our efforts to induce our employés to become interested in our business have been much of a success. Of the original eight who became stockholders, five have since sold out. Three new ones have taken their place, making at the present time six of our employés who are stockholders."

For the promotion of thrift, the Great Northern Railway Company,[1] on May 1, 1900, set aside one million dollars' worth of stock for the use of the Great Northern Employés Investment Company, so as to give its old and faithful employés an opportunity to invest their savings in a manner which will allow them to benefit through the company's dividends and by that means provide for them a safe investment and enable them to share in the company's prosperity. In order that such investments may be made in sums as low as $10, the separate company was formed for the purpose of holding shares of stock of the Great Northern Railway Company, receiving dividends thereon, and managing the details of the business. No deductions will be made for expenses of management, as the Great Northern Railway Company has agreed to bear the entire expenses of the Investment Company.

On account of the limited amount of Great Northern stock which the Investment Company will hold, and owing to the fact that the number of employés varies from time to time, it was necessary to limit the class of employés to whom the privilege of making this investment be granted.

Any one, excluding day laborers, in the service of this company for at least three years in continuous employment in good standing, whose yearly salary or wages do not exceed $3000, is entitled to subscribe to certificates issued by the Investment Company against this stock set aside for its use. Such subscriptions may be made as low as $10 or in any multiple of $10 up to but not exceeding $5000 to be held by any one employé. The dividends on this amount of stock are collected by the Investment Company and by it paid without any deductions to the holders of its certificates. This has resulted in the holders of certificates receiving 7 per cent. per annum upon their investment. The Investment Company guarantees to cash their certificates at par at any time within thirty days after notice. The certificate holder on the other hand must surrender his certificates for cancellation and redemption

[1] Great Northern Railway, St. Paul. Organized 1889. Number Employés, 39,581.

when he leaves the service of the Great Northern Railway Company.

"I am pleased to be able to advise that this plan has worked very satisfactorily," writes Louis W. Hill, President.

February 26, 1906, a circular by the treasurer of the company stated that stock to the amount of $955,000 had been subscribed for. He furthermore stated that the object of the contract between the companies mentioned was to provide a safe and permanent investment for employés of the railway company. It has been noticed that numerous certificate holders have used the Investment Company as a convenience, purchasing investment certificates and shortly thereafter cashing them and using the money in other ways, thus using the Investment Company as a means of obtaining a good rate of interest for a short time on idle funds. This is entirely contrary to the spirit under which the trust was created, and notice was given that hereafter persons redeeming investment certificates will not be permitted to take out other certificates later on. In case employés of the railway company desire to take out investment certificates it is expected that they will retain them indefinitely and while in service.

Early in May, 1906, the Illinois Central Railroad Company[1] stated that on the first day of each month the company would quote to employés, through the heads of their departments, a price at which their applications will be accepted for the purchase of Illinois Central shares during that month. An employé is offered the privilege of subscribing for one share at a time, payable by installments in sums of $5 or any multiple of $5, on the completion of which the company will deliver to him a certificate of the share registered in his name on the books of the company. He can then, if he wishes, begin the purchase of another share on the installment plan. The certificate of stock is transferable on the company's books, and entitles the owner to such dividends as may be declared by the board of directors, and to a vote in their election.

Any officer or employé making payments on this plan will be entitled to receive interest on his deposits, at the rate of 4

[1] Illinois Central Railroad Co., Chicago, Ill. Organized 1851. Number Employés, 32,121.

per cent. per annum, during the time he is paying for his share of stock, provided he does not allow 12 consecutive months to elapse without making any payment, at the expiration of which period interest will cease to accrue, and the sum to his credit will be returned to him on his application therefor.

Any officer or employé making payments on the foregoing plan, and for any reason desiring to discontinue them, can have his money returned to him with accrued interest, by making application to the head of the department in which he is employed.

An employé who has made application for a share of stock on the installment plan, is expected to make the first payment from the first wages which may be due him. In case an employé leaves the service of the company from any cause, he must then either pay in full for the share for which he has subscribed and receive a certificate therefor, or take his money with the interest which has accrued.

President J. F. Harahan writes, February 29, 1908:

"A considerable number of employés have taken advantage of this plan, and it has proven very satisfactory to all concerned."

The Thomas Devlin Manufacturing Company,[1] in the interests of mutuality, makes the following offer to its employés:

"In order to give good and faithful men a chance to advance their own interests as well as that of the company, this company will give —— one of its employés, the earnings of $1000 worth of stock for a term of five years from —— (these earnings to be ascertained and declared by the board of directors) on the following conditions:

The said —— understands and agrees:

First.—That this offer on the part of the company remains in force only so long as he gives continued and faithful service (that being the consideration for the offer).

Second.—That he agrees to allow the sum of two dollars per week to be retained by the company, towards the purchasing of the $1000 of stock of which he is to receive the earning capacity as above stated."

[1] Thomas Devlin Manufacturing Co., Philadelphia, Pa. Malleable Iron and Hardware. Organized 1902. Number Employés, 690.

Then follow the obligations on the part of the company to protect the stock for the purchaser and his heirs in the event of his death. The dividends have fluctuated from 15 per cent. to 5 per cent.

"We feel that this plan has been of advantage to us. It was suggested to us by a strike we had in our branch works, the Philadelphia Hardware and Malleable Iron Works. We have only adopted this plan in our works, the Thomas Devlin Manufacturing Company, since 1902," writes Mr. Devlin.

The employés choose two of the directors on the board of directors in the Philadelphia Hardware and Malleable Iron Works, and the majority of stockholders elect five directors. The minority of stockholders nominate their own directors, who are voted for at the regular annual meeting. In the Thomas Devlin Manufacturing Company the men are not represented on the board. In the event of the death of an employé stockholder, the company buys his stock at par, otherwise the estate might have trouble to dispose of it.

CHAPTER VII

PROFIT SHARING

OCTOBER 9, 1869, Brewster & Company,[1] carriage builders of New York, made the following proposition for a kind of industrial partnership to their employés:

"From the beginning of our next fiscal year, we offer to all persons in our employ, excepting those now having an interest in our business, a certain share of our annual profits, in addition to the regular wages, which we propose shall be no less than the highest wages paid in other similar establishments.

The share of the profits so given to labor to be divided at the end of each fiscal year among the hands, in proportion to the amount of wages which each person shall have earned during the year.

It is our purpose that labor shall share not only in the profits of our Broome Street factory, but in those of our Fifth Avenue repository also, and in all profits realized upon whatever is sold there, whether carriage or anything else.

It should be mentioned also, in order to a full understanding of our plan, that we do not propose that any member of our firm shall charge or receive any interest on his capital invested in our business, nor shall he receive any salary for his services.

The exact portion of the profits which labor shall receive as its share, to be determined on consultation with a committee, to be elected by the shop; but, in order that you may at this time have a general idea of what we think will be the amount of labor's share, we will say that in our opinion about $8000 would be a proper amount out of such a business as we did during the last fiscal year. Of course our plan may be overtaken by dull trade, and the profits reduced; but, on the

[1] Brewster & Co., New York City. Carriage and Auto Manufacturers. Organized 1856. Number Employés, 500.

other hand, having a business constantly increasing in volume and quality, we may reasonably expect that the share will be much larger, especially as we shall then have, if our plan works well, the hearty coöperation of every man in the shop.

Should a person be discharged from our establishment at any time during the year, and before his share of the profits is ascertained, his interests shall not be forfeited—provided the wages he may have earned shall amount to the sum of $100—but at the end of the fiscal year, he shall be paid the share of the profits due to his earnings.

But if any person shall voluntarily leave our employment, he shall then forfeit all claims upon labor's share of the profits, and whatever sum would have been due him on account of such profits shall be paid over to the shop fund to be managed by trustees appointed by the hands, in aid of sick and unfortunate employés of our firm, and to be used in any other manner that the hands may decide upon, and in order that this relief fund may be speedily and firmly established, we propose to set apart a share in the profits of our business during the present fiscal year, as a beginning, which we guarantee shall amount to the sum of one thousand dollars, and trust it will exceed that.

We propose also, out of the profits of our business, to employ by the year an able physician and surgeon, whose services shall be rendered free of cost to all in our employ, and to their immediate families, at his office; and who will visit without charge all whose residences are not too remote to be of convenient access. This we propose doing as soon as the necessary arrangements can be made, and without waiting for the general carrying out of the plan.

In order that the plan of participation may have the full benefit of the judgment and skill of every person interested in its success, and that all may share with us the responsibilities attending the management of the business of the shop, we propose that each department shall elect three or more persons, who shall act as a local board of control—whose duties shall include certain portions of the management necessary to their department; the care and custody of the property and interests of the firm, as well as the hands—to see that nothing is destroyed or wasted—to settle all minor questions arising in their department, and to exercise such other powers as may be delegated to them by by-laws, to be made when the new organization is completed. One member of each of these local boards to retire at the end of every quarter, but to be eligible to re-election if the hands desire to continue his services; this, in order that an incompetent or unjust member may be speedily removed from any control over the affairs of his department beyond the power of his single vote.

The chairmen of these local boards are to organize as a board of governors, and this board is to have the general control of the entire shop, and to act as a higher power than the local boards; and to this board of governors any person in the shop may appeal who may feel aggrieved by a decision of any of the local boards; and they will also act as advisers of the local boards, in case their advice is sought. And, to guard against any hasty or ill-advised action this board of governors shall elect a member of our firm as their president—not to preside over their meetings, or to take part in their deliberations—but all their decisions, before they shall be deemed laws to govern the shop, shall be submitted to such president for his approval; and should he, at any time, deem a decision unwise or unjust, he shall return it to the governors for a reconsideration; if they shall adhere to their decision by a two-thirds vote, then such decision shall be final, notwithstanding the objection of the president.

The foregoing we offer as a mere outline of a plan which we hope to see elaborated by a shop committee, acting in concert with our firm and brought into successful operation; and we feel sure that, when it shall have received your earnest consideration, few if any will doubt its feasibility.

Our object in presenting it to your notice some time in advance of the date we propose it shall go into operation is, that time shall be given to work out all the details, so that failure may be avoided. We are aware that difficulties will be met in perfecting the organization, but we are quite sure that our mutual interests in the success of the plan will enable us to overcome them.

In conclusion we wish it to be distinctly understood that in offering this plan for your consideration, we do not claim to be prompted solely by the interests of those in our employ; on the contrary, we have faith that it will serve the interests of all concerned, and are free to say that we believe we shall be gainers in proportion to your gains; and we pledge ourselves that if this experiment during the first year shall confirm us in this belief, we shall make such further concessions to labor's share as will satisfy the shop of our faith in our plan.

One word more. We make this proposition at a period of profound peace in our shop—when there are no ugly questions to be answered, or demands to be silenced by it; it is wholly a voluntary act on our part. Nor do we come to you with this offer suffering from any disaster, disappointment, or even discontent, for our business is already the largest of its kind in the United States, and our last year was in every way the most successful that we ever experienced. We do not therefore invite your coöperation in order to restore a lost or impaired business, or to make good a deficient capital; but in our prosperity and success we do it for our mutual benefit, and that together we may demonstrate that neither Labor nor Capital can ever so efficiently promote its own advantage as when it seeks it, in harmony with the other, and with generous regard for the interests of the other.

(Signed) Brewster & Co., of Broome Street."

From the foregoing it will be seen that the industrial partnership was in the hands of a board of governors. Each department of the business elected three of its own men to what was called a board of control, from which body the firm chose one man to represent the department on the board of governors, the chairman of whom was a member of Brewster & Company.

The chairman had the power of veto, but the governors could pass over his veto by a two-thirds vote. This therefore left the men in absolute power as to the rate of wages, hours of work, or any detail connected with the management of the factory. In this was found a serious defect, as the governor of each department really had more power than the foreman. Furthermore, as the board of control and therefore the governor was elective, the best men were not always selected.

In the spring of 1871, a general eight hour movement was in

the air for all trades. There was a separate union in the carriage trade which the Brewster employés generally joined and held the balance of voting power on account of their numbers. During the movement for an eight hour day this question was brought up by the board of governors, but no final settlement was reached. In the meantime, Brewster & Company told their men that they did not think it was fair to belong to the union while this question was being considered. The men refused to retire, but said they would abstain from voting. The minute this large number ceased to vote, the balance of the union declared a strike for eight hours. The Brewster men out of sympathy for their fellow workers in other houses, and not able to withstand the call of "scab," struck.

The men stopped work and sent a delegation of three to the firm, asking that their demands for eight hours be granted, a power they already had without striking. Brewster & Company replied that the sole object of the association was to get together for mutual advantage; in other words, the only gain they expected from the association was good fellowship and individual interest in details of the business, in return for which they voluntarily paid the men about $10,000 a year. They did not propose to pay this to have them strike, and by the strike the partnership was dissolved.

Their thoughtlessness could not be better shown than by striking in June, when the year's annual dividend would have been declared the first of July.

Two weeks later the men came back to work unconditionally, and naturally the partnership has never been tried again.

In talking with some of the old men still with the firm, they said that the idea was popular and the men liked it, but it was not appreciated by the majority; the reason for this was attributed to their lack of intelligence and inability to appreciate the advantages which would accrue to them at the end of the year.

Prosperity sharing is the system which Mr. H. A. Sherwin informs me is in vogue in his establishment. He attempted profit sharing in the '70's. It was continued for three or four years and dropped "for reasons which it is a little difficult to explain," but suffice it to say that the plan was not considered a success. Later they concluded that prosperity sharing was more practical.

The Hoffmann & Billings Manufacturing Company [1] have had no system of profit sharing since 1896. Previous to that time they did have a system of profit sharing which was carried on for two or three years, but was finally dropped, as it did not prove to be what they wanted. The plan at that time was to figure the amount of wages paid during the year, equivalent to capital invested, that is, in equal proportions. At the end of the year, if there was a profit, the actual capital invested was allowed 6 per cent. interest; any profits beyond this were divided in proportion among the capital invested and wages paid.

"Of course, we only had something to divide when there was a profit shown. If we happened to have a loss, the company stood that themselves, but our experience was that when we did run across a year that showed a loss, our employés were under the impression that they were being done out of a profit which did not exist, and for that reason we concluded that it was sort of a 'jug-handle' affair and quit it," reports the treasurer of the company.

The Ames Shovel and Tool Company [2] had a system of profit sharing some 14 years ago, which was satisfactory to the men while there were profits to divide, but not acceptable when there was a loss, although they did not participate in it. The system was abandoned during a strike.

Fels & Company,[3] Philadelphia, have a system that has been in use during the last seven years, and has thus far been given as a dividend to wages.

"We have had a good deal of satisfaction through it, in that it has benefited the employés and has attached them closer to

[1] Hoffmann & Billings Manufacturing Co., Milwaukee, Wis. Manufacturers of and Jobbers of Material used for Gas, Steam and Water. Established 1885. Number Employés, 350.

[2] Ames Shovel and Tool Co., St. Louis, Mo. Manufacturers Shovels. Organized 1874. Number Employés, 155.

[3] Fels & Co., Philadelphia, Pa. Soap Manufacturers. Organized 1874. Number Employés, 550.

us, but it has the unsatisfactory feature of being in a sense arbitrary, which we have not yet seen our way to overcome. We appreciate the defects in this, as in most profit sharing plans, and do not deceive ourselves in the belief that it is the solution of the problem," the firm reports.

The proprietor of the Newport Daily News[1] makes no statement to the employés, but pledges himself to divide a certain share of the profits of the paper among them.

A kind of profit sharing plan is the John G. Myers Fund,[2] established in 1903 in the name and memory of the founder of the house, who died in 1901. This is still a co-partnership in the control of Mr. Myers' family and not a corporation. This fund applies only to those who have completed fifteen years' service with the firm, which was established in 1870.

The characteristics of this plan are that—

First—It provides a continual increase in salary after the limit to which the position occupied is entitled, is passed.

Second—It compels the recipient to save most of this increase to be paid as an insurance fund to a named and approved beneficiary.

Third—It provides an additional progressive cash increase in salary proportioned to the success of the business.

When the fund was established, an amount in credits was given to each one qualified, equal to what would have accrued had the plan been in operation since 1870. At present there are 86 members, 69 men and 17 women, and the total amount standing to their credit is $82,000. The annual cost in additional credits and cash distribution is about $10,000. It is the testimony of the company:

"We have had occasion in the five years' life of the fund to observe how wise and beneficent is the insurance feature, and we are satisfied that the other benefits have largely increased the loyalty, enthusiasm and efficiency of the members."

Houghton, Mifflin & Company have a combination system of savings and profit sharing. To encourage thrift, they have

[1] Newport Daily News, Newport, R. I. Organized 1846. Number Employés, 30.

[2] John G. Myers Co., Albany, N. Y. Department Store. Organized 1870. Number Employés, 600.

opened a savings department exclusively for their own employés. Deposits may be made at any time, but may not exceed $1000 in all. Six per cent. interest is paid. In addition to the regulations of this department, each depositor's pass-book contains this notice:

"Whenever on the first of April of any year the deposits of any depositor equal or exceed $100, and remain one year thereafter, the proprietors of the Riverside Press [1] will further pay to such depositor a portion of the annual profits of their business, within one month after their accounts for the said year are made up; but this amount shall not exceed 4 per cent. additional on each $100 so deposited; and the proprietors do not absolutely guarantee more than 6 per cent. interest first above mentioned, the extent of the further payment, if any, being dependent on the profits of the business."

The firm state:

"This system was adopted by us in 1872, and has been found by all parties most satisfactory in its results. We do not issue any reports. The division of the extra percentage over six per cent. has varied from one-half to four per cent., according to the variation in the profits from time to time. In a force at the Riverside Press averaging some seven hundred, we have two hundred and eleven depositors at present."

The Baker Manufacturing Company [2] has been operating under its present system of profit sharing during the past nine years with very satisfactory results. This firm is organized with $200,000 preferred stock, fully paid up, and has issued in profit sharing during the past nine years $264,469.16. There is an authorized capital of $600,000; $400,000 of which is common stock to be issued in profit sharing.

Profits are divided on the earning power of labor and the preferred capital stock. The dividend paid to preferred capital is its earning power and the wages paid to labor are the

[1] The Riverside Press, Cambridge, Mass. Printing and Binding. Organized 1849. Number of Employés, 700.

[2] Baker Manufacturing Co., Evansville, Wis. Manufacturers Wind Mills, Iron Pumps, Gasolene Engines, Feed Grinders, etc. Organized 1873. Number Employés, 150.

earning power of labor. An employé earning $500 per annum stands equal in profit sharing with $10,000 in preferred stock earning $500 per annum.

According to the By-Laws:

"The earnings of the preferred stock shall be a dividend of 5 per cent. per annum, which shall be paid quarterly in advance.

The earnings of hour and piece labor shall be the product of the total number of hours employed during any year by the price fixed for such labor per hour. This is not to exclude piece work, but persons working by the piece shall be credited in profit sharing only with the amounts they would have earned in the same time at a fixed price per hour.

The earnings of salaried labor shall be the total amount paid in salaries during any year.

The fixing of all wages and salaries, and the hiring and discharging of employés shall be done by the general manager, superintendent, or by any such other officer as the company may designate.

All hour and piece work wages shall be paid weekly, and all salaries at the close of each month.

To determine the net profit, an inventory shall be taken January 1st each year of all assets, including sinking fund, but no accrued interest; and of all liabilities, including preferred stock, common stock, amounts credited toward the purchase of common stock and sinking fund. The net profit or loss shall be the difference between the assets and liabilities.

If there should be a net loss in any year's business there shall be no dividend on the common stock or on amounts credited toward the same, no profit sharing and an amount equal to the loss shall be drawn from the sinking fund to restore it. In case the sinking fund is not sufficient to pay the loss there shall be no profit sharing until the loss in excess of the sinking fund is fully restored."

Mr. A. S. Baker reports that during the past nine years the division of profits has averaged about 80 per cent. of the earning power of both capital and labor, making the net dividend, including profit sharing to preferred stock, an average of 9 per cent. and has increased the earnings of every profit sharer about 80 per cent. of his wages. "You will see by the foregoing that we are coming to be practically a coöperative company. The only defect that we have discovered in our plan is that it permits a man to quit the employ of the company and carry with him his common stock, which he generally offers for sale, making an outside interest that is not always in harmony with the management of the company. This, however, is a very small minority; at present not over 5 or 6 per cent. of the whole paid-up capital."

From 1884 to 1902, Mr. A. Reinle[1] followed a profit sharing plan in the conduct of his business, and found it very satisfactory, with this exception, that his men were paid in cash, while his share consisted of additional holdings of buildings, machinery and stock. In 1902 he decided that if the men were willing to share in the profits, they must share in the risk of the business, so he incorporated as Reinle, Salmon & Company, the men paying for their stock by dividends or profits as they were earned. This plan includes the heads of departments and some of the most desirable employés.

"We find," says Mr. Reinle, "that the results have been very satisfactory in every way, financially, in the dividing of responsibility, and in the economy of running the business."

A profit sharing system was adopted by the N. O. Nelson Manufacturing Company[2] in 1886, in pursuance of which interest was allowed on its capital at the usual commercial rate and the remaining profits were evenly divided between capital and labor, after setting aside 2½ per cent. for educational purposes and 5 per cent. for a provident fund. Interest was regarded as the proper wages of capital; the educational fund was for the purpose of providing a free library, while the provident fund was to be used in caring for the families of deceased employés and for such as were incapacitated for work by reason of sickness or accident. Under this plan dividends of

[1] Reinle, Salmon Co., Baltimore, Md. Manufacturers Show Cases and Store Fixtures. Organized 1902. Number Employés, 120.

[2] N. O. Nelson Manufacturing Co., St. Louis, Mo. Manufacturers of Wholesale Plumbers' Supplies. Organized 1883. Number Employés, 600.

8 and 10 per cent. were paid for a number of years. These amounts were paid in cash or in the company's stock, according to the wish of the employé, until 1890, when the rule was adopted of issuing stock for all dividends to employés. These shares were, however, redeemed at par whenever the holder for any reason desired to leave the service of the company.

In 1894 the rules were altered so that profit sharing dividends were allowed to only such employés as saved 10 per cent. of their wages when working full time and receiving full pay and invested this amount in the company's stock. The purpose of this requirement was "to offer a substantial inducement for men when in good health and having steady employment to save something for the future, and also to make the sharing in the business profits dependent on each one doing something toward it in a direct and personal way." The plan was also further modified by increasing the dividend paid on wages to 2 per cent. as against 1 per cent. on capital, and by charging the expenditures for beneficial and educational purposes directly to the expense account of the company instead of providing for them by means of a specific fund. The company stated that owing to dull times and the considerable outlays for social and industrial betterment in Leclaire, no dividend had been paid for the last six years, but that the plan has not been abandoned and that much is expected from it in the future.

Early in 1906, a banquet was given to the employés, customers and friends of N. O. Nelson, when he announced that the profit sharing system which he adopted in his business many years ago amounted to more than $108,000 in the last year. Out of this amount $17,688.80 was given to schools and charity, and the balance divided among his customers and employés.

Inclosed in the invitations sent to customers and employés was a check for the amount the recipient had drawn for his or her part, and this notice:

"St. Louis, December 30, 1906.

Dear Sir:—

I take pleasure in advising you that you are entitled to $—— of the net profits accruing from this business for the fiscal year ending November 30th, 1905, which is a dividend on your purchases in accordance with my letter of announcement to our customers dated Jan. 13th, 1905. We accordingly enclose you certificate for —— shares of stock in our company; the remaining $—— will be applied on future issues of stock to you, when other annual dividends on the gross profits of your purchases entitle you to additional stock in multiples of $50. You are privileged, however, at any time you may wish, to add enough cash to make a full share or half share. When fractional parts of a share are held on deposit until made up to half a share or more, they are not to be considered as cash items or credits on account; they cannot be applied toward the payment of your merchandise account to us. This dividend is at the rate of 25 per cent. of the gross profits we have made on your purchases during the year. About half the amount is directly from the company and the other half from my portion of the profits. In the announcement at the beginning of the year I said that the dividends would be paid in my stock at a price on which the average earnings of the last three years would yield 6 per cent. This would make the price of the stock worth something more than two for one, or $200 per share. But I prefer to issue it to the customers and the employés at $100 per share, thus giving you twice the amount that the circular promised. We leave, undivided, a reasonable surplus fund so that if the profits of next year or succeeding years should be materially less, the surplus will help to even them up. The same terms or better will be in force the coming year.

I trust it is clear to you that we in no manner use the prospective dividend to affect prices. We sell at the prices that we would if there were no profit-sharing arrangement, just as we pay the same wages and salaries that would be paid without any profit-sharing. It is nothing more nor less than taking the employés and the customers into partnership and letting them have between them almost the entire profits of the business.

The attitude of the customers and also of competitors has been entirely cordial. All seem to recognize that the principle is right, that the carrying out of it is fair and impartial, and that I am privileged to dispense with further profits for myself.

The amount of this year's dividends to customers is $53,-177.48; to employés $37.931.74 and to the provident fund

$17,668.80, making a total of $108,778.02, which is exclusive of the regular cash dividend to stockholders.

(Signed) N. O. NELSON."

What has proved to be a successful plan of profit sharing was inaugurated by the Roycroft board of directors in 1887. At first only the chief employés and general officers of the company were admitted to participation, for it was considered that these men were in a position to make the business of the concern more prosperous through special care and attention, and as an appreciation of this extra effort each participant was allowed a certain sum, depending upon the amount of salary he received and the rate of dividends allotted to stockholders; thus, if dividends were high, the participation was correspondingly high, and vice versa. In 1890 the system was enlarged so as to include foremen and assistant foremen, whose participation was based upon the foregoing method, the payments, however, being proportionately smaller. Since the latter year the plan has been somewhat extended annually among the older employés of the classes named. The company reports that it has reason to believe the system is an excellent one and attains the desired end, for it has incited greater interest in the affairs of the establishment, inducing suggestions for improvements, little economies and the exercise of more care in consuming supplies and materials.

Profit sharing was inaugurated January 1, 1901, at the Simplex Electrical Company,[1] and is still in operation.

The beneficiaries are the factory employés only, in which is included a small factory office force, but does not include the general superintendents. The main office force and sales departments, being separate from the mill, have no share in the scheme.

On January 1st each year a preliminary list is made up, including all employés who were candidates for a share, conditioned on the fact that the employé shall have been in their employ at least twelve months.

[1] Simplex Electrical Co., Boston, Mass. Manufacturers Insulated Wires and Cables. Organized 1895. Number Employés, 275.

The actual profit sharers are those who, being on the preliminary list, remain continuously in their employ until March 1st of the following year, making the minimum possible time of employment before a dividend is received of 26 months, and the difference between the number on the preliminary list and the number of actual sharers represents those persons who are either discharged or leave of their own account during a period. The estimated pay roll is obtained by multiplying by 52 a full week's pay for every person on the preliminary list. The actual pay roll is the total of the wages received during the calendar year by the actual profit sharers.

At the beginning of each year the percentage of the profits of the company which shall go to the profit sharers for that calendar year is determined, and this has occasionally been increased as the estimated pay roll has increased. After the close of the year, when the profits of the company are determined, such proportion as had previously been determined on, is the dividend to the profit sharers, and dividing this by the actual pay roll, gives the percentage of dividend which each man receives on the wages which have been paid to him during the calendar year.

The payment of dividend is made on or about March 1st for the previous calendar year, delay being necessary in order that the books of the company may be settled. In case of death during the year of any person whose name is on the preliminary list, a death benefit is paid and charged against the profit sharing account, the amount of which is discretionary, but which shall not exceed an amount equal to the previous year's rate of dividend on the actual wages while actively employed, plus the amount of wages which it is estimated the employé would have received had he been able to work for the balance of the year. In cases of sickness a certain discretionary power is exercised, treating each individual case as seems reasonable and fair to the other employés.

All of the above points are covered by a set of rules posted at the beginning of each year, and by which the firm considers itself bound to abide.

While term of service is the only official requirement for profit sharing, some care is used in watching the candidates for the profit sharing dividend, and if a man seems unworthy, there is no hesitancy in discharging him, even a short time before the dividend is to be paid.

The plan is constantly explained to the employés as being not charity, but as a business proposition enabling them to receive extra compensation for more efficient service, the amount depending upon the result of mutual efforts.

YEAR	1901	1902	1903	1904	1905	1906
Estimated Pay Roll	100.	180.41	187.47	158.50	188.48	214.85
Actual Pay Roll	74.70	104.19	108.59	111.58	159.09	182.45
Dividend %	11.05	15.	12.01	7.428	12.784	18.45
Minimum Dividend (Women)	26.86	88.77	27.95	17.87	25.05	44.68
Minimum Dividend (Men)	28.68	44.77	85.58	19.16	42.18	25.24
Maximum Dividend	109.55	188.10	158.78	87.82	182.98	258.79
Names on Preliminary List	100	186	145	154	172	212
Actual Profit Sharers	79	105	105	114	149	178
Women	5	9	6	7	7	28
Men	74	96	99	107	142	150
1901 Sharers	78	66	60	54	48	49
1902 "		105	90	79	64	60
1903 "			105	85	70	66
1904 "				117	97	85
1905 "					149	124

Estimated pay roll and actual pay roll are proportional figures only, based on 100 estimated pay rolls for 1901. The number of employés is in all cases proportional only, based on 100 names on preliminary list for 1901.

The firm reports: "The results have varied a good deal with different individuals, being as a rule very marked with the more intelligent men, and having little or no apparent effect on some. On the whole, the results, while not ideal, are reasonably satisfactory, as most of the men are jealous of any waste which they realize reduces their dividend as well as our profit, and we feel that the money which is paid out is saved or earned by extra care and diligence, and so long as the plan works as well as it has in the past, we shall continue it.

"As the percentage of the profits which is to be divided is determined at the beginning of each year, the final amount of the dividend is entirely dependent upon the success of the business, and each profit sharer is therefore a partner to that extent, and this we consider the key to the whole situation."

The Saugerties Manufacturing Company[1] began a system of profit sharing in 1901, when a dividend of 5 per cent. to labor was declared. The following amounts on a capital stock of $25,000 have been distributed:

February, '01	$ 4,085.70
" '02	4,192.16
" '03	4,393.45
" '04	4,506.30
" '05	4,657.42
" '06	4,680.39
	$26,515.42

Each year at the time of the distribution, the treasurer has enclosed the amount of the dividend accompanying it with cards of greeting.

Mr. Gillespy writes me:

"Our motive in the introduction of profit sharing was not altogether unselfish. As officials we hoped to reap benefits for our stockholders as well as for our employés. We are not as sanguine as at the beginning as to the success of the movement. We do not regret the distribution, but should feel better satisfied if we could make the division more in the line of merit. Our waiting list is not so large that we are able always to choose the best. A distribution to those only entitled to it would engender ill feelings and discontent. We are now considering whether it may not be in the interest of justice to discontinue the profit sharing plan and increase the daily wage of those entitled to the profits."

July 1, 1897, George A. Chace, Treasurer of the Bourne Mills,[2] Fall River, Mass., made the following announcement:

[1] Saugerties Manufacturing Co., Saugerties, N. Y. Manufacturers Blank Books. Organized April 24, 1895. 220 Employés.

[2] Bourne Mills, Fall River, Mass. Manufacturers Cotton Cloth. Organized 1881. Number Employés, 700.

"To the Employés of the Bourne Mills:

Eight years ago, in May, 1889, the board of directors of the Bourne Mills voted, in a generous moment, to try an experiment in profit sharing. For two years or more the business had proven profitable, handsome dividends had been paid to the stockholders, and the directors hit upon this scheme to express their good will towards their employés with some hope that it might result in mutual benefit. The action was not taken without due deliberation. The idea had been under consideration perhaps a year. The president, Hon. Jonathan Bourne, who held over half the capital stock, favored it from the first. Although 79 years old at the time, he had the clearest head among us, and, upon this subject, was fortified by years of experience as a whaling merchant, in which business it had long been a custom to offer a lay, or share of the profits, to the men who shipped for a whaling voyage. Mr. Bourne died about a month after our experiment began, and we shall never know what other plans for the advancement of the employés of this corporation he would have set forward if he had lived till this time. Ample time was allowed for the matter to become familiar to each member of the board. Edward Everett Hale and Carroll D. Wright, with others, were consulted. A copy of Dr. Hale's little book, 'How They Lived in Hampton,' was presented to each director, and some of them read it through twice. In the midst of the discussion, Mr. Gilman published his treatise on 'Profit Sharing,' and this book was taken into the board meeting to be read and freely criticised. Mr. Gilman himself has taken a cordial interest in our experiment, and has put himself to a good deal of pains to give us assistance at various times. Final action was taken by the board on May 20th, and the announcement was made to you in my letter of May 23d, 1889.

"The first trial was limited to six months, beginning July 1, 1889. The board has always been conservative and cautious in this respect; it was only after the seventh trial that it ventured to pass a vote to continue profit sharing a full year, and during the eight years it has been favorably passed upon twelve times.

"It will be brought before a new board of directors again next November, and doubtless their decision will depend upon what sort of record we make between now and then. Personally I favor the continuance of profit sharing so long as it can be made a mutual benefit.

"There is some disadvantage in a short term in profit sharing. If it had been known at the start that the project would be continued eight years, it might have been wiser to have planned a scheme to cover the whole period; and thus have saved for you a large dividend which you would receive at the end of the time; that, I believe, is the most approved theory of profit sharing from the employers' standpoint. Still, to the prudent employé, there is something to be said in favor of the short terms—the money is actually in hand and may be saved or spent at pleasure; and, really, a habit of voluntary saving is worth more than a sum of money saved for one's benefit. To promote this habit of voluntary saving, an employés' savings fund account was opened in 1891 under the authority of the directors, the object of which was to foster the habit of saving small sums with the intention that any sum of five dollars or more would be transferred to a savings bank at the convenience or desire of the depositor; any amount from five cents to fifty dollars was accepted, no one's deposits being allowed to exceed one hundred dollars, however; the account was closed a year ago for private reasons; there had been 2819 deposits amounting to $9937.28. We have reason to hope that some portion of this sum of money was saved because of the opportunity offered, and we trust that many of you have snug deposits in the savings banks through this fund, and the extra money you have received in profit sharing. We can recommend the savings banks of Fall River as among the very best in the commonwealth.

"In my letter to you eight years ago to-day, July 1, 1889, I explained briefly the principles of our plan of profit sharing, which are very simple and easy to understand, the essential points being that every employé—man, woman or child—who continues faithfully at work during any term, is entitled to a share of the profits; that the employé shall share in proportion to the dividends declared and paid to the stockholders, and that the share shall be a dividend upon the wages earned during the specified term. Our plan capitalizes your interest in the Bourne Mills at the most you can earn during a term of six months; a rate of dividend is calculated by dividing a certain percentage (not less than six nor more than ten per cent.) of the amount paid to the stockholders by the total wages, and then the amount of each individual's wages is multiplied by this rate for each one's share, or 'divvy,' as you have named it. It was estimated that this divvy might amount to a little over 2½ per cent. of your wages, while it was explained that the average dividend of all the savings banks of Massachusetts the previous five years was a little over 2 per cent. (semi-annually). The following is the list of dividends actually paid to you:

No. 1,	3 1-3 per cent.	No. 9,	3 per cent.
" 2,	3 1-2 "	" 10,	2 1-2 "
" 3,	2 1-2 "	" 11,	3 "
" 4,	3 1-3 "	" 12,	3 "
" 5,	3 1-3 "	" 13,	7 "
" 6,	3 1-2 "	" 14,	3 "
" 7,	3 2-3 "	" 15,	3 1-3 "
" 8,	3 "	" 16,	3 "

or an average semi-annual dividend for eight years of 3.375 per cent. or total of 54.00. The savings banks of Massachusetts paid the last eight years 2.035 per cent. or total of 32.56.

"You will understand that 54 per cent. means $54 on $100, that is to say, if your wages have averaged $100 for six months you have received in the eight years a bonus of $54; if you have earned an average of $200 a term you have been paid $108 extra, or if you earned as much as $300 a term you received in addition $162, and so on.

"A comparison of the month of May, 1889, with May, 1897, shows that the average pay of all employés on the pay rolls is ten per cent. greater in 1897 than it was in 1889 just before the beginning of profit sharing, notwithstanding the standard price of wages, except mule spinning, was higher then than now, and the mills were running 60 hours a week as compared with 48 hours now."

The thirty-third semi-annual dividend of 5 per cent. on wages earned was paid June 2, 1906.

January 1, 1904, the Driver-Harris Wire Company,[1] Harrison, N. J., began a system of profit sharing whereby those in their employ three years or more receive January 1st of each year 3 per cent. of salary for the year; those two years receive 2 per cent. and one year 1 per cent. This plan the sales manager reports as "quite satisfactory." He adds, "We have had several betterment features in mind for a long time, first among which are dining rooms for our men and women employés, but up to this time we have been unable to carry out our plans, owing to lack of room."

H. S. Peters Company, Dover, N. J., also have a limited form of profit sharing, where those admitted to participation in it are all employés who fill responsible positions. The amount allotted to each is dependent on the importance of the position occupied by him in the business. This plan has not yet been worked out to include all employés because the firm is doubtful as to the wisdom of such a course. The ordinary employé who has no responsibility beyond doing his regular daily task is not in a position to make such an arrangement mutually advantageous, and therefore through lack of interest, such plans almost invariably become ineffective.

At the end of the first year of the profit sharing plan begun by the Thomas G. Plant Company[2] in 1904, the firm stated that the superintendent and heads of departments had for three weeks carefully gone over the ratings of each and every member, carefully questioning the foreman in charge, and after the most thorough investigation had placed the members of each respective class in accordance with what the evidence showed he was entitled to.

Every consideration was given each member as to his value to the company, the quality of the work he produced, the amount of work done per day, neatness, manner of conducting himself as to being quiet and orderly, attendance, being at work every day and always on time. Any member who considered that he had not been classed fairly was advised to ask

[1] Driver-Harris Wire Co., Harrison, N. J. Wire Manufacturers. Organized December 23, 1898. Number Employés, 110.

[2] Thomas G. Plant Co., Boston. Manufacturers Women's Fine Shoes. 3500 Employés.

his foreman to explain fully the reasons for so classifying him.

At the outset it was stated that at the end of the year the members would be divided into four equal classes. This division was very difficult, hence for the future the members will be divided into three classes, one-quarter in Class A, one-half in Class B and one-quarter in Class C, eliminating Class D. Many good workmen lost the opportunity of a rating in the A Class by being lax in their attendance; others were prompt in their attendance, but took too little pride in the class of work they did; some did first-class work, but so little that they were of less value than if they produced a good day's work; others were so careless about their berth and person that their untidiness was a strong mark against them.

Being either noisy, disorderly or difficult to manage is a factor that bears strongly in placing members in the lower class, even though they may otherwise be first-class workmen.

For the eight months ending May 1, 1904, $50,085 were saved, and a dividend of $30,651 added to this amount by the Plant Company, making a total of $80,736 which the 1600 members of the sinking fund department had accumulated.

The foremen, heads of small departments and inspectors became members a year ago. The general division was formed the middle of September, and from that date to February 1st many new members were added. The majority of members belonging to the saving fund department have averaged thirty-one weeks.

The dividend of $30,651 was divided among the four classes as follows: $14,078 to 375 members, who were in Class A; $9125.23 to 375 members, who were considered "good," and rated under Class B; $4885.17 to those considered "fair," Class C, 395 in all; $2562.57 to the 394 people in Class D.

The following are the conditions of membership in the fund:

Deposit 10 per cent. of the weekly earnings.

Turn out first-class work.

Do a good day's work.

Look clean; be orderly; keep machine and berth clean.

Come to work on time, and at work every day unless sick or excused.

The firm state as a further incentive that in promotion,

in making changes, in giving steady employment or in discharging, preference will always be given to members of the department who are in good standing.

To create a fund for the benefit of members who may become sick, disabled or die, making assistance desirable, each adult member of the relief and saving fund department shall pay ten cents each week, and each member under 20 years of age five cents per week from his earnings.

Each member incapacitated for work shall be entitled to draw, during a period of seven weeks in one year; if 20 years of age or upwards, $7 per week, and if under 20 years of age $3.50 per week.

At the death of a member there shall be paid out of the fund to the beneficiary one hundred dollars, if the deceased member had been contributing ten cents a week to the relief fund up to the week of death, and fifty dollars if the deceased member had been contributing five cents per week to the relief fund up to the week of death.

No person shall be eligible to membership until he has been in the employ of the company for a period of three months.

It is the philosophy of the company that not one man in a hundred will form the habit of saving unless he places himself under some obligation to save. For that reason the Plant Company is most anxious to have all its desirable employés become members of the profit sharing, relief and saving fund department, so that they may form the habit of saving a part of their weekly earnings, which in time may be a sufficient amount to protect them against want.

At the Wayne Knitting Mills there is a profit sharing plan to promote harmony between the executive and operating departments by inviting free discussion and interchange of ideas. The officers wish every department manager to feel that he or she is a stockholder in the business, that on the success of the individual parts depends to a degree the success of the whole enterprise.

A certain per cent. of the profits, after all interest and other charges have been deducted, is divided among the various department heads. This per cent. is based on the annual net profits for the ten years previous, and the allotment amounts to from $5000 to $10,000 annually. These department men and women have organized themselves into a club called the T. I. Club. The share each person receives does not depend on the size of his salary, but on his efficiency, and the latter is not wholly determined by the officers, but is voted on by his brother club members. Each member of this club is asked to write his opinion of the ability of every other member, and as to whether every member is getting the most out of his particular department. The T. I. Club meets every two weeks and discusses various questions of mutual interest, and whatever tends to promote the betterment of the entire service. This work is full of interest to the management and to the employés. It has been in operation for two years, and already has had a noticeable effect in increased personal endeavor, and a hearty desire to coöperate with the officers in charge.

The success of the profit sharing plan, and the dining room project, both started largely as experiments, has been decisive enough to warrant larger plans for the future. A fund has already been established to be devoted to the erection of a separate building, which will be called "The Wayne Assembly Hall Fund." This hall will be used exclusively by employés, and will contain a dining room, with tables and lunch counters, and all the necessary equipment; a gymnasium and reading room, a bowling alley and billiard tables.

The Valentine & Bentley Silk Company [1] established a system of profit sharing with employés on January 1, 1902, the heads of departments only being admitted. A year later, on January 1st, 1903, the privilege was given to all employés to purchase on easy terms the company's gold bonds, bearing interest at the rate of 5 per cent. per annum; in addition to the 5 per cent. interest, a bonus is given to the holders of these bonds from a fund set apart for that purpose from the profits; this is placed to their accounts, and at the end of five years handed to them in cash.

Spratt's Patent (America) Limited,[2] has a system of profit

[1] The Valentine & Bentley Silk Co., Newton, N. J. Silk Manufacturers. Organized 1903. Number Employés, 300.

[2] Spratt's Patent (America) Limited. Manufacturers Foods for Dogs, Poultry and other Domestic Animals. Organized 1885. Number Employés, 95.

sharing which was put in operation at the beginning of 1903. Under the plan a percentage of the profits over and above a certain fixed sum is set aside for division among the principal employés at the end of the fiscal year, the number of beneficiaries and the amount of the allotment being at the discretion of the general manager.

At the close of 1903 on the occasion of the first year the plan was in operation, 12 employés participated in the division of profits, the dividends amounting to sums that varied from three to seven per cent. of their annual wages.

In any discussion of profit sharing or "dividends to labor," the premium plan of paying for labor should have a very prominent place. To ascertain the principles and merits of the premium plan, I requested a summarized statement from Mr. F. A. Halsey, editor of the *American Machinist,* who is the inventor of the system. In his own words,

"One of the standing objections to the premium plan is that under it the rates may be cut as under piece work, and hence it seems to be as objectionable from this standpoint as piece work. The answer is that while the system does not make rate cutting impossible, it does make it unnecessary, for under piece work the cutting of the rates is a necessity which the fairest-minded employer in the world encounters sooner or later. Under piece work the piece price and the piece cost are yoked together, and the piece cost cannot be reduced to meet reduced selling prices without cutting the piece price. Under the premium plan there is no piece price, but the piece cost and the premium earnings are so yoked together that an increase of earnings necessarily goes with a reduction of cost, and as time goes on and production increases, the employer finds his costs going down without cutting the rates. It is not pretended that the system will overcome cupidity and avarice, get blood from stones, or make philanthropists of skinflints, but it does overcome the necessity for rate-cutting, which is inherent in the piece work system, and it thus permits fair dealing, which piece work, in most lines of work, prohibits. The chief merit of the system, in fact, is that it is in accordance with the strictest principles of economics. Were it otherwise it could not stand. Its sole aim from the employer's standpoint is to produce work as cheaply as possible. The workman gives a full equivalent for every extra dollar paid him—a fuller equivalent in fact for the premium portion of his earnings than for the daily wages portion—and a partnership interest in efficient production is secured without any features savoring of charity, patronage or paternalism. The system does not make the employé a ward or protégé of the employer, but preserves his independence and his manhood, while giving him an opportunity to profit by his industry.

While we hear a great deal of the identity of the interest of employers and employés, when these interests are considered in a large sense, it is nevertheless, as a rule, tacitly assumed that between two individuals and in the matter of immediate wages the interests of the parties are antagonistic—the interests of the employer demanding low and those of the employé high wages. A moment's reflection will, however, show that while the employé desires high wages per day, the employer desires, and if he is to live, must have, low wages per unit of product, and it is obvious that if these requirements can be harmonized the assumed antagonism of interests becomes harmony instead.

The premium plan does harmonize the needs of the employé for high wages per day and of the employer for low wages per piece. It sets out to increase wages per day, but by a method that shall insure a more than proportionate increase of output, a method indeed that insures that the increase of output shall be accomplished before the increase of pay, by basing the increase of pay on the increase of output. The system is as simple in principle as this statement. It simply recognizes that the greatest spur to self-exertion is self-interest, and that no system of espionage or discipline or whip cracking can be as effective as one which honestly offers and pays hard dollars for extra work.

The premium plan is an application to production of methods long in use in connection with sales. The plan of offering a salesman a salary and a commission is closely analogous to the premium plan, and if for the salary he is expected to sell a certain minimum of goods per annum, the commission applying only to the excess above this minimum, the analogy is exact. Under the premium plan the workman is paid by the day, and for this daily pay is expected to produce a certain minimum of product, while for any excess beyond that amount he is paid a premium, the amount of this premium being based on the excess and being less per unit of product than the old wages cost. It is applicable to any class of work of which the output can be reduced to units."

Any method that pays the worker according to his merit should be satisfactory, for it is unfair that the slow, go-as-you-please workman should receive the same compensation as the quick, active employé, who uses his brains as well as his hands to increase the output. The Chambersburg Engineering Company[1] sets a price on the work to be done, paying the workman his regular day wages weekly, and when his premium work is completed he is paid one-half the difference between the price of his contract and the actual day wages paid him or the profit. When the price is set it is distinctly understood that there will be no reduction in the price unless improved machinery for reducing the cost of that particular piece is installed at the company's expense.

If the workman by his brains can devise some means or design a jig or fixture for holding his work, which will materially reduce the cost of production, the company will make this jig or fixture, if in their judgment it is practical, and will make no reduction in the price of the contract, even though it should cut the cost of production in two.

Mr. James A. Smith, secretary of the company, writes, that after 20 years' experience in paying men by piece work and by premium plans, he considers the latter by far the best system.

"We consider it," he stated, "the only fair method of compensating employés in the manufacturing business, and also the most satisfactory method from our standpoint."

In an iron foundry it was announced that after March, 1901, whenever practicable, workmen would be paid as follows:

[1] The Chambersburg Engineering Co., Chambersburg, Pa. Manufacturers Steam Hammers—Hydraulic Machinery. Organized November 29, 1897. Number Employés, 300.

1. The time within which it is expected that a job will be completed is set by the company. This is called the "time limit."

2. The workman is paid at his regular hourly rate during the time he works on the job, except as in (3), and if the time taken to do the work is less than the time limit, he is paid a premium for every hour saved. Payment will be made only for work which passes inspection. The premiums will be proportioned to the different rates of wages, as follows:

Wages Per Hour	*Premium Per Hour*
00 cents to 9.9 cents	5 cents
10 " 14.9 "	6 "
15 " 19.9 "	7 "
20 " 24.9 "	8 "
25 " 29.9 "	10 "

Example: Suppose a man's regular hour rate to be 22 cents and his corresponding premium rate 8 cents as given above. Suppose the time limit for a certain job to be fixed at 20 hours. The man will be paid 22 cents an hour for the time worked, and 8 cents an hour for all the time he can save. If he completes the job in 15 hours, thereby saving five hours, he will get 15 times 22 cents, 3.30 as wages, and 5 times 8 cents, 40 cents, as premium for saving time. His total pay for the job will be the sum of his wages and the premium, or 3.30 plus 40 cents, equal $3.70. In this particular case, it would make the man's pay amount to 24 2-3 cents an hour while on this job.

3. In case it requires the full time limit, or longer, to complete the job, the workman will receive his hour rate during the time employed, unless the work is spoiled by the workman through gross carelessness, but it is expected that, under ordinary circumstances, work will be completed within the time limit.

4. If work be spoiled and rejected but can be made right it is made right by the workman, and the time consumed is added to the job time already spent upon the job.

If any part of the work is spoiled, the time is figured the same as if all pieces had been right, and from the pay which would be due, if this were the case, shall be deducted a pro rata amount for the number of pieces spoiled.

5. If the work is not first-class, but still can be used, it is passed as second-class. The time will be figured as if all were right, and deduction made of one-half the amount of premium that would be made if the pieces were rejected.

6. Premiums and time limits will not be frequently changed; the plan is to have them continue for not less than a year. Changes thereafter may be necessitated by reductions in prices received for work, or by the introduction of new methods, tools, or machines, changes in dimension limits, or re-arrangement of shop. In other words, time limits like everything else, must be modified from time to time to conform to general business conditions and the general tendency toward more rapid and cheaper production per piece, occurring from year to year in all lines of industry, and necessitated by lower selling prices. Gross errors either way will be corrected at any time.

7. All time spent in obtaining and putting back into place jigs, fixtures, tools, and all time spent in setting tools, getting ready, taking down tools and cleaning up machines in proper condition for the next job to the satisfaction of the foreman—in fact, all time spent either directly or indirectly on the job must be charged to the time worked on the job.

The general manager informs me that the plan has been given up for the present, not so much because he did not like it, as because he was not satisfied with the man in charge. "Like everything else," he says, "it must be in charge of a good man, and a foreman who is interested and sympathetic; and the prices must be set by a man who thoroughly understands his business and is disposed to err on the low side, of course, without being unjust."

The Cincinnati Milling Machine Company[1] have had the premium plan in operation in their shop for seven years, and are quite satisfied that it has worked to the advantage both of themselves and their employés.

[1] Cincinnati Milling Machine Co. Manufacturers Milling Machines. Organized 1888. 500 Employés.

In order to set a fair average time performance on a given job, they make a careful study of the operation to be done, the speeds and feeds at which it should be handled (taking into consideration the class of skilled labor required by the nature of the job) and arrive at what they consider about a fair and average time in which the job should be done by a workman of the grade selected. If the workman reduces this time, he is then paid an extra premium beyond his daily wage rate for one-half the time saved at his regular daily wage per hour. As a concrete example: If the company sets the time for a certain operation on a given number of pieces of the same kind at 100 hours, and the workman completes the job in 80 hours, earning 20 cents per hour as his regular daily wage rate, they pay him a premium for ten hours at 20 cents per hour, or $2. So long as the time is fairly set, this acts as a very considerable inducement to the workman to increase the output.

Frequently the same workman handles the same job successively many times, and thereby acquires individual skill, which enables him readily to earn a premium. This plan puts a premium upon skill, and upon the individual fidelity, enthusiasm and industry of the workman, and renders him compensation in accordance with these factors—which the company thinks are the true basis of compensation.

On the other hand, a manufacturer can be well satisfied to pay the additional wages, provided he gets an increased output, which is the factor that ultimately governs his net cost.

In the opinion of this company, "The basis of a successful premium plan is, of course, a fair setting of the time. This time should only be changed when the conditions of the job change. It should be understood with the workman in advance that if a manufacturer contributes anything directly toward reduction in the time by supplying an improved machine, or improved jigs or fixtures, or high speed steel cutting tools where previously carbon steel tools had been used at the original setting of the time,—that then it would be perfectly proper and fair to lower the time set.

"On the other hand, this time should not be lowered by the manufacturer just because a workman, through his own individual skill, has arrived at a point where his earnings grow considerably beyond the ordinary day rate.

"There are of course a number of complexities in a premium plan which need careful study. It involves a careful taking of the time. If this time reporting is left to the workman, and if all the jobs as they follow one another are not under the premium plan, the workman, if he be dishonest, may charge his time to the non-premium job and take it off of the premium job, thereby making an extra earning illegitimately.

"Furthermore, if the time on a job has been fixed in relation to the workman earning 20 cents an hour, that time is entitled to be lowered, should a workman earning 30 cents an hour be put on the same job.

"Where the time has been fairly and consistently set, it would also seem fair that the workman's losses as against this time should be charged against his gains, although we do not do this, and, as far as we know, it is not common practice among other manufacturers employing this plan.

"However, even considering all the irregularities which may creep in, and some of the difficulties in carefully administering the premium plan, yet, where the plan is pursued under conditions above described, in our judgment it will work to the benefit of both the employer and the employés."

At the Lodge & Shipley Machine Tool Company[1] the Halsey system of premium work was introduced in 1905. The firm state that it is eminently successful from the point of view of the employé, as well as their own. In their opinion, where the system falls down or is not successful, it is generally due to a lack of liberality on the part of the employer, or to the fact that the line of work is not made in sufficient quantity for the employé to get the benefit of the gain by repetition. Quoting Mr. William Lodge, president of the company, "In most cases the employé in our establishment makes in the neighborhood of 50 per cent. more than his regular wages and under such a condition his product is doubled, for the reason that if ten hours are gained, he gets paid for five of these hours at his

[1] The Lodge & Shipley Machine Tool Co., Cincinnati, Ohio. Organized September, 1902. 500 Employés.

regular hourly rate, while the company gets the other five hours.

"It is better than piece work because in general it has been the experience throughout the whole United States, and I think I may safely say in other countries, that where the man doubles his wages under the piece work system, the employer thinks he has not been well treated prior to the time of establishing the piece work and that he is correct in cutting the prices. This is not only discouraging to the employé but results in future in choking the job, or, in other words, he will not produce enough to double his wages but will keep it down to some smaller amount, fearing that his price will be cut for the next lot of the same pieces.

"Of course it is essential that there should be the best possible coöperation between the employer and the employé. The employer must show that he takes an interest in assisting the workman to make the premium system profitable to him. I might say that since we have established this system we have never cut the price established unless we totally changed the method of doing the work by making additional appliances or adding new machinery and changing the operations which generally involve the making of costly tools."

At the Chambers Brothers Company the premium plan has been adopted in some of the departments during the last eight years. Prior to this time there was no piece work plan or any other except payment by the hour, without much regard to the actual work performed by the individual mechanic. The introduction of the premium plan met with some objections and difficulties at first, but as these were overcome, the men became pleased with the system. The manager states that much of their work is experimental, and on this the premium plan is not used, "but on routine work we consider it preferable to any system we are familiar with."

The Miller, DuBrul & Peters Manufacturing Company,[1] established the premium plan in 1903 in one department which was crowded with work, but running behind. The results were

[1] The Miller, DuBrul & Peters Manufacturing Co., Cincinnati, Ohio. Cigar and Cigarette Machinery. Organized 1873. Number Employés, 150.

very satisfactory to all concerned. The plan has since been abandoned on account of certain changed commercial conditions, whereby the work is very irregular, with no definite basis on which the premiums may be estimated. "We believe the premium plan to be a very good one, and a successful method of increasing the output for the employer and increasing the wages for the employé. The one difficulty we discovered, however, in our application of the premium system was that we made a mistake to apply it to a department as a whole, and although the results produced were satisfactory enough, still we believe the results would have been better yet had we been able to bring the system down to the individual output of each employé working under it. The employés seem to have been all very well satisfied, and had no complaints, and the premium money seemed to have been a welcome addition to their regular compensation."

The Providence Engineering Works [1] have used the premium plan of paying for labor. The pay of the workmen is increased by this system from 15 to 20 per cent., as it was found that market rates had to be paid irrespective of premiums earned by the workmen. In working out the details of the plan, a premium rate of four cents per hour was adopted for boys or men receiving 16 cents and under, and eight cents an hour for handy-men and machinists receiving over 16 cents per hour. The company makes it a point, which it regards as the backbone of the system, to allow the time limits to remain permanent, except where new tools or methods of manufacture are introduced, and as a matter of fact, they have been left the same even after the introduction of new tools and methods, except when such new tools or methods have worked a very radical change in the product. About a year ago the time limits were reset on steam engine work, which had remained unchanged for seven years previous to that time. The idea in changing the limits was more to equalize them so as to make them fairer to the workmen on various jobs, as it was found by experience that while some were high, some were also rather low, and

[1] Providence Engineering Works. Steam and Gas Engines; Steam Turbines; Automobile Parts and General Machinery. Organized 1899. Number Employés, 312.

the effort was to get a better average so as to have a more uniform increase in wage. This attempt to readjust the limits created a slight temporary disturbance which was over as soon as the true motive of the change was apparent to the men.

The superintendent of the firm reports, "The plan has worked satisfactorily from our point of view, and we think also from the workmen's point of view, as we repeatedly have requests from them for new limits to be set on work previously done by day labor."

CHAPTER VIII

HOUSING

The Peacedale Manufacturing Company,[1] founded in 1801, was incorporated in 1848. Shortly after its incorporation, the company began its first specific efforts for industrial betterment. The company tenements are plain, well built, comfortable houses, and though not especially modern in design, are always kept in excellent repair.

One cottage of eight rooms, surrounded by trees and shrubbery, rents for $8.33 per month. Another eight-room cottage in a very desirable location rents for $12.50 per month. Cottages of seven rooms rent for sums ranging from $7.50 to $10 per month. Another class of houses contains two and three tenements of varying sizes. The tenements in the two-tenement houses contain from 6 to 11 rooms each, and rent for from $4.42 to $11 per month according to location, while the tenements in the three-tenement houses contain from three to eight rooms each and rent for from $3.45 to $6.92 per month. A number of very attractive homes have also been built by employés of the company.

The population of Hopedale, Mass., is about 2000 persons, while the Draper Company, which manufactures all kinds of machinery for cotton mills, has in its employ at times as many as 3000 men. A considerable portion of these men are skilled mechanics, restless and much inclined to move away after a time. For this reason few of them care to own homes of their own, preferring to pay the moderate rent charged for the company's houses. Under these conditions the company now owns a large percentage of the dwellings in the place and plans are being prepared for about 20 additional houses to be erected in the near future.

[1] Peacedale Manufacturing Co., Peacedale, R. I. Manufacturers Woolen and Worsted Cloth. Organized 1848. Number Employés, 700.

The tract of land upon which are situated the houses for the use of the employés contains about 30 acres, and was laid out by a distinguished landscape artist, who prepared the plans for the entire work before any of the improvements were made. The company next built macadamized roads, with concrete sidewalks, put in sewer and water pipes, and obtained building plans from several different architects in order to secure variety in the construction of the houses. The buildings are all of wood, the exteriors consisting of shingles painted in various harmonious colors. Their construction is such that while all have about the same amount of room on the inside, the exteriors are so treated as to avoid monotony of appearance. Each house contains two tenements, each of which comprises a parlor or living room, a dining room, a kitchen, and a pantry and hall on the first floor, three sleeping rooms and a bath room on the second floor and a good storage room in the attic. A few have a fourth bedroom in the attic. The floors of the lower hall, the dining room, kitchen, pantry and bath room are of hard maple, the rest of the house being finished in white wood, either painted or in the natural color. Every house has a good cemented cellar, and many are furnished with gas and electric lights and other conveniences. The handsome appearance presented by these houses is greatly augmented by the well-kept lawns surrounding them, beds of bright colored flowers, neatly trimmed hedges and attractive shade trees, all contributing to the general effect.

The rentals are $3 per week for each tenement not supplied with heating apparatus, or $3.50 per week for such tenements as have furnaces. As the houses cost in round figures about $4500 each, or about $2250 for each tenement, exclusive of the land on which they stand, this price yields the company only a small income after deducting water rates, insurance, repairs and depreciation.

They provide houses that take care of about 400 families and the others are provided for in towns adjoining, where there is a surplus population. Hopedale contains first-class schools, library with reading room, roads, park system, and other desirable things all furnished by the town, and on the other hand, as the Draper Company's is the only business there, and as it and its individual largest stockholders who live there pay a very large proportion of the taxes, while some of the above are furnished under the name of the town, and others by the company, the result is the same to a certain extent in either case.

Frank J. Dutcher writes, October 25, 1907:

"As regards our conditions at the present time, we are adding a few more similar houses, and are also building 20 double houses in the town of Milford within walking distance of our works, these houses being of a little less elaborate construction and smaller size, made with the view of renting at a lower price. The new double houses that we are building here in Hopedale of similar general construction and size to those that we have written you about in the past are costing to-day, leaving out the question of land, at least $1000 each more than they did within three or four years."

The company sees that all buildings are kept in good repair, and insists upon a strict observance of proper sanitary regulations on the part of the occupants. The premises are well drained, vaults are cleaned out and ashes and garbage removed at stated periods and particular care is taken that the yards, both front and back, shall be kept in perfectly clean condition. Prizes amounting to $300 are distributed each year by the company to those tenants whose yards are kept in the best condition. The amounts thus awarded were divided as follows: One first prize, $10; twelve second prizes, $7.50 each; forty third prizes, $5 each. These prizes are based upon the general conditions of the premises, both in front and in rear of the houses, special attention being given to the care of the grass and consideration to anything else that may have been done. This plan has been in operation eight or ten years, and has proved an excellent one, for in addition to being an incentive to the tenant, it obliges a committee from the company to inspect the premises at frequent intervals, and this in itself leads to the discovery of anything that may need attention.

The first houses planned by the architects for the Ludlow Manufacturing Associates were built without sufficient regard for the requirements of the people who were to live in them, but in recent years the managers have made a careful study of plans in order to provide, at least possible cost, cottages which will meet all requirements. Each new set of cottages, as built,

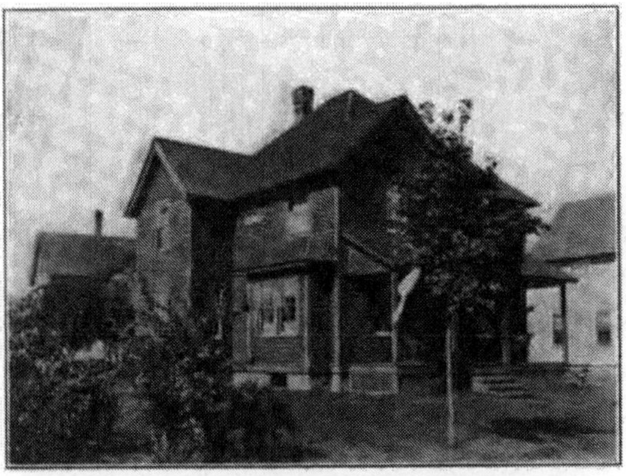

One of the Employés' Houses at the Ludlow Manufacturing Associates, Ludlow, Mass.

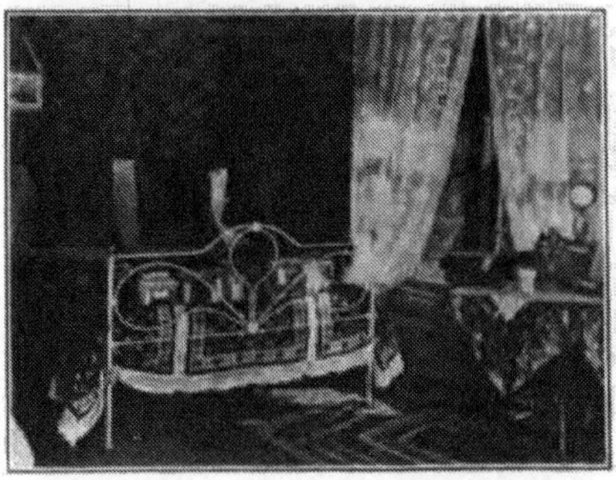

Interior of a Miner's Cottage at the Colorado Fuel and Iron Company's Mines.

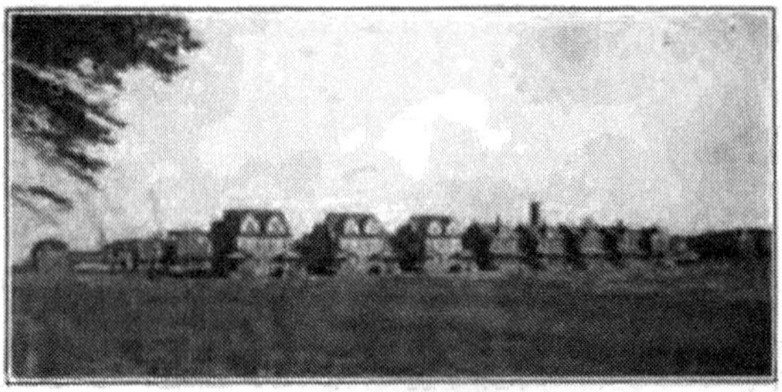

View on Sixth Avenue, Kinkora.

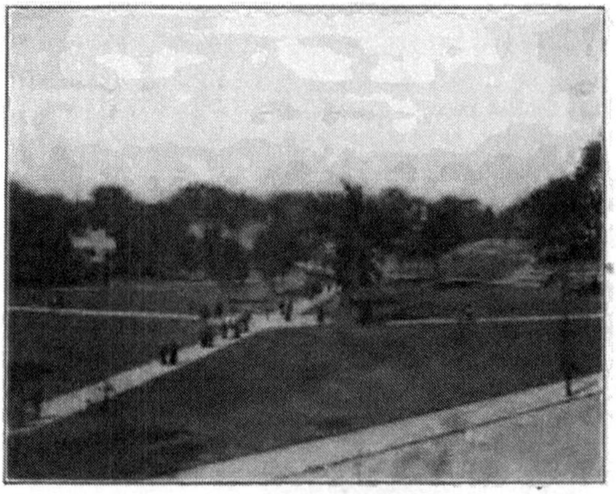

Some of the Employés' Homes Facing the Common at the Ludlow Manufacturing Associates

has been planned to remedy some defect in a previous plan, to incorporate some improvement suggested, or to lessen the cost of construction. The tenants have been asked for criticisms and suggestions, which have been acted upon when approved. Different families have different ideas. Some prefer stairs opening from the kitchen, some from a front hall, some wish the bath rooms upstairs, and others downstairs; hence a variety of plans for dwellings of substantially the same size and cost has been followed. In planning these houses the following considerations have been constantly in mind. Economy of room, economy of heating, economy of work in the care of house and children, the largest available amount of sunlight, economy of cost and simple and well proportioned outlines.

The earlier experiments made by this company in the building of homes for its working people were regarded as failures. Shortly after the acquisition of its property at Ludlow the company erected a few cottages which seem to have been planned more with reference to outside appearance than to meet the requirements of the occupants. Moreover, these houses were found to be too expensive for the class of people they were intended to shelter, and in many cases they were not properly cared for by the tenants. The company next constructed a number of large tenement houses—some accommodating as many as eight families—but they proved even more unsatisfactory than the single cottages and the plan was soon abandoned. After a careful study of the matter a second and successful attempt was made to introduce individual houses, these being simply but conveniently constructed and renting for a comparatively low sum. For several years all houses constructed by the company conformed to this general plan, with the exception of a few two-tenement houses, containing four rooms each, with separate front and rear entrances, which were built for the sake of economy in providing small flats for newly married couples.

With the large increase in population during recent years, however, it was found that the construction of so many single cottages was tending to spread the village over too large an area, and in order to economize space and also to give a choice in the selection of a home, a block of six-room and nine-room houses was built, also 24 suites of rooms, some of them over stores, and some in a separate block, each apartment or house having a bath room. It is stated that the apartments at the present time seem to be unpopular, apparently because it is the fashion in the village to have a separate cottage and operatives who have lived in flats in other villages refuse to accept a better one in Ludlow, and demand a cottage.

The houses are neat and substantial structures, of pleasing architectural design and with attractive surroundings. Almost all are two stories in height, well finished, painted within and without, and supplied with running water and other modern conveniences. A cooking range and a sink are found in the kitchen, while a large cellar furnishes a place for storing fuel and provisions. The houses are warm and comfortable, well lighted and ventilated and convenient in arrangement throughout. The monthly rental with bath varies from $6 for a four-room apartment in a large double house to $9 for an eight-room cottage. To this must be added a charge of $1.25 per month for full water privileges, making the total rent $7.25 and $10.25, respectively.

The paper mills operated by S. D. Warren & Company [1] afford employment to about 1200 persons, representing approximately 400 families. The larger part of these are now owners of their own homes, having been able to save sufficient means to build for themselves. In this they have been encouraged and helped by the company, which considers home-ownership a very important factor in promoting the welfare and contentment of the workingman.

Although most of the houses built by this company were erected a number of years ago, and consequently are lacking in some of the features possessed by more recently constructed buildings, they are, nevertheless, tasteful and conveniently arranged. One type of house built by this company is one and one-half stories in height and is built of wood with brick foundation. The interior accommodations consist of a hallway, a parlor, a dining room, and a kitchen on the first floor, and four sleeping rooms of fair size and a smaller chamber on the second floor. A porch over which the upper story projects,

[1] S. D. Warren & Co. Manufacturers Paper and Pulp. Cumberland Mills, Me. Organized 1854. Number Employés, 1200.

occupies one corner of the house. The interior is neatly papered in attractive patterns, the floors and woodwork being finished in oil or painted. The kitchen is provided with a hinged table and a sink, and each bedroom has a large clothes press. A cellar with cemented floor serves as a storeroom for fuel and provisions. In this is located the water closet, which connects with the sewer outside. Kerosene is used for lighting and coal and wood for heating and cooking. Garbage is deposited in a can provided for the purpose and is removed at stated periods. The exterior of the house is kept neat and attractive in appearance by the company, which also sees that the interior is in proper condition before a tenant moves in. If any changes or repairs are made while the tenant is occupying the building he must bear the expense.

The lot upon which this house stands has a frontage of 50 feet and is 100 feet in depth. The building occupies 720 square feet, leaving a considerable space at the side and rear for yard and garden. The rental is fixed at $9.35 per month, including full water privileges. As the value of the house is estimated at $1500, not including the land, this is considered a very moderate return to the company on the investment. The rent is calculated on the following basis:

Five per cent. of $1500 (value)	$ 75.00
Taxes	22.00
Water	10.00
Insurance	1.50
Total	$108.50

The same rule is applied in determining the rental of other houses.

Another type of house similar as to general plan and interior arrangement, but differing somewhat externally, contains two rooms on the lower floor and four chambers above. The common kitchen or living room of these houses is quite large, and they have always been quite popular with the operatives. The rental with water is $8.17 per month.

A number of dwellings owned by the employés of the company were built under the following conditions: Believing it better policy to encourage operatives to acquire homes of their own than to build and rent them, the company some years ago purchased a tract of unimproved land in the vicinity of the mills, put in sewers and other improvements, laid out streets, and sold lots to employés at a price which did not more than cover the cost of the land with its improvements. Money for the construction of houses was advanced at 4 per cent. interest, building plans were furnished free of cost, and each worthy employé was given an opportunity of securing a home, even when he had nothing to offer in the way of security. Under this plan nine houses, ranging in value from $1500 to $3000 were erected, and the scheme would probably have had a much larger development but for the fact that shortly after it was put into operation an electric road was built through the village, connecting it with Portland a few miles away. This road had the effect of concentrating the building improvements of the village along its line and rendering the company's property, which was somewhat remote, less attractive to the operatives than it would otherwise have been.

In 1895 the company owned 96 houses, with a total estimated valuation of $150,000. Of this number 12 contained four rooms, 8 five rooms, 30 six rooms, 39 seven rooms, 3 eight rooms, 3 nine rooms and 1 twelve rooms each. In addition there were two boarding houses, with 15 and 20 rooms respectively, for the accommodation of unmarried employés.

These dwellings are seldom vacant, and there is practically no loss of rental. A most generous policy is observed by the company in dealing with its tenants. Ejection is never permitted. When a tenant is sick and unable to meet his payments, he is allowed to defer them until such time as may suit his convenience. Sub-renting is not permitted, but tenants may receive boarders if they desire. The company states that houses for one family have given the greatest degree of satisfaction and that they are the ones preferred by employés.

In the early days of the Waltham Watch Company's existence many houses, mostly of modest proportions but sufficiently ample for the demands of the times, were constructed and rented to the company's employés at very reasonable prices. The company had at that time a large amount of unoccupied land, much of which had been laid out in streets and building lots, on which the houses were erected. In that way, in connection with private enterprise, sufficient accommodations were provided for the families of employés. With the growth and development of the watch industry in Waltham the demand for houses increased, and the liberal wages paid enabled many employés to build homes for themselves, and on a scale of much greater expense than those originally built, the value of many of them, including the ground, ranging from $2000 to $5000. In this way practically all of the land owned by the company was sold and built upon. Nearly all of the houses erected by the company have since been purchased either by the occupants or by those desiring investment.

Although the Waltham Watch Company does not at the present time give its attention to the building of dwellings for its employés, it has for many years maintained a large boarding house, erected for the accommodation of its unmarried female employés. The present structure is the result of additions made to the building erected by the company in 1865 for the purpose of providing comfortable housing facilities for such employés at the lowest possible cost.

The original building was two and one-half stories in height, but with the growth and development of the company's business and the introduction of modern methods of manufacture, permitting the employment of a much larger proportion of female help than formerly, the need of making a greater provision for the comfortable housing of that class of labor became apparent. To meet this need and also to insure against an unreasonable price for girls' board on the part of private boarding houses, the company greatly enlarged the old building, furnished it throughout and fixed the price for board easily within the reach of all. The "Adams House," as it is called, is a roomy four-story wooden structure, with a wide piazza in front, and surrounded by well-kept and attractive grass plots. The sleeping rooms, of which there are at present 67, are plainly but comfortably furnished, well lighted, well ventilated and heated by steam. The usual furnishings are provided: a table, a washstand, a chest of drawers with looking glass, an arm chair, a rocker and an ordinary chair, and a broad comfortable bed.

A small closet serves for keeping trunks and clothes, and on the walls, which are neatly papered, are a few pictures. Each of these rooms is occupied by two young women, who are expected to keep them in good condition, and are encouraged to adorn them with engravings, books and growing flowers. At the present time two near-by houses are leased to furnish additional dormitories for those who desire to board at the house, even though they are compelled to room outside.

The dining hall is capable of accommodating all the boarders at once. In all, meals are served to about 300 persons.

In the summer of 1907, Joseph Bancroft & Sons Company, Wilmington, opened Rockford Hall, a boarding house for the girls employed in their mills. This building is 100 feet long by 30 feet wide and three stories in height. On the first floor there are a large living room, with open fireplace, reading room, matron's office and a large dining room and kitchen. On the second and third floors are fifteen bedrooms each. Each of these bedrooms contains two single iron beds and a stationary washstand with hot and cold water. Besides the beds each room is supplied with a bureau and a rocking chair. There are bath and toilet rooms on each floor, and the whole house is lighted by electricity and heated by steam. The floors all over the house are oiled and waxed, and have rugs on them. The living room is a very attractive room, furnished with mission furniture. In the basement is provided a well-equipped laundry, which the girls have the privilege of using without extra charge.

While the John B. Stetson Company, Philadelphia, organized in 1865, does not build houses to rent to its employés, it has encouraged saving and home-building among them in the strongest possible way. For some years it has offered to its employés as a reward for efficient service shares in a building and loan association conducted under the auspices of the company, upon which money for the purchase of homes (but for no other purpose) can be borrowed at any time. These shares, which are paid for and carried to maturity by the company without any cost whatever to the holder, are designed to take the place of extra wages, and are given only to such operatives as show unusual efficiency in their work. The number of employés for whom such stock was maintained at the date of the last report was 203, the total number of shares being 1418, and the largest number held by one person 30. Twenty-eight homes have been acquired by employés under the operation of this plan. In addition to these, this association, which was organized in 1879, has been the means through which all houses have been purchased with stock maintained by employés themselves, and 24 with old shares matured, making a total of 63 homes up to the present time secured through the medium of the building and loan association. It is stated that 15 per cent. of the adult male employés of the company now own their own homes, while 289 now hold shares in the association. The total deposits of the saving fund are $35,685.98, on which interest is paid at the rate of 5 per cent.

The village of Leclaire, founded in 1890 by N. O. Nelson, occupies a tract of land containing 125 acres, adjacent to Edwardsville, Ill., and about 18 miles northeast of St. Louis, Mo. Believing that nothing contributes so greatly to the welfare and contentment of the American workingman as the possession of a comfortable home, this company endeavors to provide houses for its employés on terms that put them within the reach of all who desire them. The price charged for land, including improvements, varies from $2 to $2.50 per front foot. To this is added 6 per cent. interest dating from 1892. The company builds the houses on plans mutually agreed upon and charges for them the cost of raw material and labor, plus the average profit made by the manufacturing business. As the firm has its own planing mills and wood-working force, the net cost of a house to the purchaser is considerably less than if bought in the usual way. Payments are made monthly, the amounts varying from $12 to $20, according to the price of the house, the wages of the buyer and the size of his family. The attempt is made to provide a house for every one desiring it and to make the payments such as he can afford. The company states that no difficulty has ever been experienced in keeping up the installments. In the event the purchaser desires to remove and dispose of his property, the company voluntarily refunds the amount paid for the house, after deducting therefrom rent for the time occupied. There is no intention to provide houses for rent, except in a few cases for temporary occupancy. These bring from $8 to $12 per month.

No particular style of architecture has been adopted, but all the houses are planned to meet the requirements of good taste, economy and convenience. Electric lights, plumbing of the most approved type and an abundance of pure running water are provided. Householders are charged $5 per year for full water privileges, including sprinkling and irrigation, and 25 cents per month for lights. Nearly all of the houses are built on lots containing one-third of an acre of ground, and are placed at a sufficient distance from the street to allow for ample front yards. A large steam-heated greenhouse, maintained by the company, supplies residents with plants and flowers free of charge for beautifying the grounds surrounding their homes. The winding cinder roads, bordered with spreading shade trees, the groups of ornamental shrubbery and plants and the carefully cultivated flower beds in and about the factory grounds and parks give the place an attractiveness rarely to be found in a manufacturing community. Employés may here enjoy the advantages of a city with the freedom and economy of country life. All who wish can keep their own poultry and cow, grow their own vegetables and fruits and yet live within easy reach of their place of employment.

Although the company spares no effort to render Leclaire an attractive place in which to live, it does not require its employés to reside there. Many have homes in the adjoining town of Edwardsville, where they constitute a most important and progressive element of the population. On the other hand, a considerable number of persons living in the village are not employed by the company, being attracted thither by the numerous advantages offered all residents.

The plan of providing dwellings for their employés was first adopted by the Westinghouse Air Brake Company[1] some 12 or 13 years ago at the time of the removal of its factory from Allegheny to Wilmerding. A tract of unoccupied land adjoining the works was purchased, upon which the company

[1] Westinghouse Air Brake Co., Pittsburg, Pa. Manufacturers Air Brakes and Air Brake Apparatus. Organized 1869. Number Employés, 3000 to 4000.

constructed a number of houses very economically by making large contracts at cash prices. The houses were then sold to the employés at about cost and upon terms which enabled them to pay for the properties in monthly installments extending over a period of ten or fifteen years. In this way a number of houses were acquired by the better class of operatives; but the plan was afterwards abandoned, as it was found that the liberality of the terms induced purchases by persons who had not previously formed the habit of saving and who found it very difficult to keep up with their payments, especially during slack times. Under the plan now in force the purchaser of any property is required to pay about one-fifth of the purchase money in cash upon delivery of deed. He then executes a purchase money mortgage, payable in five years, with interest payable quarterly at the rate of 5 per cent. per annum. While no requirement is made, it is expected that the purchaser shall reduce the principal of the mortgage quarterly by such payments on account as he may be able to make. This plan enables him during hard times to keep the transaction in good shape by merely paying interest, while, on the other hand, when good wages are earned, he can discharge such part of the principal of his mortgage as he may desire.

The houses built by this company are of excellent construction and most pleasing architectural style. Among the best of the different classes of houses is a two-story brick dwelling, containing seven rooms, including the attic, renting for $22 per month. Another class of dwellings is built to accommodate two families. This is in the nature of a double house, each side having six rooms besides the attic, and renting for $18 per month. Each tenement has a hallway, a large parlor, a dining room and a kitchen on the first floor, while the second floor consists of three bedrooms, one 13 by 14 feet, the other two of fair size and a well-arranged bath room. The attic measures about 20 feet square, making a convenient place for storage purposes, while a large cellar, extending under the entire house, affords ample room below ground.

A row of brick buildings contains a number of tenements, ten in all, each having seven rooms and being provided with separate entrances both front and rear. The first story contains a hallway, a living room or parlor, a kitchen and a bath room. On the second floor are three large bed chambers, while two or more rooms are finished off in the attic. Each tenement is provided with a good cellar. The rental of these houses is $16 per month, with the exception of those on the corners, which rent for $18 a month. All of the houses are equipped with gas ranges for the use of natural gas, hot and cold water, porcelain-lined bath tubs, inside lavatories and electric light fixtures. Some have gas furnaces for heating, while others have open fireplaces for gas. All have slate roofs.

The company has also built a series of several cottage flats for the use of small families. These buildings of which seven have been erected, contain ten flats of three rooms and a bath on the first floor, and ten flats of four rooms and a bath on the second floor, with separate entrances to each. Each is provided with a good cellar and some of the more recently constructed ones have wide porches at the back. These flats are well constructed and have proved quite popular, the moderate rent asked putting them within the reach of many who could not pay the prices charged for the larger and more expensive houses.

A number of frame dwellings of different types have also been built at different times. These rent at prices ranging from $14 to $22 per month. The lots upon which these houses are located are from 30 to 40 feet in frontage and from 100 to 120 feet in depth. Practically all houses have bath rooms and a number are heated by furnaces as well as by fireplaces.

The Colorado Fuel and Iron Company, which operates a large number of coal, iron and other mines scattered throughout Wyoming, Colorado, Utah and New Mexico, in addition to rolling mills at Laramie, a huge steel plant at Pueblo and two railway systems and whose pay rolls carry the names of nearly 15,000 employés, has for a number of years been directing its efforts in a practical and intelligent manner toward bettering the condition of the vast army of people dependent on its various enterprises for support.

Among the numerous measures adopted for the accomplishment of this end, is the substitution by the company of neat and comfortable dwellings for the usual squalid and unsanitary miners' shacks. Numbers of such houses have been constructed by the company at all of its leading mining camps and manufacturing centers, forming, by their varied color and design, most picturesque and attractive villages.

At Coalbasin, in 1901, the company erected over 70 cottages. They are warm and comfortable, containing from 3 to 6 rooms, plastered and finished throughout in modern style. At Segundo about 150 houses have recently been completed. These are all plastered and neatly finished within, provided with porches and projecting eaves, and painted in varied and harmonious colors. Arranged in regular order upon streets, they appear to decided advantage by the side of the older and more poorly disposed dwellings of the place.

The group of dwellings erected at Jansen, Las Animas County, for the occupancy of the company's railway employés is also worthy of mention.

The houses usually contain from 4 to 6 rooms each, and, while very simple in arrangement and architectural effect, they are comfortable, convenient, sanitary and homelike. The price charged for rent is uniform throughout all the camps, $2 a room per month, or $8 for a 4-room house.

In a number of camps the company has erected houses for the accommodation of teachers of the public schools and kindergartens which are intended to serve as models for camp housekeepers and to furnish a center for sociological work. In these the teachers have as many rooms reserved for their use as are needed, leaving the remainder of the house to the occupancy of the family in order that the teachers may not live entirely alone. At Redstone a small cottage has been set apart as a special object lesson to employés. It is furnished throughout in inexpensive but artistic style and is designed to show how much can be accomplished in the way of making a home attractive with small outlay of time and money. "Casa Vivienda," at Pueblo, is another example of the model home. The style and size of the houses vary according to the class of employés for which they are intended.

The Cactus Inn, a two-story, 50-room bunk-house, provided with shower baths on each floor, for housing single men, was built by the Newhouse Company.[1] Separate from this is an-

[1] Newhouse Mines and Smelters. Engaged in Mining and Milling Copper. Organized 1903. Number Employés, 500.

other building, containing a dining room having a capacity to seat 100 men, a large kitchen, beneath which is a vegetable cellar and opening from the kitchen is a large bake-oven and also a large ice box built on the outside of the building. Above the kitchen are five rooms and shower bath for use of the kitchen crew. Forty-seven cottages were erected, ranging from three to six rooms each, furnished with water, shower baths and electric light; rentals varying from ten to twenty dollars per month for each.

Like other brick manufacturers, the Sayre & Fisher Company [1] was in the habit of housing its unmarried men in boarding houses with rooms containing from 60 to 80 men. In 1897 it decided to do something toward bettering their condition and erected a large cooking department equipped with every modern appliance necessary to cook by steam. Large dining and storage rooms were erected at the same time, and all these structures were lined with enameled brick and the floors laid in tiles, thus insuring the possibility of perfect cleanliness. In addition to these structures a new and very large dormitory was erected, containing 50 rooms arranged to accommodate four beds to a room. Each man is given a key to his apartment in the dormitory. On the first floor of this building is a room arranged with all necessary conveniences for washing. The walls are lined with enameled brick and floor with tile. A degree of cleanliness and personal comfort hitherto unknown in the lives of men who work at brick-making has thus been provided for the employés of this company through the medium of these improvements, and there is every reason to believe that the employés appreciate the change, and that the firm is well pleased with the results.

Each married man employed at the Briarcliff Farms [2] as far as possible is provided with a house, which he is given every inducement to keep as neat and clean as possible. The unmarried men are almost all housed in a large building called

[1] Sayre & Fisher Co., Sayreville, N. J. Manufacturers of Brick. Organized 1887. Number Employés, 1460.

[2] Briarcliff Farms, Briarcliff Manor, N. Y. Dairy Farming. Organized 1907. Number Employés, 150.

Dalmeny, which is a large dormitory for housing the single men who work on the place, and in construction is very much like the Mills Hotels in New York, after which it was modeled. The men eat in a common mess hall, have common reading and sitting rooms, and each man has a bedroom to himself, with a window in it and a place for his clothes.

It is a rule of the place, well known to all, that "cleanliness is next to godliness," and on first entering the building one is confronted with a row of wash-basins, placed invitingly for him so that he experiences the least inconvenience possible in washing his hands if they need it, and they always do.

The four mills operated by the Pelzer Manufacturing Company,[1] with 110,000 spindles and a full complement of looms, constitute one of the largest cotton manufacturing plants in the South. The number of employés approximates 2800, all of whom reside in houses which are the property of the mill corporation. These cottages, of which there are about 1000 in the place, contain an average of four rooms each. The main rooms are usually 16 feet square, while the back or shed rooms measure about 14 by 16 feet. The yards are ornamented with flowers and shrubs, and each house is provided with a plat of ground sufficiently large for gardening purposes. Tenants are required to keep their premises in good, clean condition, and prizes are offered by the company for the most attractive looking cottages and yards.

Water is supplied to employés free of charge and a large tract of meadow land is set apart for the pasturing of cows. All sanitary and street work is paid for by the company, which spares no effort to render life in the village pleasant and attractive to its inhabitants.

The rental of the houses has been fixed at 50 cents per room per month, or $2 for an ordinary cottage. This rate, it is stated, is barely sufficient to pay taxes and repairs and yields the company no return whatever on the money invested. While it is true that these dwellings are far inferior in construction to those of a representative industrial community in the North, at the same time it is claimed that they are amply sufficient

[1] Pelzer Manufacturing Co., Pelzer, S. C. Cotton Manufacturers. Organized 1881. Number Employés, 2800.

to meet the requirements of those who occupy them, the mild climate and somewhat primitive methods of life prevailing in this section rendering more elaborate housing facilities unnecessary.

Aside from its extensive manufacturing operations, begun in 1887, the Maryland Steel Company, Baltimore, has devoted much attention to the subject of providing comfortable and sanitary houses for the people in its employ. A large tract of land, embracing several hundred acres adjacent to the mill property, has been laid out in streets and building lots, upon which the company has erected about 800 houses for the accommodation of the employés. These are neat frame and brick structures, as a rule two stories or more in height and equipped with baths and underground sewerage. Artesian water of the purest quality is supplied to all the houses. A few of the buildings are of the tenement house type, but by far the greater part are individual cottages, well finished throughout and painted in attractive colors. The number of rooms varies from five to six in the smaller dwellings to twelve or fifteen in the larger, a few houses containing an even greater number of rooms. As the monthly rental of these houses averages less than $2 per room, it is seen that the company receives but a moderate return from the money invested, after deducting the necessary expenses for taxes and repairs. About 50 per cent. of the men employed in the works occupy homes which are the property of the company, the remainder coming daily by rail and trolley car from Baltimore and intervening points.

Practically all of the dwellings of the Niagara Falls Power Company,[1] about 100 in number, are occupied by officers and employés of the industries located on its lands and using the power generated by it. The architecture of these houses combines a general uniformity of design with a pleasing variety in form and detail. All are painted in the colors adopted by the company (yellow and white) and present a very attractive appearance. The rentals charged by this com-

[1] Niagara Falls Power Co., Niagara Falls, N. Y. Engaged in Developing Hydraulic and Electrical Energy and Distributing the Latter. Organized March 31, 1886. Number Employés, 190.

pany range, according to the size and construction of the houses, from $9 up.

These houses vary greatly in size and general interior arrangement, some being individual cottages containing from five to eight rooms each, with bath and cellar, and generally heated by furnace; others being in the nature of double and three-tenement houses, the former having six rooms, with bath, furnace and cellar, and the latter having five rooms without bath; while still others are designed to accommodate four families. Separate front and rear entrances are provided in all double and three-tenement houses, and all houses are furnished with electric lights, water and other modern conveniences.

The lots are generally about 115 feet deep, affording ample room for yards and lawns. All houses are placed 20 feet back from the street line, the intervening space being covered with flowers and grass. The streets are usually 50 feet in width, with macadamized roadway of 25 feet in the center and rows of shade trees on either side.

It is the intention of the company, as soon as the character of the settlement is firmly established, to give its tenants an opportunity to purchase their homes on easy terms, thus avoiding the evils which have at times resulted from the too positive application of the proprietary system.

The provision of dwelling houses for the employés of the J. B. and J. M. Cornell Company [1] was comparatively a new undertaking for this company. Prior to the removal of their works from New York City in 1898, the need of making such provision was not apparent. But with the establishment of the plant at Coldspring it was found necessary to provide more comfortable homes for the workingmen than could be found at the place, especially as practically all available houses had been taken up.

The dwellings were designed by the president of the company, Mr. J. M. Cornell, and while they were built with economy, in order that the price of rent might put them within the reach of the great mass of the employés, much care and

[1] J. B. & J. M. Cornell Co., New York City. Iron and Steel for Buildings. Organized 1847. Number Employés, 1500.

thought were given in order to secure the comfort of those for whose use they were built.

Every house has a good cellar in which is installed a furnace. The first floor consists of a hallway, parlor, dining room and kitchen, the latter containing a range and is supplied with hot and cold water. On the second floor are four large bedrooms, with closets and bath rooms with exposed plumbing. A well ventilated attic over these bedrooms insures comfort during the heated season.

The houses are all painted white for the first story, the shingles on the second story and those on the roof being stained in various and harmonious colors, so that each house is different from the others in appearance. The lots upon which they are situated measure about 50 by 80 feet each, and are ornamented with attractive flower beds and hedges in front and by trees planted between the houses. The beauty of the surroundings is much enhanced by the rows of wide-spreading shade trees bordering the highway in front.

The rent of the cottages is $12 and $15 per month. This price yields the company only about 5 per cent. on the investment. They are within easy walking distance of the company's works and are much sought after by the employés.

The first houses of the Plymouth Cordage Company contained groups of five and eight tenements under one roof, These tenements contained a living room 9 feet 11 inches by 12 feet 1 inch; kitchen 13 feet 8 inches by 14 feet 5 inches with entry 5 feet 7 inches by 9 feet 6 inches; two rooms 12 feet 1 inch by 15 feet and 14 feet 5 inches by 15 feet, both with large closets. The houses were situated within five feet of the road, allowing only a small front yard. Each house was allotted a garden, where, during the summer, the employés could raise their own vegetables. The only plumbing in these houses consisted of one sink situated in the small entry. The rent was from $1.50 to $1.75 per week. With the building of the new houses the old type was discarded, and on the new tract of land which was purchased, lots were laid off about 100 feet wide and 150 feet deep. Two-family houses were then planned and built along more modern lines. They are far more picturesque than the old ones, and lend themselves to more individual treatment.

They contain on the first floor, kitchen, 13 feet 2 inches by 16 feet 6 inches; parlor 10 feet by 12 feet 6 inches; dining room 11 feet 1 inch by 12 feet 3 inches and bathroom 5 feet by 7 feet. Upstairs, one type has four bedrooms, another three and another two. These houses are situated about 30 feet from the road, giving them sufficient lawn in front, which lends itself to adornment with flower beds or shrubbery. In the rear is the garden, also hen yards, with ample space for the clothes yard. They are built of wood and shingled, and range in rental price from $1.90 to $2.50 a week per tenement. At present a few houses are built along these lines which rent at about the same price as the old tenement blocks, $1.50 to $1.75.

In noting the advantages to the community from the location of a large industry in its midst, may be instanced the action of the Niagara Falls Power Company, which opened a large building on one of the principal thoroughfares of the village for a general store on the lower floor, while the upper story has been handsomely fitted up as a public hall, which has been placed at the service of the residents of the village. The company has also built an attractive railway station on the line of the New York Central and Hudson River Railroad and has erected a large plant for the disposal of the village sewage.

A description of the excellent drainage and sewage system of the village may be of interest, by reason of the peculiar physical conditions encountered in its construction and may offer suggestions for other new and growing communities. Quoting from an article by John Bogart:

"The tract of land upon which the village is located contains about 84 acres and is of oblong shape, being about 3000 feet long in a direction parallel with the Niagara river and about 1500 feet in width. The whole area of the village, as well as that of the land between it and the river, distant about 1000 feet at its nearest point, is very flat and slopes very slightly to the river bank. An extreme surface variation of only 4 feet was noted over the whole 84 acres of meadow land upon which the village now stands. The average level of the river is about 3 feet lower than the lower parts of the village, but the water of the river occasionally rises to very near this elevation. It was therefore impracticable to carry the drainage of these grounds to the river with sufficient fall in pipes and gutters to quickly relieve the surface from the water of rainfalls, while to conduct the requisite sub-drainage directly to the river was simply impossible. The character of the soil, which consists of a few inches of surface loam overlying a stratum of hard, tenacious clay, with rock foundation, rendered the ground heavy and sticky during wet weather, and dry and dusty at other times. These conditions had to be removed in order to provide for the smooth roads, grassy lawns, trees and flower gardens contemplated in the plans. Moreover, with the coming of the colonists, ground in such a condition would have proved a fertile field for the spread of malaria and kindred diseases. It was necessary also to provide an outlet for the sewage of the houses. As with the drainage, a direct discharge into the river was impracticable by reason of the latter's elevation. Under these circumstances a scheme was evolved by the company that has proved an entire success. The principal pipes of the drainage system follow the streets; those to convey sewage are in alleys. The latter are at a higher elevation than the drain tiles, this permitting house connection for sewage without disturbing the drainage system. The drain tiles are 2 inches in diameter, being laid about 40 feet apart and from 4 to 6 feet below the surface. They have open joints, no mortar or cement being used, but around the joints is wrapped a double thickness of cheese cloth. The 2 inch tiles deliver into lines of 3 inch tiles laid in the same way and placed generally in the streets under the grass surfaces, but so disposed as to draw the water fully from the ground under and on both sides of the paved parts. The 3 inch tiles lead at frequent intervals to receiving basins in the center of the streets, from which the effluent is conducted by lines of vitrified pipes to a large masonry well located at the sewage disposal works. From the well the drainage water is pumped directly into the outlet chamber of the disposal plant, whence it passes into two small streams flowing into the Niagara river. The whole village is underlaid by this drainage system, which has completely changed the physical and sanitary conditions of the ground, it being no longer heavy and muddy during the warm season. The level of the ground water has been lowered fully 4 feet, which is, virtually, and for all horticultural and sanitary purposes, precisely as though the whole surface had been lifted 4 feet.

"The sewage system is entirely separate and takes no storm or drainage water. The pipes, whose minimum diameter is 6 inches, have cemented joints and are flushed automatically at regular periods. Through them the sewage is conducted to a compartment in a well, whence it is pumped into an elongated tank or disposition chamber so arranged as to insure a very slow passage of the fluid. Here it is treated automatically, by the action of float valves, with milk or lime and a solution of perchloride of iron. Sedimentation and precipitation of the solids follow, floating substances being intercepted by screens. Chloride is delivered through perforated pipes near the bottom of the tank. When a certain quantity of the purified fluid has passed over a wire into a terminal tank, it flows, by siphonage, into the effluent chamber, from which, with the drainage water, it enters the stream. A second set of chambers is provided so that, while one set is in use, the deposited material in the other may be removed by a system of traveling buckets for use upon the cultivated grounds of the company. The building which shelters the well, the pumps and the disposition chambers, also contains the dynamo for the electric light service of the village."

A model cottage is situated about half a mile from a certain factory, but located in the neighborhood where many of the employés live. It is a model cottage in this regard, that each room is furnished with all the essentials of a modest simple home, such as a workman, with his wife, would expect to have at first. The price of each article is given, so that one may know exactly what it will cost. The cost of furnishing the dining room, for example, is $60.75. At the same time that the necessary furnishings are shown, comes the opportunity for the indirect surely, often the direct, teachings of a few simple æsthetic principles—that there should be an harmonious color scheme, that the furniture, while inexpensive, should correspond with the other decorations, in other words, that with the same amount of money it is possible to combine the beautiful with the useful.

The house is in charge of a woman who lives there, and is always willing and desirous of advising with the people concerning any matter which they may care to bring to her regarding their home life; in fact, she is engaged for that express purpose—a kind of house mother.

CHAPTER IX

EDUCATION

There is no doubt that employers are willing to advance their employés just as soon as they can respond to the demand for increased responsibility. Accordingly they encourage every movement which will increase the knowledge and skill of the workers, well knowing that it is to their mutual advantage. It is often necessary to initiate educational movements.

At first the village of Ludlow, Mass., contained one ungraded school with a single teacher. A large increase of operatives in 1878 required two additional teachers, whose classes were held temporarily in the church vestry. The Ludlow company then decided to build and own the schoolhouse. Accordingly, a schoolhouse containing six classrooms, a lecture hall and school parlor was built and rented to the town at the nominal sum of $100 a year. The managers had hoped to introduce instruction in cooking and sewing, but that plan was not favored by the town committee. Considerable friction arose between the corporation and the town authorities in regard to the management of the school. Finally the corporation refrained from making any attempt at improvements in the school work, but continued to give the use of the schoolhouse, and until within a few years had paid a quarter of the salaries. Two years ago the growth of the village required additional room, and an eight-room schoolhouse was built by the town. Perfect harmony now exists between the corporation and the town officers, and it is believed that suggestions from the former in regard to the management of the school would be welcomed by the town.

N. O. Nelson supports a school system which has as a fundamental principle the union of industrial training with education from books. This begins with a kindergarten, in which the children are taught, among other things, the cultivation of vegetables and flowers. Later a regular school course, supplemented by manual training, is introduced. The plan provides that boys 12 years of age shall be given light work for one hour each day in the factories or on the company's farm, for which service they receive adequate remuneration. As they grow older their hours of labor are increased and the time devoted to study correspondingly curtailed until the age of 18 is reached, when they are graduated from school and employed at full time and wages in the works of the company. Recently the plan has been adopted of admitting to the school a certain number of boys about 16 years of age, who perform manual work under the direction of teachers during half the day and devote the remaining time to study. These boys are charged nothing for tuition and are boarded at the company's expense. Boys and girls whose homes are in Leclaire or Edwardsville may attend the school without the payment of tuition fees. The school fund is endowed with $10,000 of the stock of the company, and every effort is made to provide training that will fit the pupil for the active prosecution of his chosen trade. The school building measures 40 by 50 feet and contains four large rooms and a hall. The rooms are separated by sliding partitions so that two or more can be thrown into a single hall for public gatherings, lectures and other forms of entertainment. The building also houses an excellent public library of about 1400 volumes, to which additions are constantly being made.

The system of public schools in operation at all of the leading points of the Colorado Fuel and Iron Company, maintains a uniform course of study, so that children may not be placed at a disadvantage in case of removal from one camp to another. Text books are in most cases furnished to pupils free of charge, equipment of the most approved character is provided, only the best and most capable teachers are employed and every effort is made to impart instruction of the most thorough and substantial character. Circulating art collections, reference libraries and other progressive features have been introduced into nearly all the schools, and the children have been encouraged to raise money for the purchase of pianos, books, flags, and pictures and casts for the decoration of their rooms.

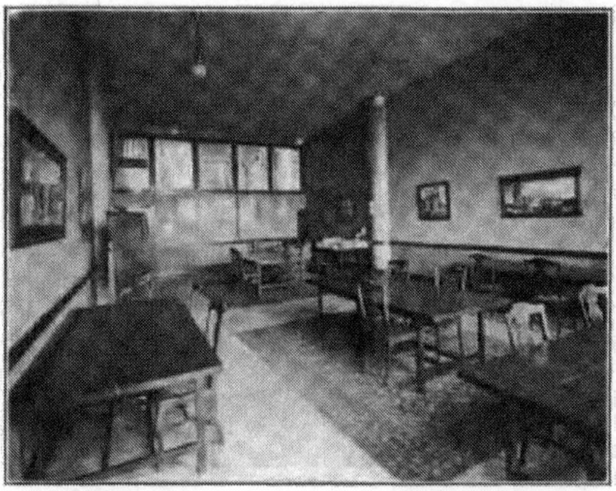

Study and Men's Rest Room at Marshall Field & Company, Chicago. The Charts in the Background Are Used for Instruction in the "Beginners' Classes."

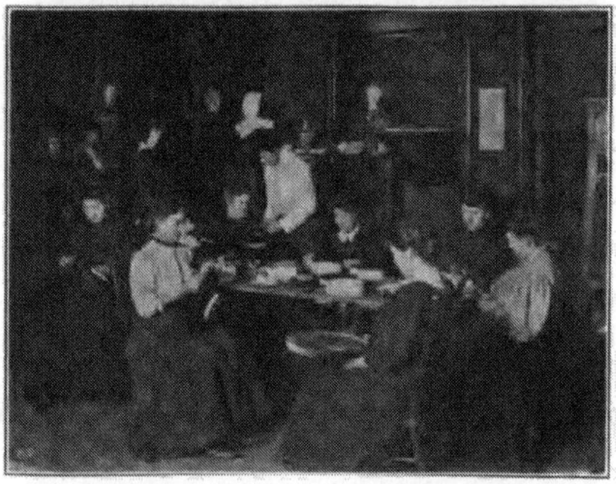

The Millinery Class at the H. J. Heinz Company.

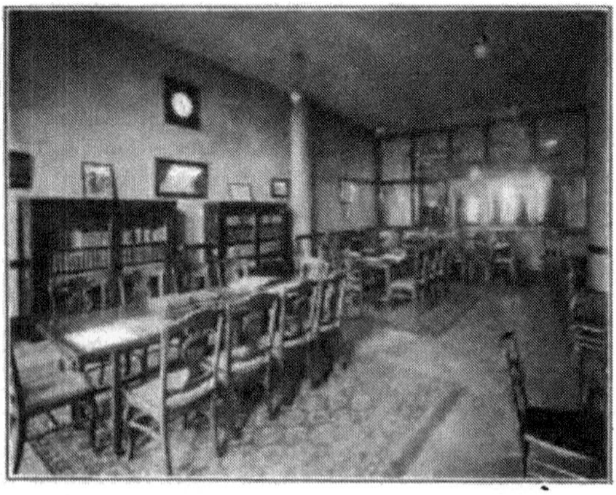

Library and Reading Room at Marshall Field & Company's, Chicago.

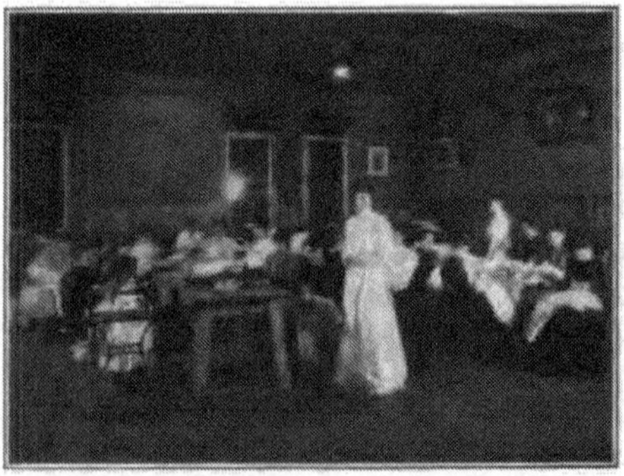

Sewing Class for the Young Ladies at the Factory of H J Heinz Company.

The school buildings are, as a rule, handsome and comfortable structures, furnished with modern appliances and well lighted and ventilated throughout. These buildings, though differing in size and in minor details of finish and ornamentation, are practically all of the same design. The schoolrooms measure about 30 by 33 feet and are calculated to seat 50 pupils each. Ceilings are 11 feet high in the lower story and 10 feet in the upper, thus providing each child with from 200 to 220 cubic feet of air. Each room has windows on the back and sides, which admit an abundance of light without injury to the eye of teacher or pupil. Folding partitions between rooms allow them to be thrown into one whenever occasion requires. Ventilation registers in the corners of each room have their flues connected with a ventilator stack in the center of the roof. A vestibule about 16 by 18 feet serves as a place for hats and coats, and rear exits on each floor afford a means of escape in case of fire.

Comfortable four-room structures have recently been completed at Primero, Segundo and Tercio. At Orient a company building has been converted into a neat and attractive schoolhouse, while at Coalbasin the building has been thoroughly remodeled and put in first-class condition throughout. At several of the newer camps company houses have been utilized for school purposes until suitable buildings could be erected. In all cases where sufficient funds for the establishment and maintenance of public schools are not available, the company willingly advances the necessary amount until the school districts can meet these expenses.

A feature of the educational system to which special emphasis is given is the kindergarten. It is recognized that this institution not only takes the child in hand at its most impressionable period, but that it furnishes a center from which radiate influences that affect the whole social betterment situation. The morning hours from 9 to 12 are devoted to the regular kindergarten work, consisting of songs, games, nature studies and various kinds of easy construction work, such as weaving rag and zephyr mats and rugs, braiding straw hats and baskets and making pieces of miniature furniture. In the afternoon the same room is utilized, under the supervision of the teacher, by classes of boys and girls engaged in weaving, basketry, carving, sewing and cooking, by physical culture clubs, mothers' clubs and other gatherings of a social or industrial nature. In the evening the room is at the disposal of adults for dances, concerts, lectures and other entertainments. A few of the kindergartens are housed in buildings erected especially for their use, but in most cases they occupy rooms in the public school.

The Pueblo Normal and Industrial School offers to teachers of the public schools and kindergartens a course of training during a portion of the summer vacation by means of which they may better equip themselves for their work. The building, which was formerly used as a hospital, has been thoroughly renovated and refitted, and, although the school is yet in the experimental stage, its good results are already becoming manifest. As an adjunct to this school there has recently been created an industrial home in which crippled employés and the widows and orphans of those who have lost their lives in the company's service are given the means of earning a livelihood. In it the young are to be given an opportunity to learn a trade, the adults to work upon whatever they can do best and to receive therefor the highest possible prices. Mattresses of excellent quality are already being turned out, and it is the intention to begin at an early date the manufacture of brooms, brushes, rugs, laces, hammocks and other articles. It is planned that the institution shall become eventually self-sustaining and, though yet in its infancy, much good is expected from its establishment. The Polytechnic club rooms are also located in this building. The membership of this club is made up largely of engineers from the Minnequa Steel Works.

In a number of the camps night schools have been established which are well attended, particularly by the foreign employés. The branches taught are the English language, reading, writing and arithmetic and in some cases history and geography. These schools are self-sustaining, each pupil being charged $1 per month to cover the cost of tuition, light and fuel. Circulating libraries have been placed in most of the communities where they are proving a powerful factor for intellectual and moral development. Each library contains fifty volumes of fiction, history, biography and travel and the boxes are exchanged often enough to keep each camp provided with a fresh supply of books.

Thus the company aids the public schools very materially by equipping them with excellent buildings and furniture and the securing of the best possible teachers. Night schools are also supported wherever the demand is manifest.

Thirteen kindergartens are also under the direct charge of this sociological department, and thus add a year to the school life of the miners' children. Special instruction is also given in domestic science and manual training. Popular lecture courses are also conducted throughout the winter months, which are designed to entertain as well as to instruct, and in which the stereopticon plays a very important part.

In 1902 a movement was started among the joint Westinghouse interests at East Pittsburg, for the social betterment of the community. A committee composed of six persons, selected from the various departments of both companies, was organized into a board of directors with full power to operate and maintain an eating house, a place of amusement and a night school.

The Casino Technical Night School began at East Pittsburg in 1902, but in the fall of 1904 it was moved to the public school building of Turtle Creek, in the heart of a valley having a population of 25,000. It is ten minutes' walk from the main entrance of the Westinghouse Electric and Manufacturing Company, the Westinghouse Machine Company at East Pittsburg and the Westinghouse Air Brake Company at Wilmerding, which employ together about 14,000 men. The rooms are large and commodious, well lighted, heated and ventilated.

The Casino Technical Night School offers for a small fee an opportunity of learning the fundamentals of engineering work. It presents an education to those who are not in a position to devote daytime to study—it enables them to secure the essentials of both the theory and the practice of engineering that they may apply these things in their daily work in the shortest possible time. The Casino student is a busy man during the day, spending little more than one-seventh as much time in school as the college student.

With the time available the students of the Casino Technical Night School do the work thoroughly as far as outlined in the catalogue, which does not purport to be a finished engineering course. It furnishes, however, a most excellent foundation in mathematics and the fundamental principles of electrical and steam engineering, upon which it is possible for one to build his own technical education. It is desired that at least some of the graduates will find the opportunity to continue their studies in some of the large technical institutions of the country. The object in attending school is to learn how to work to a better advantage to society and one's self. To learn that which best develops manly character and makes men useful to their fellow men is, in the end, the highest aim of the Casino Technical Night School.

All the courses of instruction are conducted by men who are actively engaged in practical work—men who for the most part have had a college education—men who know the kind of men wanted in the world of industry, and who are therefore able to appreciate what is best for the individual student.

During the school year a series of lectures are given on general engineering and educational topics. Arrangements are made with some of the companies in and about Pittsburg whereby classes will be permitted to visit their works and factories. As nearly as possible the inspectional visits occur on Saturday afternoons, and on such evenings as do not interfere with regular school work.

Tuition for the regular course is ten dollars a term, which is less than nine cents per lesson of one hour period. Tuition for the preparatory course is eight dollars. Each student is required to provide himself with the necessary text books, drawing instruments and stationery. Any student finding it necessary to discontinue his work during the term will be given an opportunity to personally present his case to the president, and if it is found justifiable, a proportionate rebate will be allowed.

The preparatory department is organized to give the students a better understanding of mathematics, before entering the field of more complex science. By getting a good foundation in arithmetic, the student will be better prepared to do work in physics and electricity.

The Casino Technical Night School affords the non-technical apprentices and other employés an opportunity to obtain a good theoretical training in mechanical and electrical engineering and shop practice. Workmen completing the mechanical or electrical course are considered sufficiently qualified to take up the engineering apprenticeship course. The trades apprentices are advised to pursue a course of home study or attend the Casino schools.

The course in practical engineering is designed to give a clear understanding of the operation of the various forms of the fundamental electrical apparatus together with the principles of the steam engine and a working knowledge of structure and structural materials. By completing this course the student should be well prepared to enter the field of steam and electric installation, testing, operation of power stations, wiring, inspecting, general road work and various assistantships.

The graduating student, however, should bear in mind that he is but entering the field of engineering and should not only be willing to enter practical activity at its lowest round, but should seek such opportunities for getting a broad view of his profession and for studying details and increasing his resourcefulness and self-reliance as are afforded by the various apprenticeship courses.

The manner of teaching is by text books and lectures, on which a certain amount of class recitation is expected. In problem work, much importance is put upon the developing and the stating of a problem from a collection of data or assumed conditions. In electricity, steam, chemistry and other branches, experimental work is carried on in line with the class work. In laboratory work each student makes a report upon each experiment he performs.

A small dwelling house situated at the entrance to the Plymouth Cordage Company's factory, was turned into a school building, where a kindergarten was started under the direction of a trained kindergartner. The first year the school contained about 23 scholars, the second year about 30. The third year it was necessary to engage an assistant, the number then reaching 40. The kindergarten in many ways is a great help, not only to the children, but also to the mothers, for it takes the children away from the house in the busiest part of the day, and gives the mother time to do her work unmolested, while the children return with new ideas and brighter faces. The teachers make visits about the houses and interest the mothers in the children's work. They also bring a little social life once a month when they have mothers' meetings at Harris Hall. The largest gathering of this kind occurs at Christmas time, when the children are given a Christmas tree. The proud mothers seated about the hall, seeing their little tots marching around the tree, singing and clapping their hands, begin to smile simultaneously with the children as their little faces beam with delight at the sparkling stars and trimmings of the tree.

The second step in the school was the addition of a sloyd department, in a room with ten benches. The school at first was only for the boys who worked in the mill, the other boys of the family having the advantage in the public schools. The school is carried on four evenings a week, making forty boys enrolled in the course. Later the girls became interested in the work, so a girls' class of ten was added, making fifty in all. In connection with this work there are classes in basketry and the making of cane seats for chairs.

Another branch of the industrial work is the cooking school. The children are allowed to attend the school at the age of 11 years. The school is held in the afternoon after the public schools, from 4 to 6 o'clock. Good, plain cooking is taught—how to make a dinner from cheap cuts of meat, the proper food to buy and the correct combinations to use to build up the tissues of the body and brain. The making of bread, pastry, preserves, jellies and the preparation of cereals are also touched upon. The course in cooking is three years. Generally the girls leave then and go to work in the mill.

In the government of the town of Ludlow, the industrial home of the Ludlow Manufacturing Associates (the town being similar to that of any Massachusetts village), the Associates take no part, although practically all of the village is owned by them, and the majority of the townspeople work in the mills which are also owned by the Associates. These mills produce jute and hemp yarns and twines and also jute bagging.

The Ludlow Textile School is maintained by the Associates for the purpose of training apprentices in those branches of the textile trade in which the Associates are particularly interested. It is also the aim of the school to develop desirable law-abiding citizens of the village of Ludlow.

By dividing the training of the pupils into two classes, the practical or mill part, and the theoretical or school part, the best results may be obtained. Each boy spends five hours every workday caring for some machine or performing such other work as is assigned to him in the mill. Every three months each apprentice is transferred to another machine or to other duties which represent additional stages in the process of manufacture. In this way each boy is given the opportunity of obtaining an intimate working knowledge of the work performed in every department in the mill, from the opening of the bales of fiber to the baling of the finished product.

The mill work of these apprentices is under the supervision of the regular overseers and the work performed by the boys varies in no way, with the exception already stated, from that performed by the other employés of the mill not connected with the school. Several of these overseers are members of the evening classes maintained by the Textile School. This fact has an important bearing on the treatment of the apprentices in the mill, as these overseers feel themselves to be a part of the school, and are thus directly interested in its advancement and also in the welfare of the boys while in the mill. Each pupil works five hours, or one half a day in the mill, and also attends school three hours each day. For this he receives about three-fourths pay, that is, he is paid for both mill and school work at the same rate per hour as other mill employés engaged in similar work in the mill.

There are two classes so arranged that the work performed in the mill in the morning by one class is continued by the other class in the afternoon. By this arrangement the progress of the mill work is uninterrupted. In order that all may have equal opportunities, the classes alternate in attendance, thus the class which attends the morning session of the school and works in the mill afternoons during one week would reverse this arrangement the following week.

There are but few requirements for admission. Each boy must be between the ages of fourteen and sixteen; in good physical condition; of good moral character; and must possess a fair knowledge of English and arithmetic. It is the intention to change the latter requirement to the possession of a grammar school certificate. The expense of the physical examination, which is made by a local physician, is borne by the Associates.

The term of apprenticeship will cover a period of four years and each year a new class of boys will be admitted. At present the number of boys admitted is limited to 22, divided into two classes of 11 each. Apprentices are not required to sign a contract, and may leave the employ of the Associates at any time. In any case of this sort the pupil would also be compelled to sever his connection with the school. Although the school is primarily for the training of apprentices in the textile trade, provision will be made for those pupils who show any special aptitude for drawing, carpentry or machine work.

Instruction is also given relating to the nature and uses of different fibers, and throughout the course, special emphasis is placed upon that side of each subject which is related to mill work. Much assistance in this matter is expected from a museum which is being formed. In addition to the work outlined above, a short period each day is devoted to athletic work of a systematic character.

The regular school term will hereafter commence August 1st, and continue for eleven months with a short recess at Christmas. The month of July will be spent in camp where the boys will be removed entirely, for a time, from their home surroundings.

There are a variety of movements combining the educational and the social, the lighter or recreational phase, a kind of bait to attract the attention to the serious work or to win the young people away from other attractions which are bad for them. Again in communities where there are non-Americans the educational work is the lure, with its corrective side of amusements after the lessons.

For example, in Pueblo, the Colorado Fuel and Iron Company is fast developing into a social center with its group of resident workers, what is known as the Old Hospital building, while about it are grouped boys' and men's clubs, socials, lectures, manual training, penny savings, athletic classes, night school with other social and neighborly functions. With its beautiful grounds and wide porches there is the opportunity for a real home for fifty persons. Twelve new rooms and an attractively furnished parlor have recently been added by the remodeling of the surgical and medical wards. Four of these rooms have private porches glassed and screened. A shower bath has been installed and new furniture added. The board is $4.50 per week and the rooms range from $1 to $3 per week.

The old hospital shelters the night school, the Young Men's Social and Literary Club, the C. F. and I. Jr. Club, the Penny Savings Bank, Library, the Abriendo Tennis Club, the Junior Roycrofters and is the center of many socials, lectures and entertainments during the winter.

The night school is in session three nights each week from October to May, under the instruction of three experienced teachers. All the common branches were taught and a fee of $3 per month charged. In view of the fact that the pupils are largely foreigners engaged during the day in hard manual toil at the steel works, the attendance has been regular and results encouraging. The pupils included Americans, Austrians, English, Italians, Japanese and Mexicans.

The Ludlow Manufacturing Associates of Ludlow, Mass., employ some 700 women and girls in their mills. Many nationalities are represented, the French and Scotch predominating.

Recognizing a desire for self-government among the operatives, and desiring to foster it, the management decided to establish an experimental girls' institute, which should afford useful instruction and opportunity for rational amusement.

An unoccupied office building was remodeled, providing an attractive reception room, a sewing room, a cosy office, a kitchen and in the basement a room for physical culture.

When it was announced that all who wished to learn cooking would have an opportunity to do so, and were requested to register, more girls applied than could be accommodated at one time. They were divided into three classes, each of which received a three months' course, and each division or class, on the completion of the course, gave a luncheon to husbands, brothers and sweethearts.

The general cooking instructions are as follows: The making

and care of a coal fire and the regulating of an oven, mixing bread, washing glasses, silverware, greasy dishes, egg beaters, bread-board and bowls; simmering, boiling and steaming; measuring and mixing; care of utensils used for milk; directions for making cake; buying meat, taught by means of a diagram on which are especially pointed out the best cuts for roast beef, for braised beef, for stewing and boiling; cooking inferior cuts in the best way; choosing young and tender poultry; clarifying fat and trying out lard; cleaning, skinning and boning fish. The course includes also baking bread, boiling potatoes and eggs; steaming stale bread, baking whole wheat bread and rolls; making baked and boiled custard, creaming potatoes, baking corn muffins, broiling meat, making cup cake, frying griddle cakes, baking sponge cake, cooking chicken, making soup stock and julienne soup, frying fish, broiling mutton chops, baking soda biscuit, scalloping eggs, baking potatoes, making beef stew with dumplings and baking gingerbread.

Cooking lessons were given four evenings a week. Saturday afternoons a number of Polish girls met to learn how to make American dishes. Sewing classes also were organized, though they were not so large as the cooking classes.

While the object of The Electric Club organized March, 1902, with an initial membership of one hundred and fifty, from the apprentices and engineers of the Westinghouse Electric and Manufacturing Company is largely social, yet there are so many educational advantages, that it should be described in this chapter. It seems that out of the total membership probably not ten per cent. are in a position to feel at home in the vicinity or to enjoy the many influences, privileges and opportunities of home life. The greater number have been there but a short time, and have had little opportunity for recreative society so essential to a young man's contentment and health.

The scope of the reception committee includes the bringing of the club members together socially, the provision of games for their amusement and apparatus with which they can obtain exercise and sport, the conducting of entertainments and the fostering of clubs for special purposes other than educational.

The club has proved a decided success. The members have taken an active interest in its various lines of activity, the various officers and engineers of the Electric Company have attended the club meetings and have coöperated in its work, generous financial assistance has been received from the Westinghouse Electric and Manufacturing Company and the Westinghouse Air Brake Company.

The social functions of the club are in charge of the ladies' committee; the entertainments and social gatherings under their patronage are among the most enjoyable features.

The club is also fortunate in having the local section of the American Institute of Electrical Engineers meet in the assembly hall once a month—all privileges of the meetings being extended to the members of The Electric Club.

The club has six distinct courses of lectures scheduled at present, one of which is of a general nature given by prominent officials of the company and eminent engineers and others from the outside, while the others are on purely engineering subjects given by the various engineers in the company's employ.

The excursion committee arranges excursions to the various industrial plants in and adjacent to Pittsburg on the third Saturday afternoon of each month, and in addition, special trips on shop holidays.

These trips are arranged through the courtesy of the Westinghouse Electric and Manufacturing Company, thus insuring to the members privileges in the way of guides and special exhibits that they would not otherwise enjoy. It is intended to have at the disposal of the club members pamphlets giving a general description of the plant to be visited, stating specifically the points of special interest.

These trips are of the utmost value to persons interested in engineering, and have been well attended and very successful.

In 1906 the Westinghouse Electric and Manufacturing Company made arrangements for teaching mechanical drawing to one hundred shop men, twenty men from the mechanical and electrical engineering departments volunteering their services as teachers. The one hundred students were divided into four classes of twenty-five, one class each for Mondays, Tuesdays, Thursdays and Fridays, from 6 to 8 P. M. Wednesday is set apart for a weekly lecture to the whole school. The complete course is a progressive series on mechanical drawing and the elementary principles of mechanics and machine design.

To make the work of permanent interest and value to the students, each lesson is carefully prepared and written up in the form of a sheet of instructions and advice; these sheets are neatly illustrated, and the whole lithographed on a good quality of paper. In addition to the above, each student receives the complete Westinghouse Drawing Dictionary. A section is a small group of members constituting a "self-exciting" engineering society for the discussion of apparatus, shop methods and technical subjects under the leadership of its own members. Each section pursues a definite line of work. Six sections were formed: transformers, railway work, testing, detail apparatus, road engineering, switchboards. A fixed assignment of members is made to each section in order that the work may be definite and concrete.

"Do you know that I frequently go to that store, when I really do not need to buy anything, because it is such a pleasure to be waited on by clean, intelligent and deferential young women," said a lady in commenting on a certain department store in a large city. This state of things does not come about by chance. A concerted movement for courses in salesmanship was begun, at the request of the wholesale houses and the retail stores of Boston when the Board of Education inaugurated in the winter of 1905 evening classes for the advancement of salesmen and saleswomen. These classes were held twice a week in the Bigelow School, South Boston, under the direction of Principal F. V. Thompson and were attended by about one hundred and fifty men and women.

The object of the class was to improve the students in the art of salesmanship, and with this in view all the leading houses of Boston were asked to send a member of their firm to address the class. Mr. Clark, of Jordan, Marsh & Company, was one of the most enthusiastic lecturers and his address was listened to with a great deal of interest. He spoke principally on the personality of a salesman and his duties both toward the house and the customer. Miss Hirschler, of William Filene's Sons Company, and Mr. Fitzpatrick, of Brown, Durrell

& Company, with others, also gave very interesting talks on similar subjects.

In connection with the lectures, demonstrations were given, showing the proper method of dealing with customers in the different departments. These were particularly instructive.

The class meets through the regular evening school terms on Mondays and Thursdays at eight o'clock. The Monday lecture is by a stated lecturer; that on Thursday is by a volunteer from one of the stores—the head usually of an important department who is qualified to speak from practical knowledge of the qualifications of the ideal salesman or saleswoman.

The novelty of the course lies in the conception it establishes of a really efficient salesman and salesgirl. It is the testimony of most of the writers who have made a special study of department store employés that they are often supremely uninterested and regardless of the fact that their employer's welfare is identical with their own. Such indifference is due to the lack of broad comprehensive training, as it has not been thought worth while specially to educate six-dollar-a-week people. The more difficult branches of salesmanship have indeed for a long time been understood to require special coaching. Instruction in the use of English has been the most helpful in that it adds to the effectiveness of the saleswoman, which has a direct relation to the amount of her sales.

A saleswoman who attended the course told me, "As a member of the class I would say that I feel that I derived a great deal of benefit from these lectures and think that general stores in other cities would be making no mistake in inaugurating similar classes."

Jordan and Marsh say that while personally they have not had very much interest in it, still they have reason to believe it is a good thing, and wish that all of their salespeople could and would take advantage of the lectures and instructions of the sort given at the salesmanship school.

They have had a number of pupils from the Women's Educational and Industrial Union School of Salesmanship, who have proved very satisfactory and the firm believes that instruction of this sort on salesmanship is a good thing. There is a class at present attending this school of salesmanship, and the members are divided up among a number of different stores. "We have a number of them at present. They attend the school in the forenoon, coming to us in the afternoon each day for which we pay them, and at the end of the school term coming permanently into our employ."

The third class in salesmanship offered in active coöperation with some of the Boston department stores, opened September, 1907. Positions are guaranteed to graduates by Jordan, Marsh & Company, Shepard, Norwell Company, Gilchrist Company, Wm. Filene's Sons Company, James A. Houston Company, Chandler & Company. The length of term is four months. The class meets daily from 8:30 to 5:30, giving each morning to training in the school and the afternoon to actual practice in the stores, for which the pupils receive compensation.

An advisory committee representing the above stores meets once a month in conference with the president of the Women's Educational and Industrial Union, and the director of the school.

Practical talks by representatives of the firms interested, their buyers, assistants and superintendents, are given on a variety of topics such as "The department store system and the saleswoman's place in it," "Relation of saleswoman to her firm, fellow employé, stock and customer," "Textiles and styles." The course also includes salesmanship and the discussion of experience, study of business arithmetic, practice in writing sales slips, charge slips and rapid accounts, physical culture and hygiene as means of developing wholesome, attractive personality, material, style, line and color applied to types of figure and complexion. The pupils must be at least eighteen years of age and must have a good fundamental education. Preference will be given to mature workers who have had some business experience. Only interested earnest workers, who have been approved both by the store and by the school, will be admitted. Certificates will be given to pupils who complete the course in a satisfactory manner.

The girls at the Plymouth Cordage Company's mill formed a social club seven or eight years ago, the members then numbering between eight and ten. The girls started work in sewing, courses in English and Italian and in art. From year to year the club has grown so that now there are enrolled in its membership some 80 girls, most of whom work in the mill. However, there are a few young ladies who have had the advantages of higher education who have been induced to join. They have brought in new ideas and have helped a great deal in raising the standard of the club, for they bring to bear the influence that tends to develop the character and stimulate the desire of higher ideals in life.

A woman's league at Wanamaker's, composed of a large number of women employés, was organized for social and educational purposes. It carries on classes for chorus singing, physical culture, dancing, sewing and instruction in English, German, French and the mandolin. As part of the work of the women's league, social evenings are given once a month, at which the entertainment is a lecture, reading or music, with time for sociability and dancing afterwards. The best lecturers and musicians are obtained for these gatherings.

There is a feature which may be interesting in connection with the boys, of whom a considerable number are employed by Fels & Company, Philadelphia. Their general factory work is not of such a nature as to be of use to them in case they leave for other places. They cannot make a trade of it. Thinking something was due them, opportunity has been given to every boy that showed a desire for it, of spending one quarter of his time in the machine shop, which is well equipped for the purpose. This proportion of their time with two evenings per week at mechanical drawing enables them to learn before reaching manhood, considerable about the machinist trade, and many have gone out to take advanced positions in other shops.

The Graniteville Manufacturing Company,[1] S. C., spends annually some $2000 towards the maintenance of public schools in the towns of Graniteville and Vauclause, where their mills are located.

At Proctor, the Vermont Marble Company has constructed and maintains a Y. M. C. A. building, erected at a cost of about

[1] Graniteville Manufacturing Co., Graniteville, S. C. Manufacturers Cotton Sheetings, Shirtings and Drills. Organized 1845. Number Employés, 875.

$40,000. It is fully equipped with gymnasium, baths, bowling alleys and all the other necessary features of an up-to-date Y. M. C. A. A general secretary is always in attendance. The educational committee of the Y. M. C. A. has during the past year maintained classes for the instruction of English to Swedes, Italians, Hungarians and maintained other classes for the instruction of young men along various lines of work. If there is a sufficient demand for instruction in any subject not on the regular course, it will be provided. Physical training is also given to those who desire it, under direction of the general secretary, who acts as physical director. A baseball club is always maintained in the town of Proctor. It is the policy of the company to encourage and foster a proper spirit among its employés regarding physical exercise and games.

The Metropolitan Life Insurance Company, New York, offers instruction in the higher mathematics without any expense to the home office clerical force. Many of the students have successfully passed the very rigid examinations of the Actuarial Society of America, and been admitted to membership in that organization; some of them have been offered and accepted important positions on the official staffs of other life insurance companies.

The management of the New York Switch and Crossing Company [1] stands ready to pay expenses for any employé who will take a course in any of the well known correspondence schools in which industrial science is taught. It also subscribes for a full line of industrial and mechanical publications relating to its line of business, which are distributed to all employés who desire to read them.

One large factory instituted a course of lectures on "First aid to the injured." These lectures were delivered by eminent physicians to such workmen as cared to attend, but the 26 special policemen detailed to patrol the works—men who come directly in contact with all accident cases—were required to be present. To further enlighten the employés who had signi-

[1] New York Switch and Crossing Co., Hoboken, N. J. Manufacturers Railroad Frogs and Switches. Organized May 13, 1896. Number Employés, 110.

fied their intention to continue the pursuit of knowledge of this character, with a view to putting it to effective use in the event of emergency, a small first-aid treatise was placed in their hands by the company. After they had studied this treatise for two weeks the men were subjected to an examination in order to ascertain whether they were proficient enough to be called upon to perform simple operations in surgery. Those who passed were given appropriate badges to wear, thus indicating that they were suitable persons to be summoned in instances where quick aid might be necessary. In the patrol room the company has a well stocked medicine locker and a complete set of operating instruments, and about the works it has established 15 auxiliary stations equipped with such medical supplies as may be needed quickly in accident cases.

Early in 1907 Marshall Field & Company, Chicago, organized a choral society among the employés, who gave a concert in June in the largest music hall in the city. To join this organization employés must submit to an examination; if they are unable to pass in so far as sight reading is concerned, they are referred to a sight-reading class which is held under the direction of a competent instructor in the building. They remain in this class until they are able to read at sight, when they are promoted to the choral society. The rest and music room for young ladies is much larger than formerly, and in this room the firm tries to educate them to the better class of music by occasionally introducing some special features during the lunch hour.

A band was organized at the Plymouth Cordage Company about two years ago, the company furnishing the rooms to practice in and advancing the money with which to procure many of the instruments. The band plays at all baseball games that are held on the grounds, and also plays morning and afternoon at the Labor Day show. During the winter months the band gives concerts every two weeks in Harris Hall, the proceeds of which are divided with several benefit societies, which have been organized by the employés: the United Workers' Circle of King's Daughters, the Old Colony Mutual Benefit Association and the German Brotherhood.

Through the influence of the Strawbridge & Clothier Chorus, which is composed entirely of employés of the house, there is being aroused considerable interest in the study of music, thus imparting a fairly good education in general choral work. It is regarded by some of the critics as one of the best choruses in the state. The social effect of the organization is very good, aside from its educational value. June 13, 1906, the chorus of 140 voices gave the "Legend of Don Munio," a dramatic cantata by Dudley Buck, at a concert given by the chorus for the benefit of the San Francisco sufferers. More than $2000 were raised.

For the two-fold purpose of training for expression in speech and action, and of further stimulating the spirit of fraternity within the store family, the Strawbridge & Clothier Proscenium Club was organized.

The Pelzer Company provides a course of free lectures in history and travel, accompanied by stereopticon illustrations, which has proved of great educational value.

A dancing class of five hundred and fifty members, at the National Cash Register Company, meets in two divisions each once a week. It includes both men and women. The members are generally young people, but there are some elderly and married people. Those entitled to attend are only the employés and the escorts of the young ladies. There is a membership ticket which costs fifty cents per year, and which entitles the holder to membership in any or all of the classes at the N. C. R house. The dancing class is intended for teaching grace in company, ease of manner and power of adapting one's self to social functions. It also gives a social time to those attending and a few of their friends whom they may bring with them. In fact, this really takes the place of a club house to many of the members. They are not situated so that they can entertain at home, and are improved greatly by the little social acquaintance and opportunity for acquaintance which people ought to have. Among the rights of young people growing up is the right to get acquainted, and they have a restricted opportunity within such meeting places.

At the National Cash Register Company the cooking school has 290 scholars enrolled, who are divided into two classes.

Each meets from 6 to 8 P.M. on Thursdays and Fridays in the girls' dining room, with the kitchen adjoining. The head of the domestic economy department supplies the school with every equipment in the way of both utensils and supplies. The classes are open only to the employés of the National Cash Register Company and are open to any of the women employés. Some of the pupils are the forewomen who are heads of the large departments, and include also the women who are helping at the officers' club in the kitchen, and also those in the kitchen of the big girls' dining room. The girls are taught only what will be of use to a practical housekeeper in her home. The course includes the cooking of meats, of vegetables, the preparation of soups, salads and desserts; also practical lessons in the making of pastry, pies and cake, and special attention to lessons in bread-making.

The lessons are in the form of lectures and demonstrations, and everything is cooked before the class and tasted, so that the girls may have a practical object lesson. In connection with the cooking work, girls in the factory who desire, may spend a week in the kitchen of the men's and women's dining rooms, assisting in the cooking, and as the second week's work, may cook at the officers' club. The chef of the officers' club also gives them lessons in marketing and in the choice of meats. In connection with this practical laboratory work and the lectures, the young women may have a very thorough training.

A wood carving class began in 1902. Last year there were nearly 100 girls, and this year about fifty girls and forty boys. The children draw their own designs, and do simple wood carving. The idea of this class is to teach them to begin things, to work at them and finish them, thus training the hands and the brain. The boys seem to take greater interest in this subject than the girls.

The visit of the making and recording forces of the National Cash Register Company to the World's Fair at St. Louis was a notable event. The company closed its factory for two weeks and paid part of the expenses of 2200 of its employés during their 800-mile journey to enjoy the beauties and study the resources of this Exposition.

The trip was undertaken as an education for the employés.

The great educational advantages and unequaled beauty of the Exposition appealed so strongly to the officials that all employés were advised to make the trip. To that end business was suspended to give all an opportunity of enjoying the benefits of the great exhibition. It was realized that all who went would return to their homes refreshed in spirit, full of new ideas and ready to resume their work with renewed energy. The company paid the railroad fares and admission fees to the Exposition of 1000, one-half the railroad fares of all other employés and part of the fares of all wives of M. W. W. L. members who made the trip. Every N. C. R. man and woman was given opportunity for a week's study in the world's greatest school.

In pursuance of its belief in the value of educational trips, in 1903 the National Cash Register Company sent fourteen of the leaders of the company's members of the board of directors, district managers and two factory experts to Europe on educational and business trips. The sending of these officials abroad is the realization of a plan to acquaint the men responsible for the growth of the company's business with conditions in European fields. It is the idea that such trips broaden men and enable them better to solve the problems of directing business. Believing a man is never convinced unless his wife is convinced, the company sent with the men their wives.

Nine of the officials who went to Europe were from the Dayton factory and five were district managers. The object in sending the former was to bring them into closer touch with the European organization. The sales managers were sent abroad in order that they might compare the advantages of operating in America with the disadvantages of selling in foreign territory. It was expected also that the Americans could be of considerable assistance to the European salesmen by giving them the advantage of their advice and experience.

Similar trips are awarded at intervals to department executives and workmen whose services outside their regular spheres have been of particular value. As a rule parties varying from half a dozen to twenty in number are sent to New York, Chicago, Washington, Boston or to manufacturing centers like Pittsburg, to study conditions and broaden their view points. Of course they all keep their eyes open and bring back suggestions for the betterment of machines and methods.

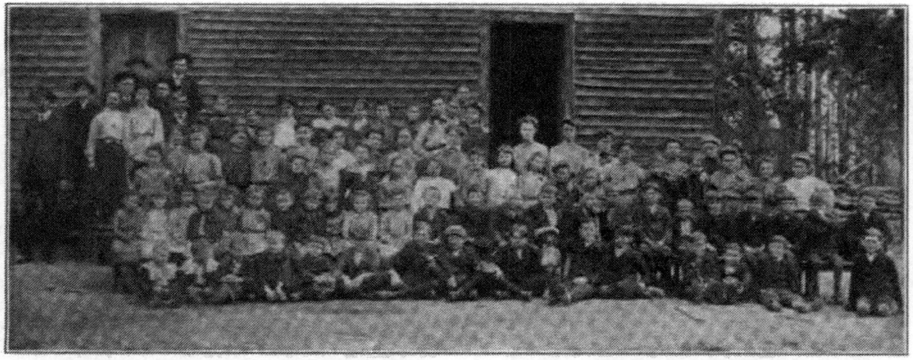

The Free Traveling Library of the Seaboard Air Line Railway. Report 67, Tucker Institute, Tucker, Georgia, T. P. Kimble, Teacher. New Room Added to School House; Black Boards Improved and Repainted; Blinds and Shades Put on and Painted; Grounds Cleared and Improved; New Trees Planted.

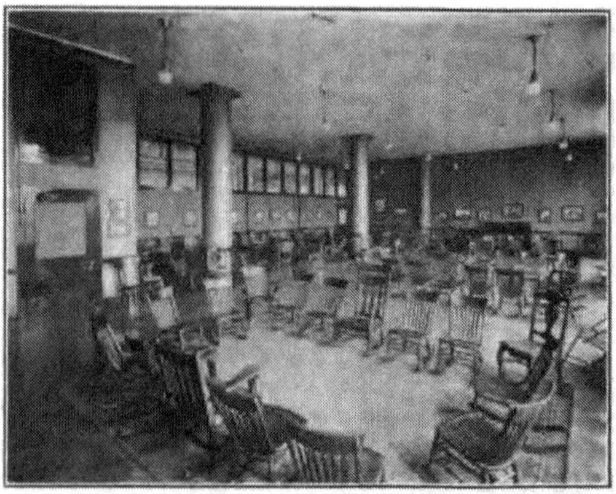

Rest and Comfort at the Noon Hour. Marshall Field & Company.

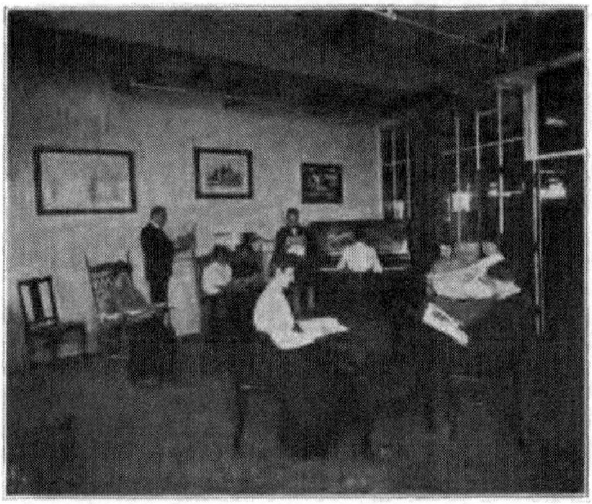

The Rest and Reading Room at the Acme White Lead and Color Works.

Twenty-five years ago, the Graniteville Manufacturing Company began to send their superintendents on educational trips. Since that time they have sent several of their other head men, and in every instance believe it has been exceedingly profitable to them as well as to the individual, because it not only enables them to keep abreast of the various departments of their business, but it brightens their ideas on every subject.

At the Acme White Lead and Color Works in Detroit, is a carefully selected library of some 1500 volumes. The room was, of course, some distance from many of the departments, especially those in other buildings. The men were always in great haste to leave the factory at noon and at night; they felt that even if they did go to the library, they would have to wait until others ahead of them were served. The company found that it was not enough to furnish the books and some one in charge of them, but the problem was how to get the books into the hands of the men. They then hit upon the device of placing in every department of the factory, on the wall, a plain wooden box marked LIBRARY, where the men leave their books on arriving at the factory in the morning and at noon. The librarian makes the collection from the boxes and then returns the desired books. By this simple administrative device the number using the library has been increased from 40 per cent. to 70 per cent.

One day the president of a factory, making a round of inspection, found that nearly all the readers were men and women from the administration building, in which the permanent library was located. Here and there a reader was found from one of the other buildings, but the percentage was exceedingly small. He at once thought that some way must be devised for bringing the books to the people, so he installed traveling libraries of selected books, magazines and newspapers for the distribution of good reading matter to employés.

Under the new plan, trucks with shelves accommodating 150 books are loaded with representative works to be found in the main library and drawn to the entrances of the various factory buildings where employés may have easy access to them during the noon hour and when the whistle blows at night.

The visits of the traveling libraries are previously announced by posted notices, and employés of all the great buildings are enabled to secure any book desired without making a special trip to the main library.

TRAVELING LIBRARIES— To facilitate distribution of books to employés, the traveling libraries will be stationed as follows:

At the main entrance of buildings Nos. 2 and 4, from 12:30 to 1 and at 5:30 on Mondays, Wednesdays and Fridays.

At the main entrance of building No. 3 and of building No. 6 for employés in buildings Nos. 3, 6, 7, 8 and 9, from 12:30 to 1 and at 5:30 on Tuesdays and Thursdays and at 12 on Saturdays.

Any book desired will be delivered by the traveling library to any of the above named stations if the librarian is notified in advance by phone.

A regular assistant also has been provided for the librarian, to facilitate the further working of the new plan of distribution, and a catalogue prepared.

Through the widened use of the library, it is possible to trace an almost direct line from the library to the suggestion box.

The men and women of this factory are coming to realize more and more that in the books in the cases on the first floor of Building No. 1, and on the shelves of the traveling libraries, lie the means to gain an education which may be denied them through adverse circumstances, or to ripen and extend the knowledge they already may possess. The means are right at hand, easy of access every working day in the year.

Means have been adopted whereby this information may be most conveniently distributed. For instance, should a skilled mechanic encounter a problem upon which he is not fully informed and has not the time to look up the information, if he will notify the librarian, the information will be located and the proper book sent him at the hour one of the traveling libraries visits his particular building.

The circulation of books for the first five days after the installation of the traveling libraries, August 22 to August 27, showed an increase of 76 per cent., as compared with the circulation on the five days prior to the installation of the new plan, August 17 to August 22.

The circulation for the period of September 1 to September 15, compared to the period of July 1 to July 15, or after the installation of the traveling libraries, showed the wonderful increase of 310 per cent. The increase was gradual each day, and the only limit to the growth of the circulation appears to be the number of books in the library. The library is open to all the office and factory employés and residents of the neighborhood. Books are issued for one week for one cent. They may be renewed for an additional week if desired.

A large newspaper is in receipt of many books, which might well be set aside for a library for the staff. This has been done by the Brooklyn Eagle,[1] which arranged that all books coming to the paper for review should go into this library, as well as magazines and weekly periodicals. The books are carefully catalogued and these catalogues are distributed among all the employés of the paper. Not only do the men and women and boys and girls of the establishment have the use of these books, but also the members of their families as well.

There are on an average 30 books a day taken out, while on Saturdays and Mondays a much larger number are called for. Whenever books are sought which are not in the library, they are immediately purchased and placed on the shelves.

Every department of the paper patronizes the library and the devil in the composing room has exactly the same privileges and the same advantage as the editor-in-chief. The president of the company, the editors of the paper and the heads of the various departments use the library in the same manner as the other employés of the establishment. There are no favorites or exceptions.

The experiment has proven very successful. It has helped to create and maintain a fine spirit throughout the entire establishment. In very many cases, owing to the intelligent suggestion of the librarian, young men have started on a systematic course of reading. There has been no philanthropy in this work and no intention of establishing a charity or benevolent

[1] The Brooklyn Daily Eagle, Brooklyn, N. Y. Organized 1841. Number Employés, 500.

institution. The management of the paper believes that it is just as essential to the growth and success of the establishment as the care of sanitary arrangements. The men and women who patronize the library become better educated, and it necessarily follows that the better educated they are, the better they will do the work that is required of them. In the case of the younger employés who are starting out on their business career and possibly undecided as to the line of work they are best fitted for, this library and its influence has been of the greatest possible benefit and help to them.

In 1902 the Santa Fé Railroad System began a series of reading rooms, which to-day number 25, with eight new ones projected for 1908, all under the supervision of a superintendent, but each having its own librarian, a man who has been in the company's service for a long time, and incapacitated for outside work. The selection of the librarian, however, is in no sense due to his unfitness for regular work, as he is required to be intellectually competent, of high character, and with a wide acquaintance among the men on that division.

The name reading room is rather a misnomer, for besides the large room containing books and periodicals there are two more, one for billiards, cards and games, and the other a bath, toilet and wash room. Bowling alleys and sleeping rooms have recently been added, and have become quite popular. Every man on the pay roll is entitled to the free use of these pleasures and conveniences. If he furnishes soap and towels, the baths are free, otherwise there is a charge of ten cents to pay the cost of laundering. Ten cents an hour is charged for the use of the billiard tables, which goes to a fund for keeping them in repair.

To draw from the library a man must sign the usual contract to replace any book lost or damaged by him.

In the selection of periodicals and books two motives control, instruction and entertainment. The illustrated and humorous magazines accomplish the latter; the literary and technical the former. There is no line of study in mechanics and the science of railroading not treated on in some form in the weekly and monthly reviews.

No effort is made to preserve these magazines by binding or

filing. The old periodicals are each week sent out to the trackmen for final use. Thus in the homes of the patient toilers at remote points these papers carry instruction and entertainment, and many children who would never see a printed page or picture are constantly receiving the benefits of the reading rooms.

Forty per cent. of the books are fiction, 15 per cent. are historical, 15 per cent. biographical, 10 per cent. technical, 10 per cent. general and the rest reference, being cyclopedias and dictionaries. Any employé has the privilege of ordering a book. If he is reading in course or interested in special study, he may ask the librarian for the required books, who reports to the superintendent of reading rooms, and the books, if they pass inspection, are at once sent. Also, if he desires books for his own private library, he may send a list to the superintendent, who buys and delivers them free anywhere on the system. The original bill with the usual trade discount is collected through the librarian. This is done to encourage the men to own their own books, and by laying aside a little each month, it teaches effectively the lesson of economy.

In addition to books and papers, they have a system of lectures and familiar talks by eminent educators and specialists. Only first-class talent has been engaged to do this work. Whenever the superintendent finds a scholar who is interested in the proposition embodied in these reading rooms, he takes him over the line and introduces him to the men. Not only the information and enthusiasm he carries, but the mere fact that the men may meet him, enlarges their views and brings them directly in contact with the intellectual life of the age.

The line is not closely drawn on amusements. There are all kinds of games, but no gambling. The billiard tables and bowling alleys are running all the time, but there never has been a quarrel in any reading room. There is no evidence that the men are angels, or fast becoming angels, and rivalries and all bad blood have not been eliminated, but the respectability of these reading rooms is entrusted to the honor of the men, and they have met the appeal as gentlemen. They can always have a bath, a game, a sleep or a book. It is their club room, their resort for pleasure and knowledge, their common meeting ground to exchange sentiments, their resting place when off duty, their one spot where they come in touch with the outer world as well as with their inner selves. The wives and daughters have access to the reading rooms on certain days, and once a week may use the baths. They have formed clubs and hold socials, and the men as a rule like to see them in the buildings.

The expense of operating these reading rooms is about $15,000 per annum, but as this increase of expense adds to the efficiency and happiness of employés, and the business can be handled more safely and economically, President Ripley considers the money wisely invested from a financial as well as humanitarian point of view.

As a most noticeable result, these reading rooms are gradually closing the gap between the executive official and the employé. It is a rare thing now to hear an employé condemn any of the officials. They act as a bond of sympathy and good will between the official and the employé. The latter realizes more and more what the former must do to hold the road together and get business, and he has dropped a spirit of criticism for one of interest and concern. The direct influence on the employés is most beneficial. It recognizes them as factors in the prosperity and success of the road, is an appeal to their intellect and conscience, and puts a premium on manhood, eliminating the idea that they are only machines. It therefore gives to each man a future built on his proper use of the present, developing a true ambition to excel, each in his department, and placing a rich master motive under each day's work. It cannot be questioned that a bath, a sleep and a book will make the trainmen more careful in reading orders and carrying them out. While it stimulates a man to make himself worthy of promotion, it also develops contentment of mind, of which hope is the mainspring, and a contented workman is a better workman for the company.

Mr. S. E. Busser, Superintendent of the Reading Rooms, writes me: [1]

"The interest has increased decidedly. We are placing sleeping rooms in all our new buildings. The entertainment feature has been developed. I am putting on this winter a

[1] November 27, 1907.

first-class musical or educational entertainment each week at every one of the reading rooms. I am getting talent from all parts of the world. Our circulating libraries are in great use and demand. The executive officials of the Santa Fé and the board are very well pleased with results. Our employés take more interest in their work. They are more reliable. They are proud of themselves and the reputation these reading rooms give them of being gentlemen and refined."

The free circulating library, the outgrowth of Colonel Anderson's desire to furnish reading matter to the section gangs along the route of the Southern Pacific Railway, is reaching a class of people who could never be benefited by the established libraries in the cities. Without it many of the railroad workmen would go for weeks and possibly months without being acquainted with late happenings, save an occasional glance at a paper thrown from the car window of a moving train, most of the passengers never thinking of the appreciation of these workmen for the papers which they might toss out of the window.

The idea of a free newspaper library for the section foremen, their families and near neighbors in the country was suggested to the general passenger agent while he was on a trip through the western part of Texas. At several places where stops were made, persons living at the isolated stations came to the windows of the car in which he and his party were, and asked for newspapers that were no longer needed in the car.

The free circulating library furnishes reading matter to the section gangs and their families, a class of people who rarely come in contact with any one outside of their immediate circle, and who would never have access to books and papers except for the Southern Pacific library.

No one unacquainted with the desolation of the life of the section hand in new and unsettled parts of Texas, and the poverty of thought and narrow outlook of their families, can fully appreciate how urgent their need is for some uplifting and educating influence.

The movement was organized in March, 1904. The plan was explained to each section foreman, and he was asked to report on the number of families in his neighborhood, who might also secure the benefit of the library.

The library is composed of donations from Southern Pacific Railway officials, contributions of papers from the newspapers in Texas and through the eastern offices in New York and Philadelphia.

The circulating library sends out packages of literature regularly, but owing to the large number of section houses and the limited supply of newspapers and periodicals, but about one package reaches a house in three weeks.

The following year the vice-president and general manager authorized an appropriation to buy Christmas books for the section children. Letters were addressed to each section foreman for information regarding the number and sex of the children, and their respective ages. About 200 books by the best authors were sent out as Christmas greetings to the children.

The library is in touch with the section houses upon the four lines of the company in Texas. There are 114 sections and through the foremen, their wives, daughters and housekeepers, about 1100 farmers' families get the benefit of the library.

That the cause of rural education is being advanced by the free traveling library of the Southern Pacific Railway is undoubted, but perhaps even more significant is the humanizing and broadening effect that it has upon the homes which it enters.

One out of many letters:

"I wish to tell you that we have derived the greatest pleasure from the perusal of the papers. They have not only given us pleasure in the mere reading of them, but as this is a lonely out-of-the-world place, they have kept us posted as to the affairs of the world, and I assure you all the section folks appreciate them."

The general passenger agent writes me (October 22, 1907):

"We find that the library has caused the public generally along our lines to assume a more friendly disposition towards our interests, especially is this so in the damage suit cases. We feel, therefore, that we are not only assisting the section men and their families and friends, but that through the library we are doing a great deal towards accomplishing closer and more friendly relations with the public at large."

The free traveling library of the Seaboard Air Line R. R., until 1899, was conducted upon the usual plan of transportation systems. About this time Mrs. Eugene B. Heard, a farseeing woman, in her Georgia home became imbued with a desire to improve conditions of families in the country districts of her native state. In the small stations and outlying districts, far from any public library, she found scores of families fond of reading, but without the means for purchasing books, or knowing just which ones to buy if the money was forthcoming. The idea of free traveling libraries on a small scale was advanced, and the Seaboard Air Line R. R. management was asked for free transportation for the boxes of books. This request met with success and every aid possible was given by the railroad, at first from purely philanthropic motives. With the generous encouragement of E. St. John, late vice-president of the Seaboard system, and voluntary coöperation of members of the industrial department organized by John T. Patrick, Mrs. Heard perfected her plans and launched an enterprise which at first seemed a doubtful experiment, but has since achieved a success beyond the most sanguine anticipations. In this case, as it frequently happens, the railroad company's generosity was "bread cast upon the water" for it was not long before the increased intelligence of the people along its lines began to benefit the company.

At first the libraries consisted chiefly of agricultural works donated by the government and contributed by friends. The unsolicited, unexpected, but gratefully appreciated gift of $1000 from Andrew Carnegie was most opportune and made it possible to place the library system at once upon a sure and safe footing. To-day 6000 books are circulated and eagerly read in the small towns and villages along the S. A. L. R. R., the enthusiasm which is aroused being proof of the timeliness of the library system. What the S. A. L. and Mrs. Heard have accomplished, can be done by any other railroad, manufacturer or department store. Nothing brings in greater returns for the outlay of time, thought and money than placing suitable books in the hands of those who will read.

From a material standpoint, the Seaboard is harvesting immense returns from the educational scheme which it has fostered. Its reputation for enlightened enterprise stands higher than ever before. So great is its popularity in Georgia, that a leading lawyer in Atlanta recently declared that he knew of several important suits for damages that had been withdrawn for the sole alleged reason that the Seaboard, defendant, was a corporation with a soul, and was doing all it could, through these "traveling libraries," to educate and improve the conditions of the people along its lines. Practically, and without a thought of direct or indirect accruing gains, Mrs. Heard in electrifying the educational pulse of the country with her own enthusiasm, has brought thousands of dollars to the Seaboard that else would have gone in some other direction. A policy of railway management that is kindly and liberal never fails to sway the popular heart, and elicits grateful appreciation.

Two series of libraries are arranged; one called the "Community," a hundred volumes suitable for rural districts, the other the "School," forty books useful in rural schools.

The school library has books of history and biography, description and travel, natural science and general literature. The sections devoted to fiction are filled with the best and most desirable collections of books, and it is said that visitors in the famous southern winter resorts find these libraries most useful and enjoyable.

In connection with the community library there is a work of village improvement carried on, and books on that subject are placed in the collection. The use of these libraries is the reward offered for efforts to improve a village or town, and a great deal has been accomplished through this work.

With the school library the same offer is made to schools in regard to improving conditions around the buildings, and seeds and designs for school gardening are given upon application, free of charge. These school gardens, 56 established in the last three years, have not only beautified the school grounds, but have proven a splendid industrial feature.

The reading table in connection with the school work, made up of leading juvenile periodicals and educational journals, has done much to foster the reading habit among the school children.

In connection with the school series, there is one called the "Lyceum," made up of the best published lectures, which, through the schools, may be given in towns where it would be difficult to get lectures. The lyceum course is very much appreciated by the patrons and has greatly assisted in making the school the social center of the community.

The use of the books is entirely without cost to town or school; but books must be replaced if lost or damaged. In each catalogue the price of the book is given. Each library may be kept six months, but only three months if it is needed in another village or school. Each library goes back to Middleton before it is sent out again. Books are taken from a library exactly as in our large ones—for seven and for fourteen days.

If a village applies for a library, the application must be signed by half a dozen citizens; if a school wishes the books, a teacher and the school trustees sign the request, and these persons are responsible for the library.

The books are in strong boxes on shelves, and securely locked, so that they are easily forwarded, each one being numbered. Reliable persons are chosen to have the care of them in all towns and villages, most of these persons being women.

Cotton mill operatives have found the books most attractive, and they soon read through one library and send for another. Children and young persons get just the sort of reading that they need, and their taste is directed and educated, great care being taken in the selection of books.

To increase their knowledge and interest in the subject of economics, banking and finance, the First National Bank of Chicago has provided a highly specialized library for its 550 employés. On the shelves there are to be found works on economics, both elementary and advanced, also "American Diplomacy," by John W. Foster; "American Commonwealth," by Bryce; works on commerce and accounting; histories of various banks, besides that of the First National Bank of Chicago; "Foreign Exchange," by Goschen, Clare and Magraff; "Theory of Credit," by H. D. McLeod; works on banking, by McLeod, Gilbart, Dunbar, Breckenridge and others; a large history of banking in all nations by well known authors—edited by the *Journal of Commerce*, New York; *Daily News* Almanacs, magazines and the Encyclopædia Britannica.

A free library and reading room, maintained by the S. D. Warren Company, is an important educational factor in the community. This contains about 4000 volumes of standard reading matter, in addition to which are found all the leading magazines and other publications. It is situated on the second floor of the building in which the company's offices are located, and is much frequented by the employés. The original cost of the library was about $5000, and some $300 a year is required to defray running expenses. A literary society, composed of women employés, meets regularly in the library.

The Pelzer Company has also established a circulating library containing 6000 volumes of approved standard literature. The library is installed in a building known as "The Lyceum," fitted up in a very tasteful and attractive manner. The main apartment of the building has been set aside as a reading room for women and in addition to the books contains about twenty-five of the leading newspapers and periodicals. Another room is reserved for the use of men, while a third room is furnished with tables and other facilities for carrying on social games. The library is open every evening from 6 o'clock until half past 10 and all day on Sunday. No charge whatever is made for its use.

A distinctly educational feature introduced by the Colorado Fuel and Iron Company is the reading room. In this is always found a number of the latest magazines, newspapers and periodicals, in addition to a reference library of maps, encyclopedias and other standard works. One of the best examples is that known as the Minnequa reading rooms, at Pueblo, where the entire second floor of a large brick building, comprising a reading room, a card and game room and two smaller rooms, is given up to the employés of the steel works as a place of recreation. At Orient and at Engle also there are well furnished reading rooms in connection with which are rooms for cards and other games. The expense of maintaining these institutions is met by means of dues, fees and subscriptions, and by the proceeds from entertainments, supplemented whenever necessary by liberal contributions from the company.

At the request of the Cleveland Hardware Company, the Public Library of Cleveland opened a branch in the factory known as the Cleveland Hardware Station; it contains 500 volumes, catalogues and all the printed matter which is used in their regular stations. One of the young ladies in the office takes care of the detail work of the library. The men bring their books in the morning, leaving them at the timekeeper's office. If they have any particular choice of books, they make out an application card, and in case the book is not in the library, the application is sent to the main library, which sends the book to the factory branch. The factory makes reports each month the same as regular stations. As a rule, the circulation amounts to about 300 books.

While it would be very hard to show any direct benefit to the company from this library, still they cannot help but consider it a good thing. It is done with practically no expense whatever to them, and they feel that any man in their employ who is inclined to read at all, should be encouraged as much as possible.

A simple but effective device consists in a small case near one of the entrances to the factory with a notice that any magazines put in this case may be taken home. Instead of throwing away the magazines around the house or offices, they are put into this case, and are usually taken home at once by the employés. This is good business, because many of the papers are technical, having a direct bearing on the business. This cannot help but benefit the men reading them.

Mr. E. C. Adams organized the nucleus of the factory library by writing to different prominent people all over the world, asking each one if he would donate a volume with his signature upon the fly leaf. This proved quite successful, and the employés secured a library of about 300 volumes, each one with the signature of some prominent person on the fly leaf.

Waltham has a large library, so that there seems to be no occasion whatever for the watch factory to have a general library of its own. It does maintain a factory library, principally technical, which is, of course, accessible to those who have occasion to use it in connection with the factory work. Some of the employés have been on the library committee, or board of trustees, for the public library, for years. In 1905 a course of study was given on literary subjects. There are local musical societies, but with these the company has no connection.

The Dodge Manufacturing Company,[1] Mishawaka, Ind., keep open doors for the heads of departments and furnish them with such reading matter as will be conducive to their betterment in that particular branch of work in which they are employed. Magazines of all classes, together with any information relating to or bearing upon the subject of economics, mechanics and engineering, are placed at their disposal. Daily papers, books of current date, and all high class in their selection, encyclopedias and books of reference are placed on library shelves.

Weekly meetings are to be held for the purpose of having a full assemblage that papers on different subjects may be read and discussed; these papers having been prepared by respective members, from three to five having been assigned for this purpose on the one subject. Writing material with the club's name will be furnished, so that members' correspondence may be carried on from their trysting place.

In 1878 the Ludlow Manufacturing Associates fitted up a few rooms in an old building as a library and reading room, with a small number of carefully selected books. In 1888 a new library was erected as a memorial to the late treasurer by his widow and children. This library building was given to the town under certain restrictions. At the same time the corporation presented to the town all the books belonging to its library and has since paid for additions of books, as well as all salary and maintenance expenses. The library now contains 7000 volumes and 55 magazines are to be found in the reading room. The patronage is fairly satisfactory and is increasing and the

[1] Dodge Manufacturing Co., Mishawaka, Ind. Manufacturers Power Transmission Machinery. Organized 1878. Number Employés, 1000.

building will probably continue to meet all the requirements of the town.

Prior to the spring of 1905 the Solvay Company contributed toward the support of a free library in their guild house, but since that time the Carnegie-Solvay Library has been opened, and the library needs of the community have been supplied through it. The company, however, continues to contribute generously toward the expenses of this institution.

For the library, the Weston Electrical Instrument Company has provided a large number of standard reference works, literary and scientific, to which are added many periodicals, scientific publications and those relating to machinery, engineering and electricity. The Weston club library, in charge of a library committee, has been made a branch of Newark's Public Library and is permitted to draw therefrom 500 volumes at a time, which are distributed on precisely the same conditions as at the public library. One of the results of thus bringing to the attention of the employés the industrial progress of the age, is that a number of them are taking scientific, engineering or mechanical courses in the Newark Technical School or in correspondence schools.

The Wanamaker library for the employés in Philadelphia, in charge of a librarian, contains about 5000 volumes.

The Potter Printing Press has a branch of the Plainfield, N. J., Public Library established in the works, from which employés are at liberty to draw books at will, subject only to ordinary library rules.

In the commercial house of Daniels & Fisher,[1] Denver, there is a school which includes in its membership as far as possible all children under the age of eighteen. They are divided into six divisions and these six divisions united into four classes, each class reciting forty minutes. The school opens at 8:30 and closes at 11:30 A.M., every day of the week except Monday. As this is a very busy day in the store, all school work, with the exception of one class of girls, is suspended.

The course of study consists of arithmetic, United States history, reading, spelling, geography and the discussion of current events. Each morning the teacher is furnished with the

[1] The Daniels & Fisher Stores Co., Denver, Colo. Dry Goods. Organized 1864. Number Employés, 803.

daily newspaper, and takes the most important topics which she can discuss with interest to the children, explaining them and answering all questions. The text books used are the property of the store. Each child is provided with the necessary books with which to prepare the lessons, and is allowed to take them home at night. The text books used are as follows: McMaster's "United States History," Belfield and Brooks' "Rational Arithmetic," Redway and Hinman's "New Natural Geography," "Stepping Stones to Literature," seventh grade.

The school room is provided with all the necessary blackboards, maps of the United States and the world and all other appliances. It is the idea of the proprietor of the store to increase gradually the usefulness of the school, and one of the proposed improvements is to establish a regular circulating library containing books of interest to the children.

All the employés between fourteen and eighteen years of age are organized into classes for systematic instruction in the usual common school branches, by Weinstock, Lubin & Company.[1]

For the young employés of the business and circulation departments a series of lectures and conferences is a part of the Brooklyn Eagle's policy. While it was not organized for social purposes, it incidentally gives them social privileges, but it is really a part of the business education of these young men. The lectures are given by experts in special lines of advertising and business work, and are followed by the answering of questions and general discussion, all of which has been of very great advantage in securing a comprehension of modern business methods.

A history class of about fifty or sixty members, begun recently, meets twice a week at the noon hour at the National Cash Register Company. The course covers the intellectual, social and moral development of Europe, commencing at the fall of Rome, down to modern times. Very little attention is paid to dates, but emphasis is given to the development.

Hochschild, Kohn & Company[1] provide educational classes

[1] Weinstock, Lubin & Co., Sacramento, Cal. Department Store. Organized 1874. Number Employés, 1000.

[1] Hochschild, Kohn & Co., Baltimore, Md. General Department Store. Organized 1897. Number Employés, 1000.

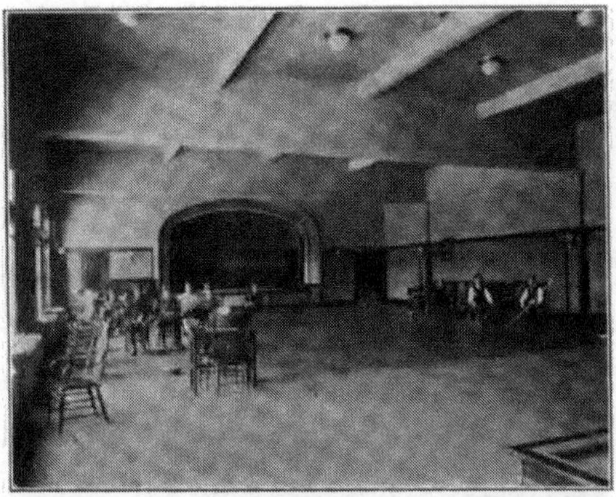

The Recreative Center for the Employés of the Chicago City Rail way Company.

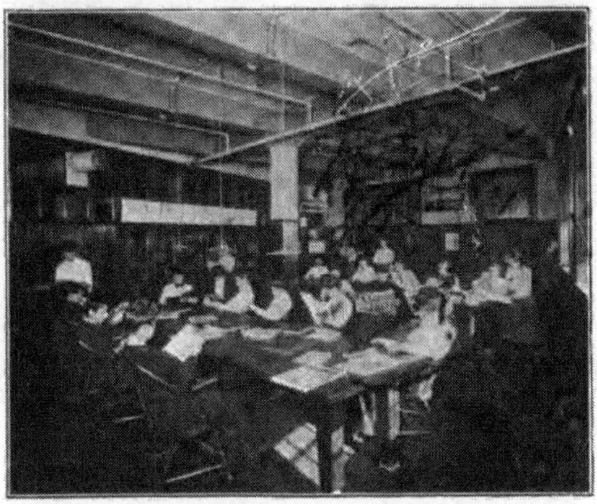

Library and Reading Room at the Thomas G. Plant Company, Boston.

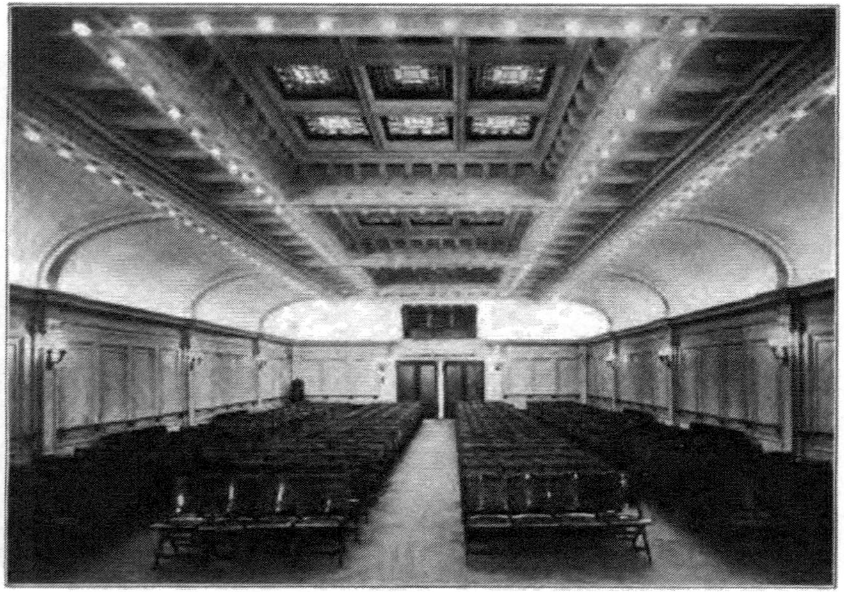

The Assembly Hall of the New York Edison Company.

for their boys, in which all between the ages of fourteen and eighteen secure twice a week, during store hours, instruction in mathematics, English, penmanship, reading, store etiquette and commercial ethics generally.

A woman's club—the "High Standard"—includes nearly all the women of office and factory of the Lowe Brothers Company, Dayton. It is a member of the Ohio State Federation of Women's Clubs. This club makes its own programs, conducts its own meetings, issues its own year book, has its own piano and, through its library committee, philanthropic committees and social committee, works for others as well as for its own members. The sessions are held in the women's dining room, on the second and fourth Wednesdays of each month from 12 M. to 1 P. M. Social evenings are arranged by the social committee.

For 1907-8, the sixth year of the club, special attention will be given to health, and a series of talks on such subjects as the importance of fresh air and sunshine, exercise, rest, recreation and food. There will be studies upon light and color, using the stereopticon, with special charts and apparatus. These lectures will be open both to members of the club and to other employés of the Lowe Brothers Company who are interested in this subject, and their friends.

Since the organization of The Broadway Department Store School, Los Angeles, in January, 1902, there have been forty-nine graduates, eight of whom graduated in 1906. Space allotted for school purposes is at the extreme end of the annex on the third floor. The room is some forty feet in width and is well lighted by a row of large windows and the school is equipped with all modern appliances. The course of study includes arithmetic, written and rapid calculations, grammar and composition, spelling, writing, physiology, civil government, current events and dictation, bookkeeping for most advanced ones and music. There are two instructors, one for music and one general instructor.

Everything is absolutely free; the time spent in school is the same as working in the store. Prizes are given at the close of the session, semi-annually, and the graduation exercises are given before the public. I learn that in every department of the establishment there are graduates of the school—filling important and very responsible positions, cashiers, typewriters, auditing clerks, receiving clerks, in the mail order and C. O. D. departments.

Mr. Letts writes me, "These boys and girls have demonstrated beyond question that owing to the training and discipline they have received through the school's instructions, they are equipped far in advance of the average department store employé. This feature of the success of our school is plainly shown in the fact that our competitors in business use every known artifice to deplete the ranks of our graduates by endeavoring to secure their services for their own aggrandizement.

"The school's expense is wholly met by the establishment, and I manifest a jealous interest in everything pertaining to the welfare and advancement of every pupil: There is no limit to my pride in the promotion of these young people, who in turn appreciate the advantages afforded by rendering faithful service."

It is not enough to provide educational facilities, but it is better to make their use so easy that there can be no excuse for failure to do so. At the T. B. Laycock Manufacturing Company's factory library, in order to reduce to a minimum the time required in obtaining books, the librarian makes frequent trips with a loaded truck through the factory and issues books to those desiring them. Many of the books in the library were contributed by the company, employés and friends; others were purchased with the money raised through entertainments given by employés. The library contains works of the ablest and best known authors, including many of the more recent publications and is in charge of a competent librarian. All employés are entitled to the privilege of the library. The card system, similar to that used in public libraries, is used.

The influence of the literary and social club is felt by the entire force; the kindly feeling existing between the company and its employés, so noticeable to visiting strangers, is in no small degree promoted by this society. Its aid committee visits the sick and looks after their necessities in time of illness.

Noonday meetings and classes for men are conducted by the Industrial Department of the Young Men's Christian Association, working through a men's noonday committee which has done much for the improvement of employés.

CHAPTER X

RECREATION

THE experience of the Celluloid Club, Newark, N. J., is so typical of conditions elsewhere, that I shall describe it in considerable detail, because there is no reason why this organization should not serve as a kind of working model, with due consideration for adaptability to local conditions. In the early life of this industry, plans for social and industrial betterment commenced, and grew with its growth; the employés being at all times inspired by a desire to cultivate every means of self help and mutual improvement. Clubs of various kinds were formed; some for athletic games and exercises, others for intellectual training and mental improvement, and still others for mutual aid in cases of distress through sickness or death. These organizations increased in number and in membership also as the Celluloid Company's business increased in magnitude and the force employed became greater.

The clubs were organized largely on departmental lines, and suffered from the incidental disadvantage of such narrow limitations not being favorable to the free extension of acquaintanceship among the company's employés. The mere departments were the centers of interest to those employed in them, instead of the entire works, of which these were but subdivisions. Things had gone on in this way for some years, the employés organizing and managing their societies as seemed to them best, without any interference whatever on the part of the employers. But the company officials had been watching the movement toward organization among its operatives with sympathetic interest, and observed much to admire and nothing to condemn, both in the purposes for which the societies were formed and in the manner in which their affairs were conducted.

Meanwhile the broader minded members of the various organizations became dissatisfied with the limitations necessarily imposed by the departmental basis on which they were formed, and soon the societies were opened to all the employés of the Celluloid Company, without reference to the part or branch of the business in which they might be employed.

This new departure produced a great expansion in the membership and also the activities of the societies; so that the question of meeting-place accommodation soon became a matter of serious difficulty. An attempt was made to secure the use of a vacant floor in one of the factory buildings, and the necessities of the situation were explained and a request to that effect preferred to the managers of the company by a committee acting on behalf of the members of the various clubs connected with the works. This application, which was the first instance in which the firm had been requested by the operatives to in any way assist them in matters relating to the organizations, was productive of important and far-reaching results. After due consideration had been given to the matter, the Celluloid Company dismissed the suggestion that any part of the factory space should be used for such purposes, as no satisfactory or suitable accommodations for the work of the organizations could be provided in that way. A further discussion of the subject, carried on between the representatives of the company and the officers of the operatives' societies, finally brought about the consolidation of all these bodies into one organization, under the expressive title "The Celluloid Club."

Instead of the privilege of using a spare floor or loft in one of the factory buildings for which they had petitioned, the company gave them, at its own expense, a club house, furnished throughout with everything required for its various uses. Its cost was $40,000. The club house is in the eastern district of Newark, within convenient walking distance of the works and of the homes of at least eighty per cent. of the operatives employed in them. In the basement are two fine, slate-floored bowling alleys, two shuffleboards, and two tunnels with targets for rifle practice.

The main entrance on the first floor is reached by a short flight of marble steps, and a fine vestibule with mosaic flooring which has the club name inserted across its width. The administration offices of the club, the café and a large billiard room are on this floor. The café furnishes lunches, and, if required, more elaborate meals are served, but only to members and the guests whom they are allowed by the by-laws of the club to introduce. Members of the club who reside a long distance from the works can have lunch served at the noon hour at a much lower rate than the same food would cost if obtained in a regular restaurant. No strong liquors are allowed in the club house, consequently none are handled in the café, but beers, ales and wines are kept in stock and served, as wanted, in moderation.

The Celluloid Company pays the taxes and insurance on the club house, but makes no regular provision towards the club's support; its theory being, to quote the words of President Marshall C. Lefferts, of the Celluloid Company, "that the club would prosper better, and inculcate a feeling of self-reliance and self respect in the employés, by letting it be felt by them that it is not a gratuity or charity offered by the company, but a club of themselves, by themselves, and for themselves.

"The company has been called upon and has met several extraordinary expenses which it felt was, perhaps, more than the club could stand, and has, through its officers, contributed prizes and subscriptions toward various plans suggested by the club."

The cost of maintaining the club is about $2225 per year. The dues, based on the present membership of 525, will yield approximately $1500; the balance of the running expenses is made up by income derived from the small fees which members pay for participation in the various games and classes.

The object of the Celluloid Club is to promote the social, moral and intellectual welfare of the employés of the Celluloid Company.

Any male employé of the Celluloid Company is eligible to membership, and may remain in the club so long as he is an employé of the company and complies with the rules. A member who has been an employé of the Celluloid Company for ten years, and who leaves the company's employ honorably, may continue his membership, but without either the privilege of voting or holding an office.

A male stockholder of the Celluloid Company may become an honorary member of the club and retain such membership so long as he remains a stockholder, with the same privileges as an active member, but without the right to vote or to hold an elective office.

The officers of the club consist of a president, vice-president, secretary, financial secretary and treasurer and a board of governors of nine. These officers, with the exception of the governors, whose term is three years, are elected for one year. No more than three members of the board of governors may be elected from one department of the company's works. All officers must be at least twenty-one years of age.

The board of governors is the controlling authority in all things relating to the club and its management. They have the care of the funds, investments and other property of the club, and exercise general supervision over everything relating to its material welfare. All bills must receive the approval of the governors, and all drafts on the treasurer be signed by them before being paid. Seven of the nine members of the broad of governors are required to form a quorum. Their power in the management of club affairs during the intervals between the club meetings is absolute; all help is employed by them and no employé can be discharged without their sanction.

The membership fee is fixed at $1, which must accompany the application for membership, and the monthly dues are twenty-five cents. A member who owes two months' dues is suspended from all privileges until he pays the arrearage. If, at the end of the third month, a member's account remains unsettled, his name may be dropped from the roll. To be reinstated, the full amount of arrearage together with a new admittance fee of $1 must be paid.

Members have the privilege of entering the club house at any time within the hours fixed by the club regulations, and making use of any of the various features or facilities therein provided; they have the privilege of introducing two guests each per week who are not eligible to active membership, but these guests cannot be taken into the club house by any other member the same week. No one under eighteen years is permitted in the club house unless accompanied by parent or guardian. Members are responsible for the acts of strangers whom they introduce into the club house.

The board of governors are required to hear and act on all

charges against members for conduct injurious to the peace, good order or reputation of the club, or other conduct unbecoming a member, and may expel, suspend or censure an accused member who is found guilty.

The club has two standing committees which are appointed annually by the president; these are the committee on entertainment and the committee on games. The committee on entertainment has the right to regulate the use of the assembly or entertainment hall, and to arrange and have sole charge of all entertainments authorized by the club that are not otherwise provided for.

For the social and intellectual culture of its employés, the John B. Stetson Company has erected at one end of the factory buildings a large assembly hall, capable of seating 2000 people; it is furnished with a grand and a parlor organ and a piano. There is also a parlor for evening social meetings. A large Sunday school, whose membership includes at times as many as 1400 persons, meets in the assembly hall.

As the number of the employés now exceeds 4800, the assembly hall mentioned above has been outgrown so far as certain occasions requiring the attendance of the whole body of employés is concerned. The company has therefore just built a new auditorium, capable of seating upwards of 5000 people, and containing a grand organ. This auditorium is especially adapted to the requirements of the Christmas celebration, which is a prominent event. On this occasion every man is given either a turkey or a hat, and every woman and girl a pair of gloves and a box of candy. To the apprentices prizes are allotted strictly in accordance with merit on the basis of quality and quantity of work and general deportment, these prizes including gold watches and chains and cash presents ranging from $5 to $20. For special merit, paid up shares in the building association, and shares in the common stock of the company are given to the most deserving. At the last Christmas celebration the following gifts were made: 358 hats, 1711 turkeys (23,500 pounds), 902 pairs of gloves, 1000 pounds of candy, 62 watches, 60 chains and fobs and the usual awards of gold pieces to apprentices, and cash presents to foremen. In addition, the cash distribution to sizers, trimmers and weavers, as a bonus for continuous and faithful service during the year, amounted to $50,000.

As a result of the numerous efforts put forth by the John B. Stetson Company for the moral and material well-being of its employés, it is claimed by the management that not only has the quality and quantity of the work done in the factory been greatly improved, but there has been a substantial increase in the company's business and profits.

One afternoon in April, 1901, the whistle at the Sherwin, Williams Paint Factory blew at 4:30 for a general assembly of the factory staff. The meeting was held in a room in the factory, flooded with sunlight from broad windows and skylights, decorated with pictures and adorned with bookcases, tables and easy chairs, and the occasion was its formal presentation to the employés, by Mr. H. A. Sherwin, the president of the company, who outlined the social policy of this new departure. "This is our club room, and we meet to-day to open it. We want every one of you to feel that it is your club room. We have been trying in many ways to help those who were laboring with us to make them more comfortable, more intelligent and happier and better men and women. This is one of them, and we hope it will be used in many ways. As we see to-day, it is not large enough for us all at once. We can have frequent meetings, however, for different purposes. Our mutual benefit society and other organizations or committees can meet here, and I know there are plans for music. There has been some suggestion of classes on matters of interest which might be a help and instruction to us all, in fact all these things are for you to develop and carry out to please yourselves. This will be a reading room and we have a good start with several of the best periodicals. This selection will grow as needed. Then we have a good library branch of our public library, and this can grow if you wish until it covers all the walls.

"We also want more pictures to educate and elevate us—in fact the company wishes to make this room just what you desire it to be. The management will welcome suggestions from any one of any plan which will give pleasure or profit to any reasonable number.

"Now you may say this is fine, but when can we get time to

enjoy it all? This we have also tried to provide for as well as we could, and beginning with Monday next the lunch time will be extended from 30 to 45 minutes, so that every day you can have at least fifteen minutes for a little pleasure and relaxation here. Now this is to make us feel better, and if we feel better we do better work.

"It is to encourage mutual sympathy and helpfulness, because the one who is interested in helping forward his associate will progress faster himself. We do not want or intend to stop in these plans for the good of every one connected with us. We want you to keep them on your mind and be ready with your suggestions of what will help you in your work. We spend one-third of our time in the factory employment—surely it is important that this one-third should be as bright and clean and comfortable and attractive as it is in our power to make it and keep the surroundings as pleasant and inspiring as we can."

December 21, 1889, nearly 2000 people assembled in the auditorium of the Steel Works Club to celebrate the opening of that institution. Many of the officials of the Illinois Steel Company and their friends came down from Chicago to take part in the exercises, and Mr. A. J. Forbes Leith, the president of the company at that time, gave the address of welcome. "My duty," Mr. Leith said, "is an agreeable one—that of opening this club house. A few years ago when the Joliet Steel Company was considering important improvements to its works an idea occurred to the officers that they were neglecting something; while they had been planning and contriving for the improvement of their mechanical forces they had omitted to provide for the repair of that other great and essential power—the flesh and blood of the men. A committee consisting of W. R. Stirling and H. S. Smith was immediately appointed, and from that day progress was made, slowly it may be, but steadily, until to-day we dedicate this grand building, due largely to the zeal and forethought of these two gentlemen, Messrs. Stirling and Smith."

It is a large stone structure built by the old Joliet Steel Company at a cost of approximately $75,000. The maintenance expenses were paid in the beginning by the old Joliet Steel Company, and are now paid by the Illinois Steel Company and other local constituent companies of the United States Steel Corporation.

The club building is leased to its members at $1 a year. The membership is confined exclusively to the employés of the corporation, who pay a nominal membership fee of $2 a year, which carries with it all the privileges of the club. It is managed by a superintendent and a board of directors, the first named appointed by the president of the Illinois Steel Company, and the latter elected by the members of the club. There are pleasant reading rooms, with more than 60 periodicals and newspapers, a large billiard room with eight tables, a well furnished and well lighted gymnasium and a hand-ball court; fine bowling alleys, a large assembly room that will seat over 900 people, a tennis court and an athletic field. There is a bath room with a swimming pool, shower and tub baths, a kitchen and card rooms, and a large reception room and three pianos.

A woman's auxiliary arranges the social functions of the club, and also sustains some benevolent features outside. Semimonthly dances given in season are participated in by the friends of the young people in Joliet who are not members of the club. From the funds derived from that and other sources, the woman's auxiliary maintains a room in one of the hospitals and extends some help to other unfortunates.

The average membership for 1907 is over 1200. Counting the members of the families who have the privileges of the club, and whose children use the gymnasium classes, there are perhaps three or four thousand who use the club. Counting those who attend its entertainment course, social functions, and who are not members of the club, it is estimated that 25 per cent. of the population of the town are within its hospitable doors sometime during the year.

The Dodge Manufacturing Company has fitted up a dining room so that when occasion demands a banquet or dinner can be served. Last year the club rooms were doubled in size. Billiard and pool tables and a kitchen were added, and very nominal dues were provided for. The management of the club rests in the hands of the members, the company making up the deficit in the treasury monthly as needed. The reading circle holds regular monthly meetings in the library, while stereopticon lectures are enjoyed bi-weekly; these usually are given by the members of the club.

It is the intention to make these quarters so persuasive in their attractions that they will be the means of bringing out all of the good, from a mechanical standpoint, that may be in one's make up. It is the sole desire and aim to place at the disposal of the employés that through which they can be bettered after factory hours.

At Redstone a beautiful club house and theater, complete in all respects, has recently been erected by the Colorado Fuel and Iron Company. Here is found a commodious lounging and drinking room, furnished with large leather-cushioned armchairs, settees and tables for serving refreshments. An ample fireplace at each end of the room gives comfort and cheer on winter evenings, and entertainment is furnished by a large Regina music box and a graphophone. All kinds of the best grade of liquors are sold here at reasonable prices, while temperance drinks, sandwiches and cakes are served at cost. Rules similar to those in force at the Coalbasin club are intended to check any tendency towards excess. Adjoining the lounging room is the large well-lighted billiard room, equipped with one convertible and two pool tables. A card and game room furnished with cards, chess, dominoes and other games, and a reading room supplied with popular magazines and newspapers, are also reached through the lounging room. On the second floor is the hall used for theatrical purposes, and provided with a full set of stage scenery, electric stage lights and other up-to-date features. In the basement are located bathrooms, toilet and dressing rooms, liquor storage rooms and the board of directors' room, and secretary's office. A furnace, also located in the basement, supplies steam heat throughout the building. On certain evenings of each month the privileges of the club are extended to the wives and daughters of members, when whist and euchre parties, billiards, pool and instrumental music and light refreshments lend interest and pleasure to the occasions. Active membership in the club may be obtained on payment of an initiation fee of $1 and six months' dues in advance, at 50 cents a month.

At Sunrise, Wyoming, and Starkville, Colo., recreation halls

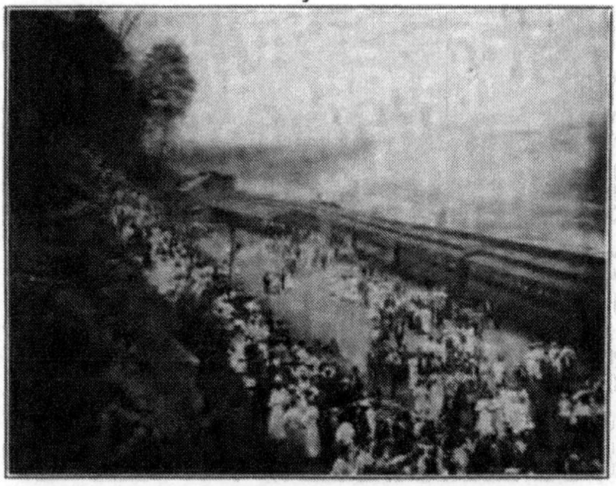

One of the Annual Outings of the H. J. Heinz Company's Employés.

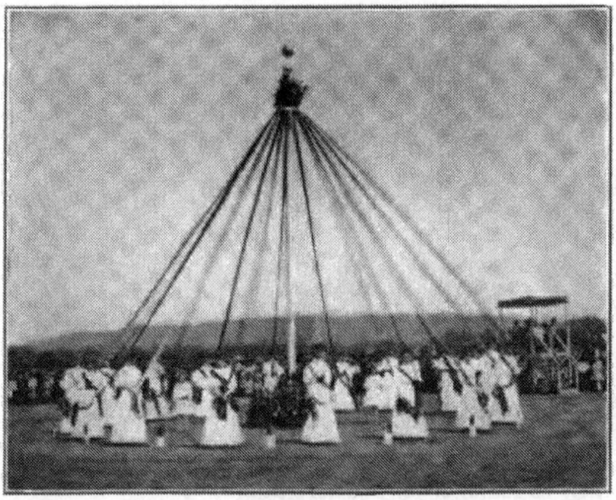

Maypole Dance at the Annual Field Day at the Remington Typewriter Works.

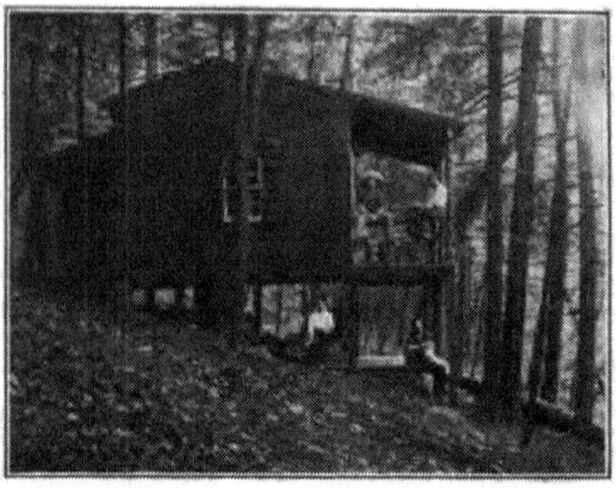

A Summer Camp of the Boys' Club of the Curtis Publishing Company.

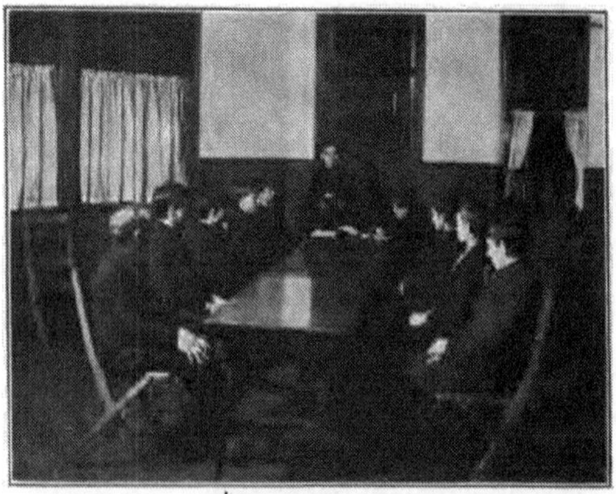

One Way of Getting Boys off the Street. A Business Meeting of the Boys' Club at the Cuovode House, a Social and Industrial Settlement at the H. J. Heinz Company's Factory.

have been built, in which the men may congregate to read, chat, smoke and play games. The hall at Sunrise is equipped with a stage and an alcove used as a library. At the latter place the building, which is popularly known as "Harmony Hall," contains two large rooms, one used for kindergarten, the other for library and recreative purposes, and two smaller apartments utilized as kitchen and cloak room. These buildings are quite popular with the employés and many socials, musicales and other entertainments take place within their walls.

Boys' and girls' clubs are also contributing to the social development of the various communities. These clubs meet once a week and engage in games, dances, contests, gymnastics and various kinds of musical and literary exercises. In the boys' clubs military drills and athletics are quite popular, while the girls' special attention is given to cooking and sewing and other practical domestic work. The attendance upon these clubs is most encouraging and much practical work is being accomplished by them. Classes in household and domestic economy have also been organized among the women of most of the camps.

Except for some studio space for art book work, the central Roycroft building is devoted entirely to intellectual, æsthetic and social opportunities. One wing constitutes the "chapel," as it is called, where as a rule on Saturday and Sunday evenings, and frequently at other times, concerts, lectures or talks are given either by some one connected with the institution, or often by talent from abroad. The chapel is at the same time an art gallery with walls covered with paintings largely the work of the Roycrofters' own artists.

In the tower room of the chapel on the first floor is a small library of books, many of them home products. In the second story are rooms where evening classes are held, all open to employés without expense save that each must purchase his own books. All the instructors are workers in the shop, and there are classes in modern languages, literature, history and designing, with exercises in debating. A special feature is made of music, in charge of a musical director from outside. Instruction in voice and piano is offered employés free, and those who undertake such study are permitted to take a half-hour daily in working time for practice or lessons. Besides pianos in the Phalanstery and chapel, there are two others in the main work building, all for the use of employés, and frequently utilized in recreation hours for dancing. A band, glee and mandolin clubs are maintained among the employés, the company having paid one-half the cost of instruments and advanced the other half to be paid back out of the proceeds of concerts.

Club room facilities and places for social intercourse abound. All the buildings are open at all times and employés are encouraged to use them freely. The large reception hall in the chapel building is ample for large gatherings and the Phalanstery rest room and many of the workrooms are attractive for smaller social meetings. It is the constant aim, in fact, to cultivate the feeling that the Roycroft Shop is for the workers, not simply as a work place where a living may be earned, but as a center for recreation, culture and social intercourse.

The recreation room at the Joseph Bancroft & Sons Company, for use at the noon hour, has a reading table supplied with papers and periodicals, which may be taken away and passed on to others.

The Glendale Elastic Fabrics Company[1] reports that it has a very excellent class of help. There is plenty of work, and all are industrious. The great majority of people own their own homes and show great interest in them and much care for them. The Glendale company does not patronize the help, or seek to gain advertising from anything they do in their interest; they try to assist other corporations in the town to provide places that people may get out doors and enjoy themselves, and in this way draw many idle people from the saloons. All the work of this nature is done by the employés themselves.

There was great need for several years for the provision of suitable recreation rooms for men and boys of the community in general, but no plan which was entirely satisfactory was hit upon for some time. Since, the problem has been dealt with by separate agencies, and the need has been met to a considerable degree. The Glendale company made changes in the firemen's hall to adapt it to social purposes. The West Boylston

[1] Glendale Elastic Fabrics Co., Easthampton, Mass. Manufacturers Elastic Fabrics. Organized 1863. Number Employés, 800.

Company also gave substantial encouragement to a social club at Hampton Mills. The enlargement of Glendale Hall will make the addition the main building, and give opportunity for commodious side rooms in the old part. The addition will contain a hall 72 by 32 feet, with stage, and the present hall will be converted into gymnasium, kitchen and committee rooms. These efforts of separate organizations on behalf of suitable recreation for those in which they severally have cause for special interest are in the right direction and have accomplished much.

A club room for the drivers and circulation department employés, who have long waits between runs, was opened by the Brooklyn Eagle. It occupies a large room on the top floor of a new stable building at the rear of the Eagle building, where magazines and weekly papers are kept on file, and where checkers, chess, cards and other non-gambling games are permitted. This is much appreciated by the men, who find it more pleasant to hang around the club room than in a nearby saloon. In building the new Eagle building, which was finished in 1904, great care was taken to provide the employés with commodious dressing rooms, iron lockers and especially a number of shower baths which were installed and are much used by the employés of the mechanical departments in summer.

For several years the Denver City Tramway Company [1] has furnished its trainmen wholesome recreation and amusement, by assisting them to equip their club rooms with gymnasium apparatus, billiard tables, bath rooms, books, papers and magazines. At each division headquarters a large room is devoted to the use of the men for club purposes and social intercourse. The men have caught the spirit and most of them are very keen promoters of their respective clubs. In this way a splendid rivalry has sprung up, which tends to keep the members active, and to improve the character of the entertainments. Dances, card parties, athletic contests and social gatherings are of frequent occurrence. Once in the summer season, each club gives a picnic up in the mountains. These functions take

[1] Denver City Tramway Co., Denver, Colo. Organized 1888. Number of Employés, 1394.

a majority of the men away from the division, but their runs are cheerfully filled by extra and regular men from other divisions; so that the public suffers no inconvenience. The men have shown their appreciation of the efforts to provide them entertainment; the company feels that the betterment work has served to improve the moral atmosphere of the divisions and helps them to keep a cleaner and more wholesome set of trainmen.

R. D. Wood furnishes a hall for the men to use as they may wish for lodge purposes; it contains a cooking school for the instruction of the wives and daughters of employés, which is conducted under competent management. Sewing lessons are given; the science of housekeeping is also taught, and the building so maintained as to be available for the many uses which the convenience of the village population may require from time to time. The workmen are left absolutely free to use or not to use these facilities as may seem best to them, for there is not the slightest pressure placed upon them in favor of either course. Mr. Wood believes that any other course would tend to bring about strained and unnatural relations between people who must work together.

In the enlargement of the plant of the Iron Clad Company, Brooklyn, a library association was planned to give the employés of the company a place in which they could read and amuse themselves. The library is tastefully decorated in red and fitted with mission furniture. A piano and billiard table, all kinds of games, the latest books and magazines, give the employés every opportunity for recreation after business hours. A committee of entertainment provides a bi-weekly evening of music and recitation. The recreation committee has purchased a farm which will be maintained as a summer home where the employés can spend their vacations. The products of the farm, such as milk, eggs and butter, will be shipped to Brooklyn, N. Y., and utilized for the daily lunch served in the dining room for the use of the employés.

In connection with the association is an educational committee, which has meetings for literary discussions and classes in mechanics, electricity, stenography, bookkeeping and millinery. Tournaments in pool, pinochle, euchre and pingpong are played every evening. In the basement of the building there are shower baths, a bowling alley and gymnasium. Sunday being visitors' day the relatives and friends of the employés are made cordially welcome. Entertainments are provided for them in the shape of music and lectures. Outsiders have been very willing to help by offering their services free to conduct these lectures and some of the most prominent people in New York have attended several of the social functions.

The Cactus Club house was built by the Newhouse Mines and Smelters Company for the use of its employés at Newhouse, Utah.

The building is of the bungalow type, and is one of the most attractive in the town. It contains a reading room, billiard room, ball room, barber's shop and bar. The only liquor sold in the town is dispensed here. The membership includes the business men of the town, mine and mill superintendents and all employés of the company who are eligible and who may be elected by ballot. The object of the club is to promote good fellowship and to provide a place of entertainment for its members, their families and friends. The club is entirely independent of the company and is managed exclusively by its officers and a committee of members. The club pays to the company a monthly rent of $100 for the property. The club has been so successful from every standpoint that the members have lately constructed, out of the funds of the club, an opera house capable of seating 300 persons, a café, restaurant and grill room, with 12 bedrooms on the second floor for transient guests.

The Lynchburg Cotton Mill Company desired to provide a social center, where the operatives could spend some of their leisure pleasantly and profitably.

For this purpose they provided a hall fitted with reading and writing rooms, smoking room, lunch room, bath rooms, rest room and an assembly hall. The privileges of the center will be extended free of all charge to those residing on the property of the company, and also to those who work in the mills, whether they reside on the company's property or not, the hall being exclusively for the recreation, pleasure and improvement of the employés and tenants of the company.

Howland Croft, Sons & Company[1] have provided a piece of ground in the immediate vicinity of their plant, which covers one entire city block, 400 by 225 feet; this has been laid out for the purpose of cricket playing and for other forms of athletic exercises. They have also created a club house thereon, containing baths, reading and recreation rooms, with other features usually found in such buildings. The club house is two stories in height; the first floor contains dressing rooms, lockers, baths, and reading rooms. The second floor is fitted up for the purpose of meetings and receptions. The building has an open porch on the first and a balcony on the second floor, for the purpose of viewing the games and contests that take place in the field. The grounds, club house and everything they contain are under the absolute control and management of a club composed of the company's employés.

There is a fully equipped gymnasium in the home office building of the Metropolitan Life Insurance Company, with shower baths for the free use of such of the clerks as desire to avail themselves of it either before or after office hours. One day of each week the gymnasium is given over to the women. They also have the use during the lunch period of a large reception hall adjoining the lunch room, in which there is a piano and where dancing is encouraged. Those who prefer to exercise in the open air have the privilege of using the roof of the building during the lunch period.

When the first library was started in 1878, a room fitted with various small games was set apart by the Ludlow Manufacturing Associates as a smoking room, but the attendance became so disorderly that after several forcible ejections the room was closed. During the succeeding years the general tone of the village improved, and in 1895 the attempt was again made. An unused part of a new mill was fitted with bowling alleys, pool tables and other games. At this time an organization was formed which still continues. This association of the

[1] Howland Croft, Sons & Co., Camden, N. J. Manufacturers of Worsted Yarns. Organized 1880. Number Employés, 510.

employés, known as the men's club, has its board of directors, and many of the heads of departments of the corporation have taken an active interest in its development, thereby giving stability and continuity to the movement. In 1898 the association was crowded out of its quarters, as the space was needed for mill purposes; but on the completion of the building now occupied the whole upper floor was reserved and equipped for permanent social rooms. The association has been actively interested in athletics, and has always insisted upon clean sports and gentlemanly behavior. During the last year the corporation has laid out an athletic field of about six acres, containing a quarter-mile running track, and fields for baseball and football; all enclosed by a high board fence. This will be under the control of the athletic association. In addition to the social rooms occupied by the association the corporation has, for the past three years, furnished space for gymnastic and basket ball work in the mill buildings. The discipline of self-control, and the demand for fair play in all sports, has had an influence in every department of town and home life. Men learn to work together by coöperating in team work and in social activity, and success in athletics has fostered a pride in the village which will help in other lines.

The preamble states that the more general the use made by the people of Ludlow of the property entrusted to the care of this association, the more nearly will the design of the donors be realized, and the greater will be their satisfaction.

To this end the rules for its use are framed on as broad and liberal lines as its proper maintenance will permit, with the single idea of meeting the needs as well as the inclination of all, and giving every one interested opportunity to do something toward the well-being of the community.

HOUSE AND FIELD RULES

The Stevens Memorial will be open from 2 P.M to 11 P.M., or such other hours as may be determined by the directors. Members, associates and visitors will use the south entrance; the north entrance being reserved, except on special occasions, for women and girls, under supervision of the social secretary and the members of the institute.

On Saturday and after six o'clock other days, the reading

and game rooms will be reserved for men and boys, except on nights set apart by the directors as ladies' nights, when members may introduce women or girl friends. Gentlemen will not smoke on these occasions and boys under 17 years of age must not smoke in the building at any time.

The gymnasium and swimming pool are reserved for women and girls Mondays, Wednesdays and Fridays, and for men and boys Tuesdays, Thursdays and Saturdays, except on such occasions as either of them may be required for special purposes. The reading, social and class rooms and swimming pool will be open during such hours on Sunday afternoon as the directors may find desirable.

Gymnasium and swimming pool cards will be issued to associates on payment of 25 cents every three months. An additional payment of 10 cents every three months will secure the use of a locker. Associates having no gymnasium cards will pay five cents for each admission to it or to the swimming pool. Towels may be hired, but each one must provide his own bathing dress.

School children under instructors may be admitted to the gymnasium and swimming pool on stated afternoons; their cards of admission will cost 5 cents a month for each child under fourteen years of age, and 10 cents a month for those over fourteen. These cards will provide for afternoon admission only and the mothers of the children may in all cases accompany them as visitors. Boys and girls over fourteen years of age attending school and having regular institute or associate gymnasium cards, can use them for afternoons as well as evenings.

Cards must be produced when called for by the doorkeeper, janitor or other official in attendance, either of whom may in their discretion exclude any one temporarily for misconduct, while repeated misbehavior brought under notice of directors may result in permanent exclusion.

The directors shall decide for what games or apparatus a charge shall be made, and will fix such charge, which will be the same to all except visitors, who shall pay approximately double rates.

There shall be no gambling of any description and every one shall pay for his own games.

Any member or associate may introduce a visitor to the men's rooms, notifying the janitor or other official in attendance, who will exercise their discretion in the matter, but frequent visits by persons who could secure cards if they so desired will not be permitted. This does not apply to girl or women friends of members or associates or ladies' nights.

The social or class rooms will be available at all times when the building is open, and when not required for the work of the girls' institute, may be used for banquets, club meetings or other special purposes at discretion of property committee.

The directors may from time to time set apart certain evenings for competition between teams selected or challenged, and on these occasions such teams shall have exclusive use of apparatus reserved during the competition. Notice of such competition shall, however, be posted on the bulletin board two days in advance.

Any member, associate or visitor having cause for complaint, or suggestion to offer, by presenting the same in writing to any director or other official shall insure its receiving due consideration.

The Acme White Lead and Color Company has secured suitable grounds near the factory, and put them into shape. Membership in the Acme Athletic Association will be open to all employés in return for their dues of 20 cents per month. The dues will be utilized exclusively for the purchase and maintenance of supplies and equipment for the different games taken up. There are no salaried officials in this organization. The games will include baseball, tennis, outdoor basket ball, quoits, lacrosse and football, and in winter they will endeavor to provide some indoor games.

There is no doubt of the growing interest in this association, evinced by its members and outsiders. They expect to be able to prove conclusively that this is a good thing from every standpoint, and the results attained in better health and spirits, hence more proficient work, will more than warrant the time and trouble expended in bringing the Acme Athletic Association up to a highly satisfactory condition.

The objects of the Acme Athletic Association are:

1. The encouragement and maintenance of athletic sports.

2. The beneficial effects to be derived by its members from healthful outdoor exercises.

3. The promotion of good fellowship, closer acquaintance and general good will among the employés.

4. The advancement of the interests of the Acme White Lead and Color Works by assisting in promoting coöperation among its employés by creating a feeling of good will towards the men.

L. O. Koven & Brother[1] have recently purchased a piece of land adjoining the main factory building. This land is being graded, and will be fitted up with seats under the trees and also with grounds for games; here the men may spend their leisure time when they are disposed to do so.

In Pueblo there is a large baseball ground for the use of employés of the hospital and steel works and three tennis courts, also a hall used by the steel workers and friends for social functions and dances during the winter.

The school houses in the mining camps are built with a hall on the upper floor specially designed for amateur theatricals, social entertainments and dances and popular lectures.

A croquet lawn and tennis ground is frequently used, not only during the noon recess, but after business hours also, in a Detroit paint factory.

At the Briarcliff farms in the summer, baseball is the diversion which chiefly appeals; high ideals are the basis of that sport. Finely graded grounds, wire-screened grand stand and the best of properties throughout, are supplied without cost through an association which in turn secures public patronage in return for its guaranty of clean sport. No player is paid, and the signature to certain articles is required of every team member, and the team accepts no cash above expenses in meeting the few dates made away from home, while it secures the fastest and best-mannered teams for games at home which its finances will permit in guarantees. And while it takes on amateur, academy and semi-professional opponents alike, it was not defeated during 1907. Play is scheduled for Sat-

[1] L. O. Koven & Brothers, Jersey City, N. J. Sheet and Plate Steel Work. Organized 1881. Number Employés, 160.

urdays and holidays only, and no gambling or rowdyism is permitted on the grounds.

"We believe that to win fairly and be considerate towards the loser are among the finest possibilities of baseball; and that to prove a good loser is even more difficult. *But win or lose, let us be gentlemen.*"

Athletic and outdoor sports are given special encouragement at Pelzer's. The employés have organized several baseball teams which have been uniformed and otherwise aided by the company. A fine bicycle race track has been kept up, upon which the members of the Smyth Wheel Club give exhibitions of fancy riding and compete for prizes offered by the company. The Smyth Rifles, also named in honor of the president of the corporation, possess the distinction of being the only military organization in any of the South Carolina mills. This company is composed entirely of young men operatives and is a part of the regular State militia. There is also a brass band fully equipped with fine instruments and numbering 36 members which constitutes the band of the regiment to which the company belongs. These organizations participate in the annual encampment of the State forces and are assisted by the corporation in all necessary ways. Then there is a large recreation park, well laid out and provided with summer houses, a large dance floor and a roller skating pavilion. In the park a swimming pool, more than 100 feet long, with dressing rooms adjoining, offers a form of most wholesome recreation.

For the purpose of encouraging physical culture through outdoor sports among its employés and their children, the Solvay Process Company has enclosed a five-acre plot close to the office building. This model athletic field has a tennis court and a running track, and a portion of the space is used for the popular game of baseball. There are not at present any special health and safety arrangements at the works, aside from what are required by law, but the company has erected a gymnasium for the employés and their children on the athletic field, where gymnastic classes are held under a competent teacher. The gymnasium is fitted up with all the appliances pertaining to a building of this kind, and is furnished also with a system of shower baths.

The United States Shoe Company has reserved land for recreation grounds for the use of an athletic club, baseball team and cricket club, composed of employés. The annual field day of the employés is now one of the events of the year. In all the matters mentioned the management are interested, and coöperate with the employés. The men have organized a band of twenty-five pieces. They give their services to charitable functions, and have had a series of concerts for the benefit of the relief association.

The Electric Club of the Westinghouse Electric and Manufacturing Company maintains nine tennis courts, glee and mandolin clubs; and with the assistance of the wives of officials social entertainments and dances are frequently given.

All employés on monthly salary are allowed two weeks' vacation with pay. Saturday half-holiday is the universal custom with Westinghouse interests. An annual picnic is held under the auspices of the Westinghouse Beneficial Association.

In 1870 the Conant Thread Company of Rhode Island furnished the transportation for their employés to one of the shore resorts on Narragansett Bay. The employés were not paid, with the exception of those on salary, for the excursion day, nor were they consulted as to the nature or place of the excursion. Ever since the company has paid for the dinner on the day of the excursion.

In 1905 a coöperative outing was arranged by the Men's Welfare League of the National Cash Register Company for 1700 employés, their families and friends, who spent eight days in camp at Port Huron, Mich. August was selected for the outing because the factory was closed for two weeks. The outing was managed by the league, which assumed all the details of the task of transporting the campers over 500 miles, housing them for nine nights, feeding and amusing them—all at a cost remarkably low. The entire necessary expense of the outing amounted to $7.80 per person, of which $5.20 was for railroad fare and tent hire, while $2.60 was for meals. The meals cost ten cents each.

The campers left Dayton on Monday, July 31, on three special excursion trains of ten cars each. On arriving at camp,

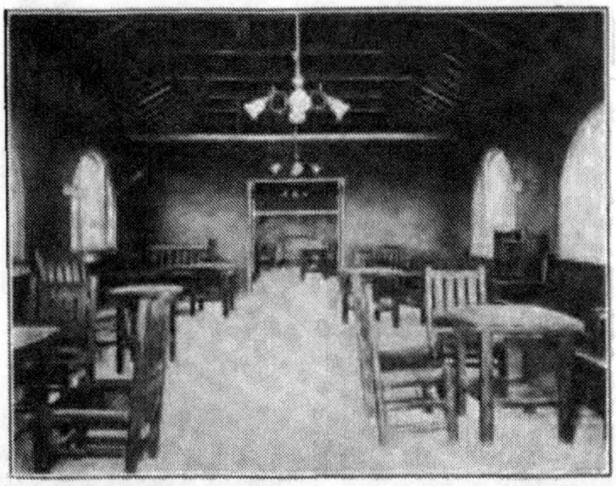

Recreation Hall for the Convalescents at One of the Colorado Fuel and Iron Company's Hospitals.

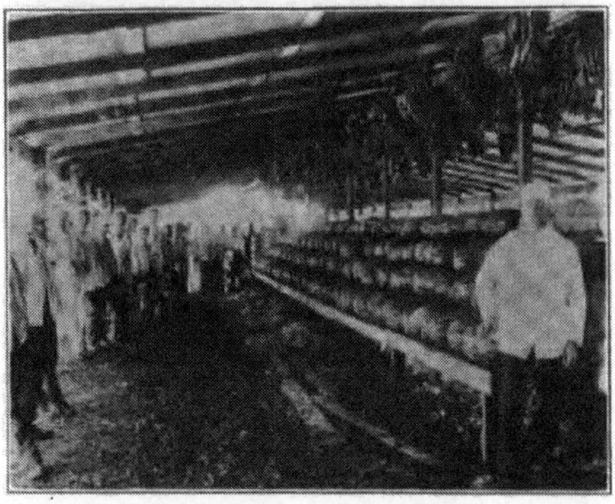

How Cæsar Cone Prepared for the Annual Picnic of His Employés of the Proximity Manufacturing Company, Greensboro, Ga.

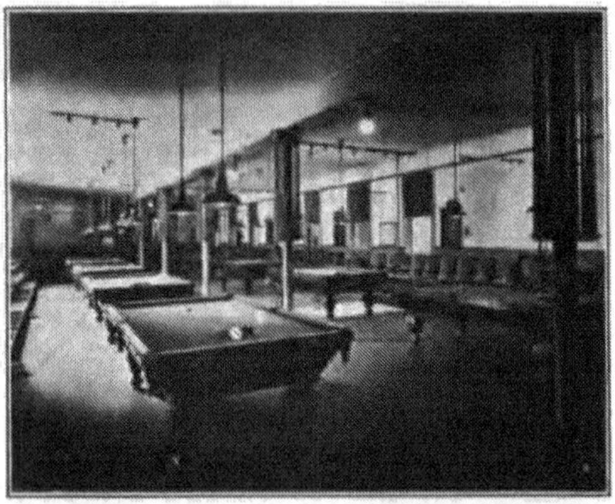

Billiard and Pool Room at the Casino of the Westinghouse Electric and Manufacturing Company.

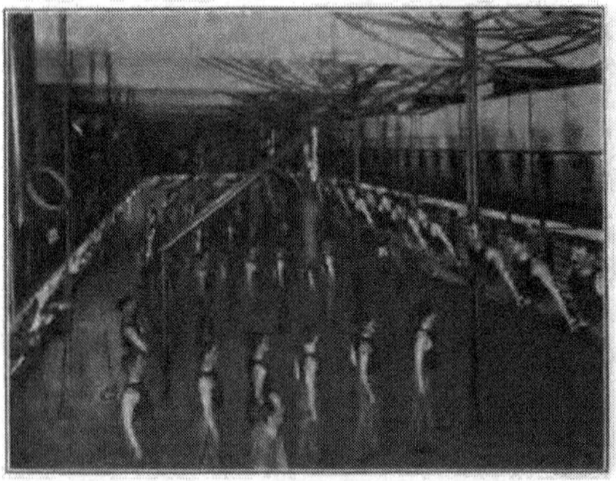

Setting-up Drill at the Thomas G. Plant Company.

supper was all ready for the campers. It was prepared and served under the direction of the head of the domestic economy department, by forty N. C. R. cooks and waitresses who had been sent to Port Huron two days before. The 900 seats in the big dining tent were quickly filled and the tired and hungry campers enjoyed their first camp meal.

The camp was laid out in a well-wooded grove on the bank of Lake Huron. The tents were arranged in rows along streets, each tent being numbered to correspond with a map from which the campers selected their accommodations before leaving Dayton. Most of the campers' baggage, which had been sent on ahead, was on the ground when the excursionists arrived.

During the vacation period, the workers lived in tents, swam and rowed and sailed, rambled through the woods, or danced.

Adjoining the big dining tent was located the cook tent, where the food was prepared and served. Along the front of this tent extended a counter with a railing just outside of it. At meal time the people, after presenting their meal checks to representatives of the league, marched along between the counter and railing, receiving their portion of food from the waitresses behind the counter.

Although the camp was in the woods away from the city, it had many of the conveniences of city life. A street car line ran along one side; electric light and water supply were furnished free by the city of Port Huron. A post-office was established in the "Headquarters Tent," at the center of the camp, and mail was received three times daily. A nurses' headquarters, a doctor's office and a barber shop were located upon the grounds. Both of the factory nurses were at the camp to care for any who were ill. Considering the number of campers the cases of sickness were very few and none serious.

The outing camp for 1905 was so successful that it was decided to repeat the plan. For 1906 the annual camp of the Men's Welfare League was held at Michigan City, Indiana, on the shores of Lake Michigan.

Special rates were again made in accord with the following announcement:

ROUND TRIP FARE FOR OUTING IS $2

The N. C. R. Company believes in vacations. The officers of the company have shown their desire to have employés go on the M. W. L. outing to Michigan City by offering to pay $1.75 toward the railroad fare of each employé and members of each employé's immediate family.

This will make the round trip fare $2.

Tickets may be bought from the Men's Welfare League.

The following shows who will be eligible to take advantage of the company's offer:

Married Men. A married man may have one ticket for himself, one for his wife and one for each of his children. If the children go on half fare, the company will stand half of the $1.75 toward that fare. No other member of a married man's family will be eligible.

Single Men. Tickets will be sold to unmarried men as follows: One for each man, one for his mother, father or sister. Under no circumstances will he be permitted to buy more than one extra ticket.

Other members of the immediate family of any employé may take advantage of the $10 rate for the outing.

The rate for meals in camp, tents, etc., will remain at $3.75, as at first announced, making total expense for the outing to each employé $5.75.

In illustration of the care in providing for all details,—the officers of the league expect to set up a tent at the factory of the same size and quality as those to be used in camp, in order that every one may gain a fair idea of the accommodations to be offered.

In 1904, when Mr. Patterson, President of the National Cash Register Company, knew that he was to spend the summer in Europe, he gave orders that his private grounds should be placed at the disposal of his employés, for a series of summer picnics and outings. The men's league was intrusted with the responsibility of the details. The first picnic was held during the middle of July; until the last of August, on three or four nights each week, Far Hills was the scene of some form of social entertainment. Lawn parties, picnics, fêtes, in all eighteen entertainments were given, and each of the 3800 factory employés attended at least one affair, while many were present on several occasions.

Wanamaker maintains at Island Heights, N. J., camping grounds and a headquarters house. The boys enjoy an annual encampment at this place, and the house is used by such of the women employés as care to arrange club outings there during their vacation. All employés receive two weeks' vacation with pay.

July 4th, 1906, an outing was given by the Cones of Greensboro, N. C., to their employés at the Proximity White Oak and Revolution cotton mills. Notwithstanding the rain five thousand people attended in a beautiful grove near the White Oak mill. A covered stand 200 feet long by 40 wide was erected in the center of the grove where the main lunch was served, consisting of chicken, ham, mutton, sausages, cheese and preserve sandwiches, with pickles, tomatoes and other relishes. The bill of fare included 2200 loaves of bread, 650 pounds of cake, 2000 fried chickens, 1000 pounds of ham, 600 pounds of lamb and 500 dozen hard-boiled eggs. Everything else was on a like scale.

Near the main stand was an avenue of 16 smaller stands, ranging from 15 to 60 feet in length, where ice cream, watermelons, lemonade, oranges, bananas, peanuts and cigars were served. The elaborate provision made for the water supply show the thoroughness with which everything was prepared. A deep well reaching 100 feet into solid rock was bored, and a pumping engine kept going throughout the day lifting the water into a 500 gallon tank which was erected for the occasion. The water was piped from this tank to the various stands and drinking stations.

A large dance stand had at one end a raised platform, built as a theater with curtain and dressing rooms. Here the various speeches were delivered in the morning, and in the afternoon a minstrel performance was given by a volunteer troup composed entirely of employés of the mill.

Mr. James Bangle, superintendent of the Proximity plant, stepped forward, and, in the name of the employés, presented each of the Messrs. Cone with a beautiful gold-handled umbrella. To purchase these gifts a voluntary subscription was taken up in the mill, and every employé, without a single exception, contributed. No one was allowed to give more than five cents.

After the speaking, $100 in prizes were awarded the residents of Proximity and White Oak villages for the prettiest front yards.

The Proximity band, an organization composed entirely of employés of the mills, furnished music throughout the day. Additional music for the dancing was supplied by a volunteer string band organized in the mills.

One stand that attracted much attention was specially characteristic of the kindness and forethought of the managers of these mills in looking after the comfort of their people. A babies' pavilion was erected with covered roof and curtained sides. Two rows of cots were set up and here the village mothers might leave their tired little ones to sleep in charge of a lady attendant who was one of their own number. Plenty of milk was provided for their nourishment. Another bit of social betterment consisted in sending baskets of sandwiches, cake and fruit to those who were sick and could not attend the picnic.

The third annual picnic was held in 1907 on the same scale, under the management of Bernard Cone. In his words of welcome, Cæsar Cone stated that the mill owners were glad of an opportunity of giving their people a day's outing, and hoped that every one would enjoy the occasion. They were much gratified at the cordial support given the management by their employés in the past, but as a still further incentive to steady work, it had been decided to offer certain prizes. From then until the end of the year a careful record would be kept, and every employé who did not miss a day's work would be presented with a five-dollar bill; those who missed one day would get four dollars; those who missed two days three dollars, and so on down the line, ending with a certificate of merit to those who missed not more than five days.

The Strawbridge & Clothier Company, at their own expense, provide an annual outing for the various athletic organizations and other groups of their employés.

The Vogler Manufacturing Company grants a full noon

hour, and has recently purchased a billiard table for the use of the employés.

At West Rutland and Center Rutland the Proctor Company has established club houses for recreation purposes. These are carried on similarly to the Y. M. C. A. at Proctor, but are not under the auspices of the general board, and their members do not have the privilege of Y. M. C. A. members.

A unique feature on the recreation side at the Hamilton and Milwaukee works of the International Harvester Company are the out-of-door impromptu concerts at the noon hour by the members of the brass band, the men who play being allowed an extra hour for dinner. Athletics are promoted with much favor at most of the works; baseball, football and bowling are general activities, and some "spirit of the game" is evidenced at the Chicago general office, when the men get out to play ball at noon, or on Saturday afternoons. A neighboring gymnasium has been accessible to the young women of the Chicago general office, and the social secretary is promoting an interest in physical training among the office employés. A gun club and a camera club interest a number of factory and office employés, and form a source of out-of-door as well as indoor recreation and education.

CHAPTER XI

COMMUNAL OR SOCIAL BETTERMENT

It is interesting to note that when an employer begins some form of industrial betterment for the individuals in his own employ, the scope of his work widens out so as to include the community, thus adding to industrial, social betterment. In this way the community receives from the industrialists who are mindful of their social and civic obligations, churches, schools, memorial halls, libraries, parks, playgrounds, town halls, gymnasiums and other institutions.

In the village community of Peacedale the organizations are not generally in the hands of the manufacturing company as such, but have been in most cases started and to a great extent carried along by the owners of that property. The fact that the stockholders of the corporation have always lived there and been a part of the village life itself has proved a valuable element in growth. As early as 1854 the village children were taught singing on weekday afternoons, and gathered into Sunday school on Sunday by one of the mill owners and his wife. In 1856 a building was put up with accommodations for the library founded some two years earlier, a reading room and a hall, in which a church was organized. These rooms were used until 1872, when the church was built, and till 1891, when the library was moved to its present quarters. Most of the organizations are thus village rather than company matters, but at the same time the company, its owners and employés practically make up the village.

The Hazard Memorial at Peacedale, R. I., was erected in 1891 to the memory of Rowland Gibson Hazard. It contains a library of 10,000 volumes, a hall seating 600 people, several class rooms and a gymnasium. The building, of stone and wood, is an important part of the village architecture, and was deeded by the sons of Mr. Hazard to trustees to hold in perpetuity for the use of the whole community. The hall is not let to any traveling show, organization or entertainments that are not considered by the trustees to be for the best interests of the village. The rental is always nominal. Its cost was between $40,000 and $50,000.

The library is maintained in the interests of the whole town, and is managed by a board of directors representing the different villages. It is used principally by Peacedale and Wakefield, and in the summer is drawn upon by Narragansett Pier and other nearby summer resorts. It is entirely free. It has not only the library proper but a reading room, which is open during the summer season until eight o'clock every night. The library is supported by voluntary funds and contributions; the town has once or twice made an appropriation to buy books, and the state contributes an annual sum for the same purpose.

In the basement of the memorial building there is a gymnasium used by the boys' club, several bath and dressing rooms, and a room utilized by the young men as a smoking and reading room. For the privileges of the gymnasium, baths and reading rooms each member pays $2.50 per annum. A few magazines and papers are taken regularly for this club and others supplied from the library upstairs. The work is under the charge of the superintendent of the building.

In the memorial several local circles of the King's Daughters' society, which are branches of the regular organization of that name, hold their meetings. About 150 women and girls belong to these circles. One circle owns a sick room outfit, bedside table, rolling chair and other articles of use in sickness, which are loaned as occasion requires to the needy and suffering in the village.

The village supports a literary society which meets every two weeks during the season from October to May. It is regularly organized with a president, secretary, treasurer and other officers. The entertainments are not wholly of a literary character, but consist of lectures, concerts, dramatic performances and light operas. They are largely contributed by local talent, but lecturers are frequently hired from outside, and one concert of the choral society is included as a regular number in the literary society's course. One night a year is devoted to what is called the South County Magazine, which is rather a unique production. Though called a magazine, it is manuscript, and read at the meeting, and illustrated by living pictures, tableaux and drawings. The membership consists of all of those who buy season tickets. The charges amount to about 15 cents per night.

The village also maintains a "Neighborhood Guild," which conducts, under the care of a competent teacher, several classes each day in sewing, cooking and home nursing. A nominal fee is charged for instruction in each of these branches, and the work is proving very successful. A class in carpentry is also taught once a week by a competent man, at a nominal fee.

These several societies afford an opportunity for much useful and pleasant work. They tie the village together and tend to raise the general tone of the community. The owners of the property feel that the efforts which they have made, extending now over a long series of years, have aided in bringing about a cordial feeling among all parties who work for the company, and in raising the general morale of the village.

The choral society, organized some years ago, has grown to be one of the leading features of Peacedale. A conductor comes from Providence once a week during the season, and there is a chorus of 75 to 100 voices who make up the membership of the society. They give their concerts each year, among the productions such music as "The Creation," "The Messiah," "Elijah," Rossini's "Stabat Mater," Sullivan's "Golden Legend," also about one hundred other works. This choral society has not only helped the village itself by giving concerts and affording the singers of the place an opportunity, but it has an indirect value in developing the local musical talent, as shown in an excellent church choir, and especially in another feature of Peacedale—the "Sunday Musics." The choral society is formally organized, has a president, treasurer and board of directors. The members pay $3 each per annum. There is an admission fee to the concerts, but the whole sum realized from these sources is not sufficient to carry on the work, so the deficiency is made up by the owners of the mill property.

A few years ago the "Sunday Musics" were begun by Miss Hazard and her sister, who simply went into the hall on a Sunday afternoon and played and sang for fifteen or twenty minutes, while a few people from the outside straggled in.

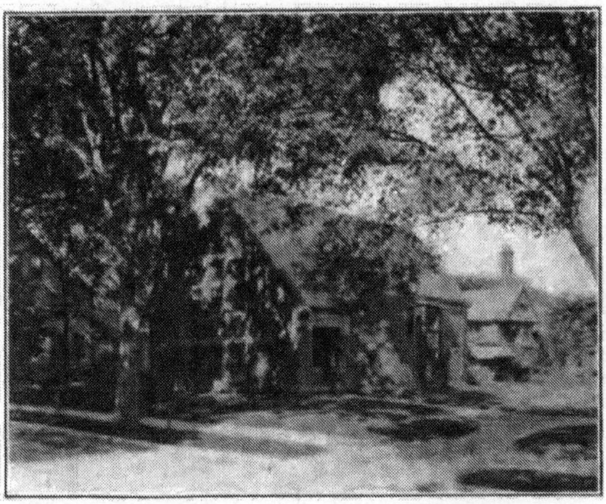

The Hubbard Memorial at the Ludlow Manufacturing Associates.

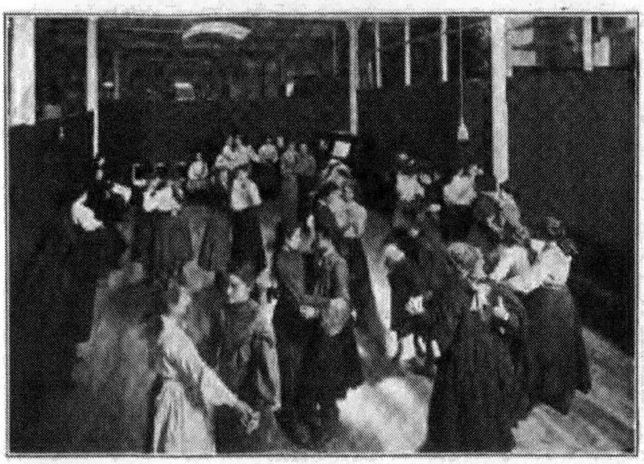

Recreation Room at Siegel-Cooper's New York Store. An Instructress Teaches Physical Culture and Dancing, the Firm Giving the Girls Fifteen Minutes Daily for This Purpose. In This Group Are Cash Girls, Packers and Markers.

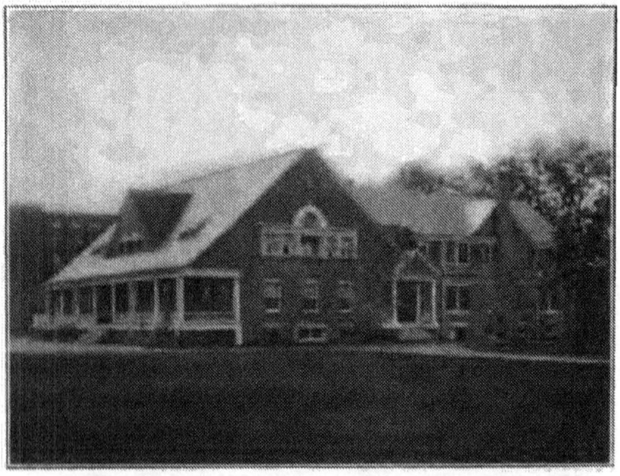

The Casino, the Social Center at the Gorham Manufacturing Company.

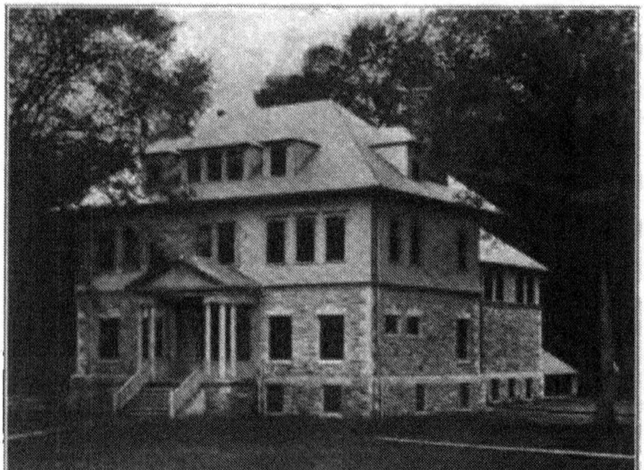

The Young Men's Christian Association Operated for the Proctor Manufacturing Company.

From that it has grown to be an informal concert each Sunday afternoon for the season, from Christmas until Easter. The several Sundays during the time are allotted to musical people in the village and town, and each one provides a program of from half an hour to an hour. The music is not wholly sacred. The concerts are attractive to the people of the village and town, who come in large numbers, and the hall very frequently contains from 250 to 500 or 600 people on a pleasant Sunday afternoon. The musicians are almost entirely local, although once in a while a first-class performer from the outside is engaged. There is no formal organization, and no charge of any sort connected with this work.

In passing a factory where there is a general appearance of neatness and good order, one is at once impressed, and contrasts it with the many places he has seen, down at the heel, the yards heaped up with rubbish, a repository for unused boxes and the scrap pile. Neatness about a factory gives an impression of prosperity; if to this is added a little decoration of vines and flowers about the grounds and premises, the community at once receives a benefit. Instead of a junk heap the factory becomes a garden spot. Many an employer is desirous of improving the general appearance of his plant, but is hampered by the conditions under which his factory was laid out years ago when no thought was given to the external adornment. Were he to build a new factory, he would now consider it good business to provide pleasant surroundings.

If at first their plans do not include expansion, industrialists are forced to a limited output, or are obliged to purchase new sites. "If my business had stayed in the city, I could never have employed more than 500 people at the very outside," remarked a large industrialist to me, as he described the new site of hundreds of acres for his factory where he has room for any possible expansion. To-day he employs upwards of 4000 people.

Thus the Gorham Company, finding it impossible to extend their plant located in the heart of the city of Providence, in removing their business to Elmwood, about three miles distant, purchased a considerable tract of land at a cost much less than it could have been obtained in the heart of the city. The site was chosen not only with a view to future expansion, but to give the employés attractive surroundings. A part of the site fringes a pond; wooded slopes, ravine banks, masses of rock and foliage offer the finest water and landscape views. To these natural effects already provided, winding roadways and paths, broad sweeps of lawn and beautiful trees give the surroundings the appearance of a park.

Not only does the community benefit by this attractiveness, but the employés instinctively are impressed and stimulated to improve their home grounds. Frequently the employer coöperates.

In order to add to the attractions of the village of Ludlow, Mass., in 1892 a hall was built for the local lodge of Masons. The upper story was arranged for the sole use of the order, and was fitted up in a manner to meet all their requirements, while the lower floor was arranged for social gatherings of the Masons and other societies or fraternities in the village. This building has proved quite popular, and has added much to the social life of the village.

A savings bank was started in 1888. The Ludlow Manufacturing Associates furnished a room, free of rent, and paid the salary of the treasurer of the bank. One or two leading men of the company also acted as trustees, but were in no other way connected with the bank. After a few years the bank was able to pay all its expenses, and now has deposits of about $220,000, and occupies a very neat bank office of its own.

Situated on Onondaga Lake, and contiguous to Syracuse, is the small village of Solvay, where the Solvay Process Company has for many years carried on the manufacture of soda and by-products. Its property extends over some 70 acres, mostly along the shores of the lake, and about 2500 persons are employed in its works and quarries. The interest of company and town are identical, two-thirds of the village tax being paid by the corporation; the well-being of the inhabitants in general and of the employés in particular, always has been a matter of thoughtful consideration on the part of the management of this large manufacturing establishment.

When, in 1886, the company instituted a sewing school for

young girls, principally children of the workmen, in a room of its office building, it was of the opinion that this plan of beginning at the foundation would prove to be a more effective way of establishing reciprocal relations with its employés, ultimately uplifting them socially and ethically, than through any direct effort among the men themselves. Experience has demonstrated that this conclusion was correct, for considerable good has been accomplished along these lines, a number of those who were pupils in the early years now having families and homes, in which is being put into daily practice the knowledge they acquired in the classes attended by them in childhood. At the outset the attendance in the sewing school was small, but in the course of time it developed so rapidly in numbers that it outgrew its original quarters, and the company, desiring to provide sufficient space to properly conduct this work, besides having in prospect the introduction of other industrial, educational and social features, constructed and furnished at large expense a commodious guild house, to which is attached a guild hall, containing modern improvements including electric lighting, a stage equipped with all the accessories for amateur theatricals, dressing rooms, a coat room for men and a cloak room for women. The main floor of the assembly room in the guild hall will seat 600 auditors, and a large gallery at one end of the room will accommodate an additional number of people. The hall is frequently used for concerts, entertainments and lectures, given under the auspices of the company, which usually charges the villagers an entrance fee of five cents, this nominal price of admission adding to the value of and interest in these events. The basement of the guild house, in which are billiard and pool tables, is devoted to club purposes by men employed in the clerical and other departments. On the first floor are class rooms, a circulating library and a kitchen equipped with a range, culinary utensils and two long tables, on each of which are installed five small gas stoves for the use of cooking classes. The company has also built a club house on the grounds for its office force, comprising chemists, civil engineers and draughtsmen. Near the latter building is a dormitory for women employed in the restaurant and guild house. These structures are far removed from the works, and in summer are surrounded by artistically arranged flower gardens and neatly trimmed grass lawns.

For the purpose of encouraging physical culture through outdoor sports among its employés and their children, the company has enclosed a five-acre plot close to the office building. This model athletic field has a tennis court and a running track, and a portion of the space is used for the popular game of baseball.

A certain amount of money is set aside by the company for the partial support of the children's classes, but each member of a class pays five cents per lesson. Teachers are employed, only a minor portion of the service being voluntary. On alternate Monday afternoons the Willing Circle, composed of the wives and sisters of the clerks in the employ of the company, convenes in the guild house, where its members outline the best methods of developing and strengthening the work that comes within their province. Three cooking classes, which have a membership of 12 young women in each class, whose ages range from 16 to 20 years, receive instruction each week. Plain and fancy dishes are prepared, and at the end of the year there is an exhibition of the work performed by the pupils. On the same evening the Knights of St. John, consisting of 32 boys, have a drill in the guild hall. The Solvay Circle meets on alternate Wednesday afternoons in the guild house, and on every Wednesday evening the dancing class of 160 boys and girls occupy the floor of the guild hall. The first class of this kind was organized in 1890. Prior to that year dancing parties held in Solvay and vicinity were boisterous affairs, but shortly after the company added this feature to its program there was a noticeable improvement in the manners of the younger element in the community, and in the dancing class of the present day a well-behaved set of youths is invariably found. The sewing school, with an average attendance of 175 girls, is divided into classes in the guild hall every Friday afternoon, each class being under the supervision of a competent teacher. The course is graded, and tuition free. Lessons in dressmaking are given to a class of young women on Friday evenings. Once a year the Solvay Willing, and other circles of the Solvay Guild, combine, and in December hold a bazaar in the assembly hall, which is beautifully decorated for the occasion.

The proceeds are placed in a special fund that aids the various philanthropic undertakings.

The Dodge Manufacturing Company of Mishawaka furnish their employés with club rooms, which are equipped with such reading matter as would be conducive to their betterment as citizens or make them more efficient workers. Magazines, daily papers, encyclopedias and books of reference on economics, mechanics, etc., are to be found on the library shelves.

Another interesting case of town development appeared in 1886, when the Apollo Iron and Steel Company obtained control of a plant at Apollo, a small industrial town about 40 miles from Pittsburg. Prudence and good management compelled annual extension, but the firm were always at a disadvantage in that they could not build with a plan. The buildings were old, were too small, so that it was almost useless to put in modern machinery; however, the business grew steadily until the issue was no longer to be dodged, "Shall we remake Apollo, or shall we begin from the very bottom a new town, which may be planned along lines of the most progressive, social and industrial development?" The latter course was decided on.

In 1895 the new town to be known as Vandergrift consisted of acres of fields and meadows, beautifully situated on the broad sweep of river, with a background of wooded hills. While the new mills were building it was imperative that homes for the workingmen should also be built, so that, just as soon as the mills were completed and in operation, the force could go to work without the loss of a single day. It was no small undertaking to house comfortably a thousand workingmen and their families. The company displayed wisdom and forethought in planning a town which should have the most improved system of sanitation and pure and ample water supply, paved streets and concrete sidewalks, gas and electricity.

In the first place the physical basis of the town was planned on the lines of natural beauty by Mr. H. L. Olmsted; accordingly winding streets, a village green or common, frequent open spaces for shrubs and flowers, relieved the stiffness and ugliness of the ordinary town.

A constant water supply was secured by artesian wells on the hills; a complete system of sewers and drains made the town clean, for cleanliness meant health; the streets were brick paved, the sidewalks concreted and little triangular spaces were planted with shrubbery. With their splendid water supply there is no need for wells, which are often the cause of malaria and typhoid fever; in fact, there are no wells. Then, too, each house is provided with bath room and water closet, doing away with unsightly outbuildings. Vandergrift is not merely a mill town; nearly every man owns his own house, and time is devoted to taking care of its people by its people.

The president, Mr. George McMurtry, stated that they already had good men when they began Vandergrift, but they needed more. He knew of no way so sure for getting a steady supply of good men, after giving them work and paying them well, as to help them a little. In his judgment no other help is so wise as giving the men a chance to help themselves. Based on this social and industrial philosophy, residence lots, averaging 25 by 125 feet, were offered at $750 to $1050 for inside and $1500 to $2500 for corner lots. This price was based on the average sales in Apollo from 1890 to 1895. While these prices were high, it must be borne in mind that all improvements, viz., paved streets and sidewalks, water and gas connections and sewer connections made on every lot are included in the initial cost. The owner, therefore, has no additional expense of assessments for improvements that are needed at uncertain periods and unknown rates, since at Vandergrift the only additional expense is that of the house. The only restriction which the deed contains is that no liquor shall be sold on the premises for 99 years. This practice of selling land without restriction to the employés will be watched with much interest, because it is contrary to the usual practice.

A school with accommodations for 200 pupils was built by the company. A bank with a capital of $50,000 was organized. A large tract in the center of the town was given for a village green, and a smaller tract for a hospital and a casino. In addition the company was very liberal in providing for the spiritual and moral needs of the town by giving any religious denomination the land, and by contributing half of $15,000, which sum was fixed as the minimum cost for construction of the edifice. There are now five churches in Vandergrift.

While the churches provided for a large amount of social

intercourse, the company felt the necessity of providing for the larger social needs of the community, especially in the winter season. The casino built, at an expense of $30,000, contains an auditorium and a stage. In one wing of the building are the library and reading rooms, and in the other, rooms for the local magistrates and court rooms. The ground floor of one wing is used by the fire department.

The founder and presiding spirit of the Roycroft Shop, at East Aurora, N. Y., Elbert Hubbard, seeks the highest development of the worker by means of work under the most inspiring conditions, not only as best for the worker himself but as securing from him the best service.

This principle has been applied in a village with something less than 2000 population, which aside from the Roycroft Shop is almost entirely an agricultural community. Except for a few skilled workmen as heads of departments and instructors, the surrounding farms have furnished all the Roycroft workers, many of whom are boys and girls, and practically all of whom are without knowledge of a trade but have acquired all their skill at the work entirely within the shop. The principle has been found to be "a wise business policy" asserts Mr. Hubbard, who stated in 1902 that upon an investment of about $250,000, a net profit of over $200,000 in seven years had been realized. One fact must be borne in mind, however, in judging of this "social and industrial experiment," as it has been called by its author. The business, chiefly artistic bookmaking and publishing, is outside the field of sharp price competition, and, owing to the special reputation of its founder and head, enjoys a certain monopoly in its market.

The property of the Lynchburg cotton mill consists of 130 acres. The mills are situated on the bottom land next to the creek, while the houses of the operatives occupy the hillside above, and are built on either side of wide streets, making a good-sized village. The houses, which are comfortable and home-like, have recently been painted and the company is having the streets graded and planted with shade trees; where necessary, retaining walls are being built, terraces laid off, low places filled, and grass is being sown everywhere. Above the village is a beautiful grove in which in the summer religious services are held, while in bad weather the church close by is used. Not far off is the school, in which teaching goes on day and night, in charge of the Salvation Army, the company paying the light, fuel, books and supplies. This mill is seeking the improvement, mental, physical and spiritual, of its employés, those in charge of it expecting to reap their reward by having their help better satisfied with their surroundings and thus more to be depended upon, and giving more satisfactory service at the big plant, which is nearly always more or less short of operatives.

It has been the aim of the Maryland Steel Company to make Sparrow's Point an attractive and healthful place of residence for its employés. The broad streets laid out at right angles, and lined with shade trees, are kept in repair by the management, which has also provided electric lights, schoolhouses, a fire department and police force, as well as a thorough system of public sanitation. The various religious denominations have handsome and commodious houses of worship on lots donated by the company. A free kindergarten was opened in 1892. Another department of the public school system is the manual training school, in which more than 160 boys are learning the rudiments of mechanical work and drawing. There is also a school of domestic science, with sewing and cooking classes for the girls.

The town of Pelzer, in which the factories of the Pelzer Company are located, contains a population of about 6000 persons, all of whom are more or less dependent for their livelihood upon the mills. The town is not incorporated, but is held as private property by the mill corporation, which owns every house and every foot of land in the place. No home ownership is allowed, the policy of the company being one of absolute industrial control, coupled with a large regard for the general welfare of its employés. There are five churches, neat and commodious in construction and well attended by the operatives. In the matter of providing educational facilities for its employés, the company has taken an advanced position. Two well equipped schools, with kindergarten departments annexed, are maintained. These are open 10 months in the year and are absolutely free to all residents of the place. There are also night classes for those whose work prevents their attending the day sessions. As a condition of obtaining employment in the mills, parents are required to sign an agreement in which the clause is inserted: "I do agree that all children, members of my family between the ages of 5 and 12 years, shall enter the school maintained by said company at Pelzer, and shall attend every school day during the school session, unless prevented by sickness or other unavoidable causes." In addition to this, each child who attends school a month without absence receives a prize of 10 cents. As there is no compulsory school law in South Carolina, and the length of the public school term is not more than four months per year, the comparative educational advantages offered at Pelzer appear very great. As an evidence of the great good being accomplished by these schools, it may be said that when they were first started probably 75 per cent. of the adult population of the place could not read or write. Now this percentage has been reduced to 15 or 20, and the illiterates are chiefly newcomers from the rural districts nearby. About $5000 is expended annually by the company in the maintenance of the schools.

The Indiana Steel Company, one of the subsidiary companies of the United States Steel Corporation, is now building a town of its own, Gary. It is incorporated, contains approximately 12 square miles, fronting the shore of Lake Michigan for a distance of seven miles, and is distant 25 miles from the center of Chicago. It is expected that other large plants will be constructed in Gary by companies allied in interest with the Indiana Steel Company. To assist in the building up of a city of homes for the employés of the Indiana Steel Company, to secure as far as possible good pavements, pure water, proper sewerage and drainage and the best possible conditions for the health and comfort of the residents of the town, the Gary Land Company has been organized. It desires that the employés of the mill shall own their own homes, and that all who wish to reside in the town shall assist in building it up as rapidly as possible and along lines that will furnish wholesome surroundings to every one.

It has fixed prices on the lots which it offers for sale as

low as possible consistent with the cost of the land and improvements, and with no desire of making a profit.

The company has built 500 modern dwelling houses, in addition to one hotel building, containing 40 rooms, one restaurant building, two modern lodging houses and one school house, with a capacity for approximately 500 pupils. An interurban electric line passing through Gary from South Bend, Ind., to Chicago, is under construction and is expected to be in operation by July 1st.

The first subdivision contains some 800 acres, divided into 4000 lots, the majority of which are 25 feet by 125 feet and some 30 feet by 150 feet. The most of the streets are 60 feet in width. The principal street running north and south is 100 feet in width, and the principal street running east and west is 80 feet in width, both paved with concrete blocks. The remaining streets are now being paved with macadam. The sewer system in the first subdivision consists of a discharge main 96 inches in diameter, with lateral branches 60 inches, 54 inches and 36 inches in diameter. A water supply system, with 91,000 lineal feet of water pipe laid, has been installed, and a competent water supply is being furnished from driven wells with temporary pumps. There is under construction a permanent water works pumping station and water tunnel, 72 inches in diameter, 15,000 feet in length, extending into Lake Michigan 7000 feet from the present shore line. Provision has been made for the installation of a water purifying system in connection with this plant, should it be necessary. A gas works with a capacity of 300,000 cubic feet of artificial gas per day is in operation.

Manufacturers realize that their workmen of to-day are growing older and must be replaced by the younger element which is growing up. Frequently the ranks are recruited from their sons and daughters. The more an employer can show the mothers that he takes a personal interest in their families the greater will be his influence over the children when the time comes for them to seek work. In this way the personal relationship between him and his workers is maintained.

One industrialist who has always tried to cultivate friendly relations with and endeavored to be on good terms with the people composing the tenement population, on Decoration and

Labor days of each year collects fifty to one hundred children who live nearest to the works, and sends them on an outing free of expense to them or their parents. Sometimes they are carried by trolley cars, and at other times they are taken out to the woods in some suburb of the city in the company's wagons. Refreshments are provided in abundance and all expenses are paid. The company is very much pleased with the results of this plan, as the interest and friendliness of the children of the neighborhood are secured and property otherwise unprotected is cheerfully taken care of by them.

For the steel works' employés in Pueblo a neighborhood house was established in the grove, as a social center for the residents of that community, many of whom are foreigners. The company encourages this work, and is represented on its board of management.

The McAden Mills built a library for the use of its employés, and the income from stocks and bonds left by Giles M. McAden in his will, is used for the maintenance. The library will of course be for the public good and use of the town of McAdenville.

One employer in order to coöperate with the people in the neighborhood of his factory, formed an improvement association. By means of lantern slide talks he showed graphically how a few vines and flowers would cover and beautify fences and sheds; the backyards cleared from rubbish and transformed into gardens, the front yards made beautiful with turf and flowers, and the decorative effect of porch and window boxes. To follow up this picture teaching, he engaged a landscape gardener, whose services were freely at the command of all. An additional stimulus of cash prizes was offered for those who made the most marked improvement. In a short time this neighborhood, from being known as a by-word and a reproach, became one of the show places of the city. The whole tone of the community was raised, and the value of property more than doubled.

Ten years ago this factory was a comparatively small affair, its building little different from those of similar use; its surroundings as unattractive as usually gather around machine shops and foundries. The region of the city in which it was located was undeveloped and not desirable for residence. Back-yards and dump piles of rubbish were the visions upon which the operatives gazed. In remedying this the management sent to the best landscape gardener in the country, with a result that to-day there are few parks which offer more beauties to the eye than the pictures framed before the eyes of the workmen. Broad open lawns, properly arranged shrubbery, garden windows and vine-covered walls are now seen on every hand.

In order to encourage the beautifying of homes and surroundings the company has adopted the plan of awarding prizes to those of its tenants whose yards and lawns are kept in the best condition. In 1902 the prizes offered were as follows: For ground as a whole, first prize, $25; second, $20; third, $15; fourth, $10, and three prizes of $5 each. Special prizes: For best work in flower culture, $10; for best work in vegetable culture, $10; for best lawn, $5; for best window or porch box, $5. A number of smaller prizes were also distributed among those whom the judges decided to be worthy of them. Competition for these prizes is not restricted to the company's employés, but is open to all residents of the village in which the works are located.

For several years the Draper Company of Hopedale, Mass., has offered prizes for the best kept premises, including the back as well as the front yard. The practice of stimulating the individual householder by means of cash incentives is growing among industrialists, who thus advance the whole tone of the community. The offer of the Draper Company is comprehensive and so characteristic of this kind of civic encouragement that their circular is printed in full:

TO THE TENANTS OF THE DRAPER COMPANY

The committee on yard prizes has had placed at its disposal the sum of $300, to be distributed for the year 1908 as follows, among the tenants living in houses belonging to the company in Hopedale:

One First Prize, $10.

Twelve Second Prizes, $7.50 each.

Forty-two Third Prizes, $5 each.

These prizes will be awarded on the condition of the premises for the season, and the yards will be inspected by the committee from time to time.

While shrubs and flowers will be given favorable consideration in judging the relative merits of competing tenements, a display of flowers will not offset a slackly kept lawn or an untidy back yard.

All vaults will be cleaned at the expense of the company and ashes carted away as soon as practicable. After this cleaning has been done, tenants will make use of the garbage cans provided for the reception of decaying matter, and ashes can be thrown into the same receptacle. These cans will be emptied at the company's expense as usual. After the final cleaning in the fall, ashes are not to be kept in the cans, and the cans are to be stored under cover.

An additional sum of $75 will be distributed among the tenants of the company living in the houses on Prospect Heights, Milford. This sum may be reduced according to the number of tenants occupying the premises during the season. It will be divided into First, Second and Third Prizes, on about the same basis as the distribution above indicated among the other tenants.

Prizes will be awarded in November.

The experiment was tried in 1906 of ornamenting the store front of Strawbridge & Clothier's with window boxes. "What a happy thought," has been exclaimed so many times, as the trailing vines and the bright blossoms have brought visions of the green and restful country to the town-tired eyes, toil-worn brains and weary hearts of the thousands of workers within the store, while the passers-by have been gladdened and surprised by the beauty of vine and flower in the heart of the city.

By many, the improvement of factory surroundings, its adornment by vines and flowers, is considered pure sentiment. But I claim that it has a direct commercial value. Illustrating concretely: In conversation with a foreman whose office window overlooked a vista of beautiful green lawn with beds of flowers and shrubbery, I inquired what was the effect of all this on him. "Well, it is like this," he said. "The other day I didn't feel at all well and thought I'd knock off and go home.

Happening to glance from my window on the beautiful outlook, I said to myself, 'Why not rest here a while instead of going home?' The quiet and restfulness of the scene seemed to work wonders. After an hour I felt strong enough to go on with my work." If this man had gone home the company would have lost his services for the day, and his whole department would have suffered.

When Walter W. Law retired from active business in New York and decided that he would devote his energies to an occupation that would keep him out of doors, he bought a tract of 225 acres near Scarboro, and called it Briarcliff Manor. The Manor now comprises 6000 acres. This Aladdin-like growth is but the realization of a comprehensive plan that was in Mr. Law's mind from the very first.

With the development of the farms as a dominating influence, the Manor is now a village of enlarged boundaries, with a greater population than ever before, and with the character of that population similarly raised. As the community grew, new and imperative needs were met in the provision of safe and ample water and sewage service and the building of modern roadways. For the same reason, new service factors were logically called into being in a place isolated from industrial market centers. Then came a hotel. In its train came stables, iron, wheelwright, paint, upholstery and repair shops, associated with the surveying, engineering and construction departments. A print shop was fitted for most up-to-date requirements, where the *Briarcliff Outlook* is published monthly, and where all the printing of the community is handled.

The policy of Briarcliff Farms is to encourage among its men the building of their own homes and aid them financially in doing so, the unmarried men boarding here and there throughout the village.

The trend of effort is to provide homes for the men and families in small individual cottages, rather than in large buildings, and to encourage in all possible ways neatness of premises and tidiness and beauty in all quarters. Restrictions are still imposed against the entrance of liquor dealers and all other undesirable property holders, influences which would hamper the effect of a splendid school growth within the village.

In the efforts of the Ludlow Associates for the betterment of the working and living conditions of its employés, its treasurer, Charles W. Hubbard, states that it has been the aim of the corporation to make the village an attractive place in which to live. Apart from philanthropic motives, the managers believe that by so doing they will be able to attract a superior class of operatives. When the present corporation first purchased the property there were but two streets, containing a church, a single-room schoolhouse and a few old-fashioned tenements. During the last thirty years the corporation has built four miles of good streets, and has partly constructed at its own expense, the water works, gas works and electric light plant, lighting the village streets without charge. It has provided and now owns the church, one of the schoolhouses, the Masonic hall and all except a few of the houses in the village. The original intention was to encourage private ownership of cottages, but after several sales were made this was deemed undesirable, except in the case of small farms outside of the village. While the original purchaser might be satisfactory, the property was liable to pass into undesirable hands, and the enforcing of restrictions as to pig pens, hen yards and other nuisances might be resented. The cottages sold have been bought back as opportunity offered.

A firm like the Plymouth Cordage Company which has found that its industrial betterment is a success in that its employés and the community coöperate by meeting them halfway is willing when it sees an opportunity to benefit others, to improve it. The thought occurred to them that where the property fronted the shore of Plymouth Bay, a bathing beach could be opened for the enjoyment of the people. The slope of the land made it necessary to build it out and restrain it by a parapet wall. This made a splendid playground for the children, where they could dig in the sand and enjoy the fresh breezes of the ocean without wetting their feet and dresses. On Sunday afternoons whole families may be seen enjoying themselves—the father and mother taking a dip while the little ones are busy making sand houses on the beach. On several Sundays there were from 600 to 700 people spending the afternoon watching the bathers as they dove and swam about. There are two bath houses, one for the men and boys, the other for the women and girls. The company furnishes suits for the bathers at the low rental of one cent per suit; also towels at one cent each. Suits are also on sale at wholesale prices. The bath houses are in charge of an experienced man, who teaches the boys and girls to swim, dive and float. During the last two summers there have been more than 9000 baths taken. The beach is usually lined with young people every afternoon, except Saturday.

On Saturday afternoon the interest of the crowd centers around the ball field, which is situated back of the office building. Every Saturday afternoon, weather permitting, a game is held between the factory club and a visiting team. The team has been growing stronger each year, winning the majority of the games played. The games were witnessed by 700 to 800 people, and are free, with the exception that they give what they think they can afford to help defray the expenses of the visiting team.

At the Central Carolina Fair held in Greensboro in October, 1906, there was an industrial betterment exhibit from the people of the Proximity and White Oak mills, when there were displayed specimens of the work made in the school, cooking, sewing and basketry classes, garden classes and original articles of various kinds made by the Proximity folk. This exhibit filled a booth 50 by 15 feet, and excited considerable favorable comment. It was a matter of astonishment to the up-town neighbors that these people could produce such excellent work. Even Mr. Cone, who was familiar with what was going on, when the exhibit was installed was greatly surprised and pleased at the creditable display. There were dresses made by girls under 16 years which would have been a credit to professional dressmakers, and in the general competition with Greensboro and the surrounding country people, the factory folk captured 19 prizes out of 23 articles listed for competition.

The Waltham Watch Company maintains three parks, situated opposite the factory, which are for public use, although under the control of the company. In one of these is a band stand, where evening concerts are given by the Waltham Watch Company Band. In connection with the factory proper, lawns, courts and three fountains are provided for the enjoyment and pleasure of the employés.

The Roycrofters believe that attractive surroundings are a good thing for the workers and also for the community. Exteriorly are well kept lawns, shade trees and flower beds, which combined with the old English style of architecture of the half dozen buildings—three of them built of stone—and the location in the residence portion of the village, give the place the appearance of a school or college rather than a factory. Within, save in press room, carpenter and blacksmith shops, which are perforce plainer, are curtains and draperies at doors and windows, pictures and busts adorning walls or fireplace mantels, with rugs and antique furniture, more suggestive of a well-furnished library than a workshop.

A croquet lawn and tennis ground is frequently used, not only during the noon recess, but after business hours also, at a Detroit paint factory.

A boys' garden may seem insignificant in a discussion of what an employer may do for the betterment of the community in which his factory is located, and yet the establishment of little gardens in a factory neighborhood was the means of improvement in values to the extent of $30,000. In 1897 an employer found that his foremen preferred to go away from the immediate neighborhood for their homes. Not being able to account for the fact, he gave the problem careful study. "Upon investigation," he said, "we found that the boys gave the neighborhood its bad reputation, and that they had cost the property owners within a radius of four blocks of the factory $30,000 in depreciation of their land. Studying further, we soon found that these boys had been made bad by idleness. Then, too, the wide windows of the new factory drew the fire of the boys of the neighborhood. They smashed the panes and damaged the machinery. They pulled the flowers, trampled down the grass and tore up the shrubbery." The proprietor called the boys together and told them about his boyhood on a farm, when he had helped to plow the ground on which his factory now stands. He challenged their interest, and said that he would set aside a tract of land, where each boy might have his own little garden. The company furnished the tools, seeds and a competent instructor, each boy pledging himself to obey simple rules and pay ten cents each month. The product of the gardens was to belong to each little farmer, for use in his own home or for sale. Prizes of medals, cash, educational trips and diplomas are given by the company. The boys were enthusiastic from the start, and soon forgot the delights of window-breaking. These boys' gardens have grown each year. One year there were seventy-two gardens, and the young farmers harvested nearly ten tons of vegetables.

A gymnastic class for girls under thirteen is open to any resident of South Park, which is the general city district in which a large Ohio factory is located. There are about seventy-five or one hundred pupils in this class, which meets Saturday mornings in one of the factory buildings. Simple gymnastic exercises are given, to teach the children correct posture and bodily grace. There is also a boys' gymnastic class of about forty members under thirteen years of age.

Many a community is unprovided with halls large enough for conventions, mass meetings or other gatherings at which the greater part of the inhabitants desire to attend. At the Natural Food Company, Niagara Falls, a spacious convention hall has been provided, with a seating capacity of 1000. It has a stage, is magnificently lighted and contains every facility for effective and satisfactory demonstrative work. As a meeting place for societies it is most advantageous, and that it is often used for this purpose attests the popular appreciation of the public-spirited generosity of the company, who gave it to the societies free of charge.

A communal movement was the recent organization by the Ludlow Manufacturing Associates of the village of Ludlow, of a series of dinners at which representative working men and village officials take part. At the first dinner Hon. Carroll D. Wright made the address. The second dinner was held in January, 1908, at the Stevens Memorial building. Covers were laid for 170, which included all the heads of departments and their assistants, the managing trustees of the Ludlow Manufacturing Associates and invited guests.

A city benefit asociation is a form of communal betterment which had its start as an organization among the related industries of vehicle making in Flint, Mich., which is known as "The Vehicle City," where the chief industries center about the vehicle and its constituent parts.

For six years there have been a Vehicle Benefit Association and a Vehicle Club, which have been elements of great importance in the ever increasing magnitude of vehicle industries and the consequent increasing list of employés. The benefit association was the first to be organized. Its plan contemplates a fund for maintenance of any employé who is incapacitated by sickness or accident, and it provides a payment of funeral expenses in case of death. Later on, as the insurance membership grew, it naturally developed into a fraternity, or a club. The managements of the different factories were glad to foster and encourage an institution of this character, and in 1901 they equipped a suite of club rooms at a considerable expense, and turned them over to the benefit association as its permanent home.

The club rooms consist of an executive office, reading rooms, billiard rooms, bowling alleys, card rooms, a gymnasium and a fine equipment of baths. From time to time additions have been made to the various departments of the work, until the club is now by far the best equipped of any organization of that character in the city.

The dues for the insurance department are ten cents a week, and for club membership the same amount. There are no fees for admission; a workman may waive his membership when he is unemployed, and can avail himself of the benefits upon again taking up his work, without additional expense. He is assured of a revenue for 18 weeks a year during sickness, or as the result of an accident, and is not in any way restricted as to his medical attendance.

The benefit department has paid out $23,000 for sick and accident benefits, and over $1500 for funeral expenses. For the same period the management expenses have been a trifle over $5000.

Membership in the benefit association is nearly 1500, and the membership of the club is 600. The employés manage the institution entirely among themselves, hold their annual and stated meetings, elect their own officers, devise and approve their own by-laws and conduct all of their own affairs.

John Roebling's Sons[1] needed a new site for the increasing expansion of their business, whose main plant is located at Trenton. Except at prohibitive prices no more land could be bought adjoining the mills. Accordingly, a site a mile below Kinkora on the Delaware proved to be the one most satisfactory. The erection of rolling mills there was, however, the least of the problems confronting the Roeblings.

Kinkora itself is but little more than a hamlet, without facilities to house and otherwise provide for a small army of workmen, and even such as it is, it is a mile distant from the site of the new city. The time and expense involved in compelling the employés to travel between Trenton and the new mills below Kinkora put that out of the question as a place for the men to live in. Something radically different had to be done, and it is as a solution of this purely business problem that the new city was evolved.

"Having determined upon Kinkora as the site for the expansion of our mills, we were forced to build houses for the men to live in who will be employed there," is the simple explanation of the Roeblings. "Inasmuch as we had to build houses anyway, we are building as well as we know how, and incidentally are providing some other things for the benefit of our employés. The rentals will pay interest on the investment. We do not ask or expect any other returns, and we certainly are not posing as idealists or reformers."

Kinkora, or "Roebling," as it is more likely to be known, lies between the Delaware river and the Pennsylvania Railroad tracks, on a tract of 237 acres. Originally little more than an arid waste of sand, it is being transformed by grading, sodding, irrigation and the planting of trees into a city beautiful.

In spending some $4,000,000, they are doing this only because business forces them to do so. It is not to avoid labor troubles—they have had none of more than trifling importance in the sixty years since the first little wire plant was built in Trenton.

The village is located on the south bank of the Delaware river about ten miles below Trenton, on a comparatively level tract about 40 feet above the stream. The streets are 100 feet

[1] John A. Roebling's Sons Co., Trenton, N. J. Manufacturers of Steel and Wire. Organized 1876. Number Employés, 8000.

and 80 feet wide, parallel and perpendicular to the bank of the river, lying in a nearly east and west and north and south direction. The wider streets have a parkway through the center, with a driveway on either side. All the streets have been planted with maple trees on both sides, and all the space in front of houses not occupied by the roadway and sidewalks, has been cultivated in grass. Ten foot alleys are run through the center of all blocks from which collections of ashes and garbage may be made, and for the accommodation of delivery wagons. All houses except types Nos. 1 and 6 are on lots 30 feet wide by 100 feet deep. The type No. 1 houses are on lots 16 feet by 100 feet deep and the type No. 6 houses are on lots 20 feet by 120 feet deep. All back yards are fenced off by a wire netting fence four feet high, with strong framework and heavy galvanized netting. The sidewalks are of crushed stone bounded with yellow pine curbing. The drives are paved with macadam and are 20 feet wide on the 100 feet streets where there are two drives, and 30 feet wide on the 80 feet streets, where there is but one drive. The land adjoining the river front is devoted to park purposes and is laid off with walks and cultivated in grass, which with its natural growth of trees makes an attractive and restful place of retreat, commanding a fine view of the river, with ample provision of seats.

The village is supplied with a system of water works with fire hydrants on every block, and a standpipe pressure sufficient for fire protection. This water system is also extended to every house and supplies an unlimited amount of filtered water which costs the tenant nothing beyond the price of his rent.

A separate system of sewers is in operation to which every house is connected, even the cheapest dwellings being provided with kitchen sinks and sanitary water closets.

Illuminating gas is supplied to the village from the main supply of an outside corporation, but the company owns its own street mains and supplies every house at $1 per thousand cubic feet.

The company maintains a general store conducted on a cash basis, or where accounts may be settled weekly. It also maintains a licensed hotel where a bar, billiard room and bowling alleys are run for the benefit of the men, and where transients may be comfortably accommodated. There are also a hotel for single men, where good board and a single room may be had cheap; a public hall for dances, entertainments, meetings and religious services; an emergency hospital fully equipped for accidents; a graded school for the children and a fire department with volunteer membership. Bread is made in a model bakery, and there is a small prison for the temporary detention of unlawful persons. The streets are lighted by arc lamps, and all public buildings and the better classes of houses are lighted by incandescent lamps, electrical energy being furnished by the company at a very low rate.

The ownership and management of the whole property is strictly a private enterprise in the hands of the company, and it is not the present intention to dispose of any property to employés. The village is not incorporated, which leaves its administration entirely to its owners.

There are 312 houses thus far constructed and they embrace ten different types. They are all of brick with slate roofs and of first class construction. The rents of the various types are based on the costs of each, and are so proportioned that the interest on the original investment is but a small amount after deducting the cost of operation.

Type No. 1 has four rooms, shed extension, two stories; attic not finished; built in blocks of ten; yellow pine trim; finished natural; rent,[1] $8.50.

No. 2 has seven rooms, including shed kitchen, semi-detached; two stories and an attic; yellow pine trim; finished natural; rent, $9.50.

No. 3: Eight rooms, bath, vestibule and reception hall; semi-detached; cypress trim; finished natural; steam heat. Two stories and attic; rent, $15.

No. 4: Six rooms, bath and shed extension; semi-detached; yellow pine trim; finished natural; steam heat. Two stories and attic; rent, $12.

No. 5: Nine rooms, bath, butler's pantry, shed extension, vestibule and reception hall, semi-detached; cypress trim; finished natural; steam heat; electric lights. Two stories and attic; laundry in cellar; rent, $20.

No. 6: Ten rooms and bath; eight houses in block, 20 feet

[1] All rental rates are by the month.

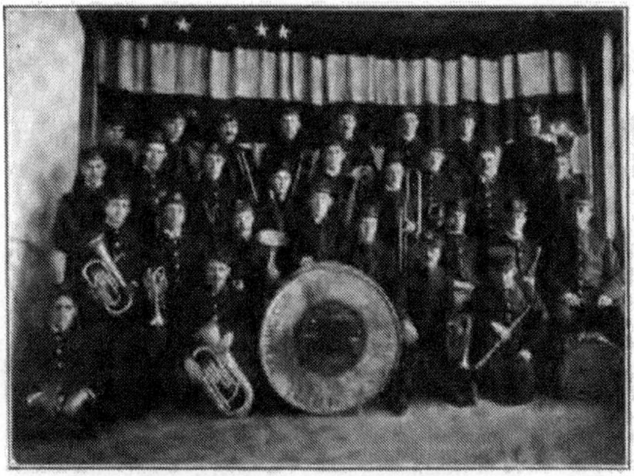

The Remington Typewriter Company's Band.

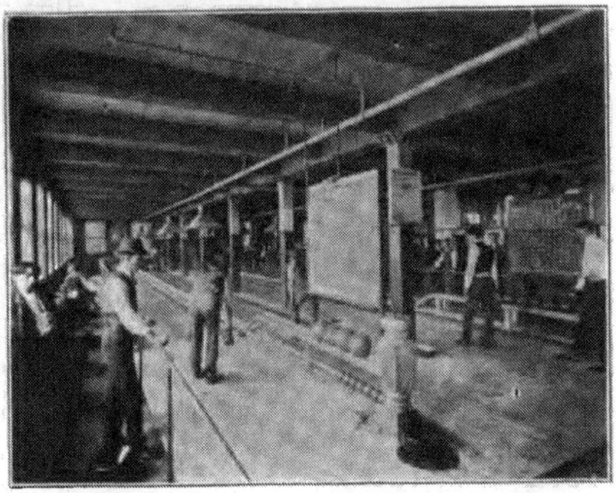

Recreation at the Thomas G. Plant Company, Boston.

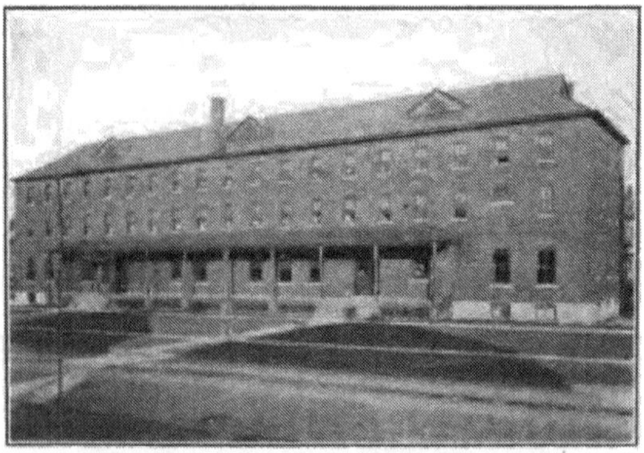

The Workingmen's Hotel at Kinkora, the Industrial Commonwealth Built by the John A. Roebling's Sons Company.

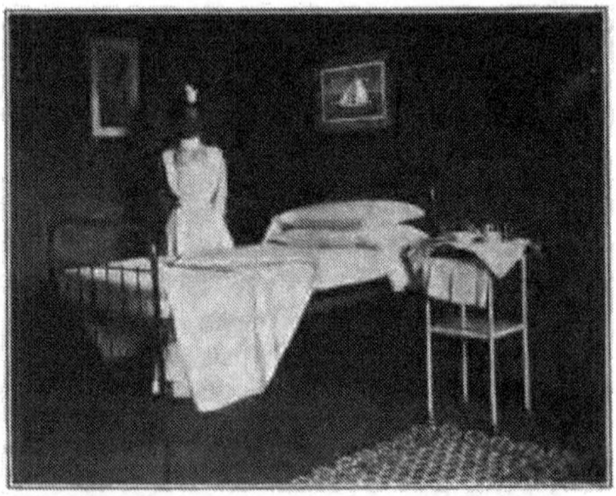

One of the Bedrooms at the Minnequa Hospital of the Colorado Fuel and Iron Company.

wide each; yellow pine trim; finished natural; electric lights; steam heat; three stories; laundry in cellar; rent, $20.

No. 7: Eight rooms, bath, butler's pantry, reception hall and vestibule, semi-detached; cypress trim, natural finish; steam heat, electric lights. Two stories and attic; laundry in cellar; rent, $20.

No. 8: Eight rooms; bath, reception hall and vestibule, semi-detached; cypress trim; finished natural; steam heat; electric lights. Two stories and attic; laundry in cellar; rent, $20 per month.

No. 9: Eight rooms; bath, reception hall and vestibule, semi-detached; cypress trim; natural finish; steam heat, electric lights. Two stories and attic; rent, $18.

No. 10: Eleven rooms; bath, reception hall, butler's pantry; detached cottage; cypress trim; natural finish; hot water heat; electric lights. Two stories and attic; laundry in cellar; rent, $25.

At Homestead, Pa., a movement which enlisted one-sixth of the population, a number equal to one-fifth of the possible membership in the organization, is succeeding in touching the community. One side of the work, the music hall, with its organ recitals, choruses, lectures and other entertainments, has attracted a total attendance during the last year equivalent to every man, woman and child attending ten times. In 1898 the Carnegie Library was organized, with four departments, the library, the library club, the educational department and the music hall.

One object of the library is to "make provision for the student." In addition to a large circulating library, a reference collection is provided for more definite research. When these conveniences are not sufficient, educational classes are conducted to give the student the benefit of more definite instruction and guidance in the pursuit of knowledge. As a rule the subjects taught are those contributing toward his daily occupation. The æsthetic and artistic sides of life are developed by the musical features included in this department.

The only tuition required to join the educational classes is membership in the Carnegie Library Club during the school term from October to March inclusive; a quarterly rate of $1 or $2 in all. A deposit of $2 is required at the beginning of the term. One dollar will be returned if the student attends seventy-five per cent. of the possible sessions. The remaining dollar will be applied on the club dues for the second quarter. The outfit for students in the mechanical drawing class is furnished at cost; instruments, uniforms and music are furnished for the band, and music for the orchestra. The text-books used may be borrowed from the library for the season.

All classes meet at 7:30 o'clock, P. M. In the mechanical drawing course the instructor is the assistant mechanical engineer of the Homestead Steel Works. As most of the students in this class fill positions in the mills the work pursued is most practical. A student graduating from this class is capable of entering a higher class in the Carnegie Technical Schools or if he secures a position in the mills is able to render valuable service as an apprentice. A number of students have been selected from this class to fill positions in the mills. No promise, however, is made that any student will be given a position at any time.

COMMON BRANCHES

Reading, writing, arithmetic, spelling, United States History, grammar and geography.

The instruction in this class, for the most part, is individual. That is, a student gets personal instruction, and is in position to take one or more studies and progress as rapidly as he is able.

HIGHER BRANCHES

Algebra, geometry, trigonometry, Latin and physics.

The branches taught in this class, like those in the class in common branches, depend somewhat on the demand of the students.

METALLURGY

The iron ores, fuels, fluxes, refractories, the blast furnace, pig iron, foundry practice, open hearth process and Bessemer process, under the instruction of a metallurgist steel works instructor.

While a knowledge of chemistry would be an aid to a student in this class, it is not an entrance requirement. Out of the 35 students that attended last year a few had a meager knowledge of chemistry. This is a rare opportunity to get a comprehensive idea of the manufacture of iron and steel.

FIRST AID TO THE INJURED

Accidents, asphyxia, drowning, burns, scalds, bites, poisons, emergencies, alcoholism, fractures and preventive medicine.

The instructor is the surgeon of the Homestead Steel Works. It is just the kind of a class that the average housewife should attend. The doctor is pleased to have any one listen to one lecture as a sample. If the work done does not appeal to him, he need not come again.

SLAVISH-ENGLISH

Mr. R. Hofen, instructor, manager foreign department, Monongahela Trust Company.

Mr. Hofen speaks fluently several foreign languages and is perfectly able to meet any demands the foreign membership may make. A notice of this class printed in Slavish can be had upon application.

The Carnegie Library Band is conducted as an amateur organization. Any man having sufficient musical ability to pass Prof. Thompson's examination is eligible to membership, club membership being the only dues required. There are at present thirty members.

The orchestra like the band is an amateur organization, and is conducted as an educational feature. A musical standard is necessary, and this may be ascertained by consulting the director. The orchestra had a membership of thirty last year.

The work done in the strings class is largely for beginners. Lessons are given on the violin, mandolin and guitar. As the students become proficient they are enrolled in the Carnegie Library Mandolin and Guitar Club. In this way they are taught to play in concert, and are given an opportunity to play before the public. There were 42 students last year.

A voice and ability to read music are required of applicants to enter the Homestead Library male chorus class. The membership during last year was 45.

ORATORIO

If sufficient interest is manifested in an oratorio Prof. D. J. George will drill the chorus for this purpose. If the singers in the vicinity, including the male chorus, can be united in this grand musical effort, it is believed it will be one of the most delightful efforts of the year on the part of the educational committee. The talent will be selected.

The children's chorus has come to be a permanent feature. Last year the chorus numbered 80. Only those having fairly good voices will be admitted. A fair test, however, will be given any child that applies. There are no dues for joining the oratorio or children's chorus. The chorus gives two entertainments this season, one in January and the other in March. The committee also plans to have the children sing at the annual exhibition of the educational department.

The library possesses one of the finest organs in the county. It is the desire of the committee on education to have the people in this community receive the most possible good from it. While the organ may be used on other occasions, arrangements have been made to give one recital for adults and one for the children.

It was the policy of the management of the Carnegie Library to give the citizens of the community an opportunity for physical development. Through the agency of the library club the means for perfect physical development are supplied; the library and educational work contributes toward the mental; and the music hall, with its entertainments and lectures, contributes toward the moral and ethical.

According to the prospectus, it is the object of the physical department to furnish to the members the best possible opportunity for the development of sound, active, enduring bodies, thus enabling them to pursue their vocations to the best advantage.

It seems unnecessary to state that it is impossible to keep in a healthy condition, much less a vigorous one, without taking sufficient bodily exercise.

There is no more effective nor convenient way of securing this vigorous, driving force than by making good use of a well-appointed gymnasium during the winter months.

To the boy or girl the gymnasium affords the opportunity to secure the proper unfolding of his or her physical capacity and beauty, and counteracts the many physical defects and unnatural conditions to which he or she is subjected in ordinary school life.

To the student it offers healthful and effective recreation from mental application, securing and maintaining the physical stamina so necessary to his safety and success.

To the young man of the office and counting room it affords opportunity for healthful relief from physical and mental strain, furnishing recreation and correcting deformities caused by his pursuit.

To ladies it affords a much needed opportunity for recreation and health-giving exercise. Here, clad in an unhampering costume, they find it a pleasure to go through exercises that build up the physique symmetrically, improve the carriage and keep the body in a vigorous, healthy condition.

To the mechanic, and business or professional man it offers a means of healthful recreation and relaxation so necessary to prevent blood stagnation during the winter months.

To the young man more ambitious along the physical line it offers an opportunity to become a gymnast of the utmost proficiency.

Recreation figures largely in the work of the institution. Basketball, indoor baseball and other games are conducted after the class periods.

The inexperienced need not hesitate to enter the classes at any time. Provision is always made for them, and the director will always be glad to consult with them as to the best method of beginning work.

Parents may feel assured that their children receive the best of treatment, and that only exercises that will positively benefit them are taught in the classes.

A cordial invitation is extended to parents to visit the gymnasium and witness the class drills.

Classes are conducted to piano music.

It is the aim of the management to encourage all scientific games and games of skill, and to eliminate all games of mere chance. The billiard room is exceptionally large, well-ventilated and cheerful. There are six billiard tables and four pool tables. Time cards are issued in order of application, entitling the holder to the use of the table for a half hour, with no extra charge for the use of tables. The game room is equipped with shuffleboard, portable bowling alley, carom boards and an assortment of other games, which may be obtained at the office.

In the parlor will be found easy chairs, rockers, reading tables, papers, magazines and books. The game room and parlor is open for boys on Wednesday evenings from 6:30 until 8 o'clock.

The tenth annual report in 1907 states that the library has increased its circulation at an average rate of 23,000 a year; the club has grown from an average monthly membership of 458 the first year to 1095; the first season in the educational work, including the band, in 1900, had an attendance of 2450, compared with 7000; the use of the music hall has grown from an attendance of 15,000 to 22,000 in 1906 and 29,500 in 1907. All this has been accomplished with no increase in endowment but an increase in income from the club and music hall corresponding with the increase in members and use respectively. "No one person is responsible for these results. The entire personnel of the library deserves the high honor of serving this community in their respective capacities, and the praise of the constituents of the institution for having done a great thing well."

CHAPTER XII

DOES IT PAY?

The preceding chapters tell the story of the various forms of industrial betterment undertaken by industrialists employing all the way from 5 up to 210,000 persons.

At this point I desire to supplement the working experience in factory, mill and workshop by the testimony of typical industrialists stating their attitude toward industrial betterment.

This study shows that in any great movement extending over a territory so vast as the United States, and dealing with such a complexity of nationalities, local conditions and personal prejudices of both capital and labor, the failures have been comparatively few; it tells the story of the way in which the various forms of mutuality have lessened the elemental friction between the employer and the employed. The fact that employers of upwards of one and a half million people who have come within the scope of this study are carrying on some form of betterment, is an evidence that they are not throwing their money away; in other words, they consider it good business. Apart from the mere commercial, there are other motives characterizing the industrial relations of to-day. As Carroll D. Wright observes:

"The rich and powerful employer, with the adjuncts of education and great business training, holds in his influence something more than the means of a subsistence for those he employs; he holds their moral well-being in his keeping, in so far as it is in his power to hold their morals. He is something more than a producer; he is an instrument of God for the upbuilding of the race."

Regarding the practicability or desirability of a policy of industrial betterment by an industrialist, whether he employ few or many workers, I quote from the letter of a prominent industrialist recently received:

"The fact of the matter is, we have considerably curtailed our work along the line of industrial betterment, and while we used to do considerable of it at one time, we are not quite as enthusiastic over it now, and are sort of lukewarm along this line at the present time, and are therefore not quite as much interested in it as we used to be.

"We went into it quite extensively. Whether it was that our people were a class of foreigners who did not seem to appreciate the work that we attempted to do, or whether their appreciation was misunderstood by us, I do not know. I feel perfectly convinced in my own mind, as do all of our people here who are watching the experiment, at least so far as we are concerned, that it was a mistake to continue it; in fact, a mistake to have started it, and while we have never regretted that we made the experiment, we have satisfied ourselves that as far at least as we are concerned, we shall never again make the attempt. There seems to be some invisible line between the employés in our factory and the office employés. We believe among our office people these little things that we did here from time to time were fully appreciated; we still continue that part of our work, and we have no doubt we shall continue to carry it on and perhaps increase it if we have the opportunity, but as far as our employés outside of the office are concerned, we have fully made up our mind that it will be a matter strictly of business with us without any show of sentiment in any way whatever. In other words, we shall buy our labor as we buy our material, and we are thoroughly convinced in our own minds that those who sell us their labor will give us as little as they possibly can for what they sell us without regard to whether or not we attempt to go more than our half of the way on some of these things outside of those which money can buy."

This was a manly straightforward statement from a man who was competent to judge, after a careful experience in his own mill. Desiring the opinion of an industrialist who was fully committed to a policy of industrial betterment, I asked him for his comments. Quoting from his reply: "Your correspondent says, 'We went into it, as you know, quite extensively.' This, to my mind, is a great mistake. Industrial betterment should be gone into very cautiously and not overdone. Let the employés themselves, as it were, show a desire for something more, and a willingness to help to accomplish it, also their appreciation for what has been done for them. I can quite believe it would be very easy to wreck industrial betterment work by overdoing it.

"I can see where a mistake was made in not getting their factory and office employés together. Your correspondent says, 'There seems to be an invisible line between the employés in the factory and the office employés.' This is a very dangerous condition in industrial betterment work, and one that will certainly retard it as long as it exists. I am very sorry to see them say, 'We still continue that part of the work that relates to the office staff, and shall perhaps increase it, if we have the opportunity, but so far as the employés outside of the office are concerned, we have fully made up our minds that it will be a matter of business with us without any show of sentiment in any way whatever.' My criticism of this sentence would be that this will only widen the breach and the factory employés will be very much harder to handle than they have been in the past. Perhaps a little experience along this line would be helpful. About five years ago when the writer made up his mind that there was too much friction among the departments and something ought to be done to eliminate it and inaugurate a better system of doing business without the friction, he called the heads and sub-heads together and talked over the matter with them. At the first meeting there were only about 18 persons present, and they were very much impressed with the meeting. Within 24 hours after that meeting, those in charge who had been antagonistic towards each other commenced to get closer together and compare notes, and it did not take them long to see that both parties were to blame. This meeting did so much good that we called another a week later. There were about 28 persons present, and the result was the same as at the previous meeting, but the output of the factory increased almost immediately. Then the next week we had another meeting of the same people, with the addition of ten or twelve more, bringing all heads and sub-heads together, about forty people. The result of these meetings was that all commenced to work together to better the conditions in the factory. The heads of departments were shown that they were responsible for the friction that existed, and should do their best to eliminate it. They did so, and substituted courteous, kind treatment for direct orders as given out by a boss. In three months the factory output increased $28,000. Now there was one thing we pointed out at these meetings as well as the friction in the factory, and that was that there was an invisible line, as your correspondent states, between the factory employés and the office staff, or between one department and another. The writer talked very strongly to them and showed them that there was no difference between the employés in their positions; they all worked in a factory, and it was their duty to try and keep down any feeling that the office staff was better than the factory. We appealed to their better nature, and I am happy to say we got the results. Our people to-day are all one, and it does not make any difference what part of the factory they work in. I believe candidly that if your correspondent would call together all his office people and have two or three good talks with them, and show them it is their duty to help along the firm by endorsing the industrial betterment work, and that they should be willing to go out among the employés and show their interest in them at all times, much good would be done. If the office employés are not willing to do this, I would say without hesitation that they are not entitled to have any benefits from industrial betterment, because they are working for their own selfish selves, and are not lightening the burden of the firm by whom they are employed, but on the contrary, they are making it harder for them to manage their factory help. I hope this criticism is not too severe, and I am convinced that this is right.

"Another clause in your correspondent's letter, in which he says they will buy labor as they buy material in future. We have just made some figures which show a very interesting state of affairs, and what industrial betterment will do for a business as well as for employés. We went into this work because we thought something was due our employés. The question of whether it would pay the firm or not was of secondary consideration, and we have kept that in the background at all times, believing that what we are doing for our people was only what they were entitled to receive at our hands. We have just figured up the first five months previous to the time when we commenced our industrial betterment work. In certain departments, piece-workers numbered 268. In these same departments piece-workers to-day, after three years of industrial betterment work, number 188; but the 188 have drawn the same amount of money as the 268 did for the same time. That is the record for the piece-workers. Now as to the time-workers: for the same length of time, under the same conditions, we find we have been able to increase their salaries and wages just 52½ per cent. in three years. Our business is larger than it was three years ago; altogether we employ about one hundred less to do the work than we did formerly. This has been accomplished by working nine hours a day and five and one-half days per week, instead of ten hours a day and six days a week. This is a direct proof that industrial betterment is better than buying labor same as they do materials. Now understand we do not profess to be perfect here in industrial betterment work, or to know much about it, but we have conscientiously tried to help our employés for the past three years, and we have worked together as one body, and have produced excellent results for the employés."

W. D. Forbes, of W. D. Forbes Company, writes:

"I have given this matter of industrial betterment the very greatest attention, and am firmly convinced that there is an enormous amount of misdirected and unwise treatment of employés under the guise of betterment. In a speech before some workmen of the most intelligent class I was most vigorously applauded when I made the statement that employés would be much better off if the employers who were able to make so much money out of their enterprises as to give recreation halls, dancing pavilions and all sorts of things of that nature would, instead of doing so, advance the pay a small percentage and let the workman pay for such entertainments himself.

"The things that are done by our company are without pressure of any kind from any source. They are simply a free will offering to the good and welfare of its employés, given in recognition of the moral obligation devolving upon employers to consider the reasonable interests and desires of the workmen, so far as the practical rules of business and the efficient operation of industry permits this to be done.

"I do not decry for a moment sanitary conditions, in fact, I would insist on them being enforced by State authorities, but I decry this idea of feeding oranges to men when they prefer to have the money for the oranges, apples, bananas or whatever is wanted. That this coddling system as suggested is unsatisfactory as far as preventing union conflicts is clearly shown in the case of a certain company who provided everything, but still had labor troubles."

Gould & Eberhardt, Newark, N. J., have no form of industrial betterment except an employés' mutual benefit association, managed and controlled entirely by workmen. The firm has nothing to do with it excepting in an advisory capacity when requested to do so by the men. A shop library composed principally of technical books is provided, but is not very well patronized. The firm reports: "We do not believe that it helps the man to give him something for nothing, nor do we believe that he wants it. We have seen in a great many instances throughout the country where various plans of this kind have been tried, that the men rather resent it, and come to look upon it as a charity which is not desired. We believe in giving a man a chance to earn his recreations, rather than provide them for him gratis, and we feel that all plans worked out on the basis of giving the man something for nothing are bound to fail, for the very reason that it can be nothing other than more or less of a charitable distribution, and that the American workman is above anything of this nature.

"We, however, do believe in providing him with clean surroundings, well lighted and ventilated working rooms, wash basins with hot and cold water so that he may leave the factory in clean condition, or any other so-called betterment which might have to do directly with his work; but beyond this we do not attempt to go."

Hale Bros. (Inc.) of San Francisco, where is located one of their six department stores on the Pacific Coast, report:

"Whatever we have done has been charged up to the expense account as the money was expended, and we have kept no track of what it has cost us, so that it is impossible for us to compare it from a definite and tangible gain basis in the abstract. We do believe, however, that all industrial betterment work results in more efficient employés, thereby being an indirect gain to the employer. We have been operating on the eight-hour day for more than three years, and cannot find that it has reduced our sales or net profits, but on the other hand the shorter work day has resulted in better health for our employés."

"April 15, 1908.

I have your letter of April 15, addressed to Mr. Patterson, making inquiry regarding our welfare work. Recently we have abandoned considerable of this work, although not in its entirety. We will continue to do some of this work as long as it is appreciated, but not on the same large scale as heretofore.

Yours very truly

(Signed) WM. PFLUM,
Vice President and General Manager."

Fels & Company, Philadelphia, write me: "We have regulated our relations with the employés on the principle of doing what logically and practically belongs to the relationship of employer and employé. We think there are very few employers who can safely go into the private life of their people, and have studiously refrained from providing many things which are furnished by other establishments. Our aim has been to pay good wages, and provide for fairly short hours, hygienic conditions and pleasant surroundings, at the same time requiring respectful treatment of all persons in the establishment."

"The policy which has long governed us in our relation to our employés is and has been such as to call for very little direct specific work in the line of industrial betterment," reports Mr. E. A. Marsh, general superintendent of the Waltham Watch Company. "Our plans and endeavors for the comfort and welfare of our people have been going on more than forty years—long before the term industrial betterment was heard of. We have always regarded it as work which was profitable, inasmuch as it tends to the comfort and enjoyment of our people. We are strong believers in the fact that external conditions have a great moral effect. We have a class of people that we believe can hardly be equaled in connection with any of the manufacturing establishments in the country. Many of them are members of the City government; two of them have held the office of Mayor, and for many years two chiefs of the city fire department were our employés, and many of our people are members of the City fire department. Some of our people have left our employment to engage in professional work, and have become doctors, lawyers, editors, ministers and members of the legislature.

"Naturally people of this class are entitled to a higher scale of wages than obtain in ordinary industrial establishments, and it is a fact that our company has always paid a higher rate of wages than any other watch factory in the world. These things being so, the natural result is that we have a class of well-to-do people of independent spirit, and who neither require nor desire assistance in the form which is often given. We do not believe in nor practice 'Paternalism.' Nevertheless, it is our policy and constant aim to create pleasant surroundings for our people, for aside from any humanitarian sentiment, which we do not at all disclaim, we are confident that the moral effect of the attractive conditions which we aim to establish is such as to constitute a wise business policy, particularly in our line of manufacturing.

"A good many centuries ago the statement was made that 'Godliness is profitable,' and while the original assertion had an individual application, it may be no violence to the original maxim to assert its truth as applied to *business*, at least to the extent of asserting that 'it pays to be considerate.'"

The President of Walter Baker & Co., Ltd., testifies: "While this business has been managed on lines which have been highly satisfactory both to the proprietors and their employés, I cannot readily point to any special form of what you designate as industrial betterment work. The house of Walter Baker & Co. was established in 1780, on the river Neponset in the town of Dorchester, Mass. The business has been carried on continuously ever since on the site on which it was originally begun—the plant being enlarged from time to time to meet the requirements of a steady increase in volume. During this long period of 128 years the company has never failed to meet all of its obligations promptly; there has never been a strike among the employés or any interference or discontent with the management of the business. The proprietors have exercised much care in the selection of the men and women placed on their pay rolls. They have required their employés to be sober, industrious and cleanly in their habits, regular in the discharge of their duties, and respectful to their employers and associates. The health and comfort of the mill hands have been carefully looked after during working hours. The utmost care has been exercised to prevent injury from machinery or from negligence of fellow workers; and in the very rare instances in which injuries have been sustained adequate provision has been made for the relief of the sufferers. The proprietors have never interfered with the home life of those in their service; nor have they undertaken to provide for their education or amusement. Most of the well meant schemes of employers to help their employés by providing homes, food, instruction and amusement have ended unhappily for both parties. Our long experience has shown that the best and most lasting service can be secured by looking after the comfort and welfare of the work people during the working hours and leaving them free to seek the life they wish to live outside. If they live in a way that unfits them for good service to us they have to pay the penalty. They are weakened instead of strengthened by having the responsibility for their way of living assumed by their employers."

Under the system thus briefly described, which has been pursued by the Baker Company for over a century and a quarter, the business has risen to be the largest of its kind in the world—that is to say, the company uses more crude cocoa in the manufacture of its great variety of preparations for food and drink than any other concern in Europe or America.

C. W. Post writes:

"When I think back of the experiences that some individuals have had in their efforts to do what is known as 'welfare' work and educational work more or less of the 'Lady Bountiful' plan, I feel like expressing myself rather vigorously. I know how almost the very soul has been cut out of some sweet-minded men who have undertaken this kind of work. They have learned to their cost that patronizing and coddling grown men and women is not looked favorably upon by the Infinite Power which governs us all, and it certainly punishes transgression of this written law in that respect. It is intended by the Creator that mankind obtain 'welfare' as the result of service and oftentimes good hard service. It is not to be fed to him in a silver spoon and his chin held up while he takes it."

At the opening of the improvements at their factory, the management of the Acme White Lead and Color Works stated:

"Industrial betterment is far-reaching, and involves something more than business success, because it affects the moral and material welfare of the community as a whole.

It is frequently said that betterment work along industrial lines has its origin, not in the desire for public good, but in selfishness—that sentiment has no place in business. This, in our view and experience, is a very grave error. Self-interest has certainly to be considered, as but few men are in business, carrying the burden with its endless cares and worries, because they love it; but rather to provide a competence for themselves and those dependent on them. But while this is so, we hold it to be also true that business men, as a rule, are largely influenced by sentiment or kindly feeling. A business policy that eliminates sentiment, we judge to be *not* a good policy, and we know whereof we speak.

There are things, precious things, that money can never buy. It can and does purchase perfunctory service, but it cannot and does not purchase loyalty and good will, without which no service is worth the having.

There are contributory causes for our business success, but they are invoked by the system of management which recognizes in every other man, a man and a brother. This explains why we have more than the usual number of old employés whose service is nearly coeval with the life of the firm. Our management has faith in the personal equation—the magnetism which draws and retains the services of competent assistants. They fight and win battles. They face all kinds of difficulties with the steadiness of veterans and they relieve of a burden which otherwise would become intolerable.

Good will is a mighty factor in business life, but it must be sincere, for unless a man has that good will in his own heart, he will certainly fail to inspire it in others. He can fool himself, but is not likely to successfully fool others.

Management may be either harsh or beneficent. The former rarely pays, and the latter rarely fails. The rank and file are always and particularly worth a little extra consideration.

Anything which tends to ameliorate the condition of factory life, without impairing efficiency or discipline, is within the scope of Acme management, and possibly reveals the secret you are looking for or answers the questions you have asked."

A decade ago when there was a decided impulse towards some form of improvement, it was undertaken not through altruism but through necessity. The awakened intelligence of workmen began to voice itself in expressions that something more than wages was due them. Hitherto they had accepted their surroundings without demur. To allay this feeling of smothered discontent, the industrialist was forced into attempts at betterment; he felt this step was necessary to hold his labor. Is it any surprise that some failures followed these attempts? Others, actuated by humanitarian principles, proved successful; they were willing to go slow for the sake of winning the confidence, disarming the suspicion and overcoming the accumulated prejudices of their workmen. All these attempts founded on mutuality endured; it was team work by capital and labor.

In the early manifestations of this new industrialism a little more than a decade ago, no particular name was given it. In 1898, as a result of my studies of the labor problem, I felt that this new movement should have a distinctive name, and suggested that of "Industrial Betterment." This was generally adopted, and quickly found a place in the literature of the day. Later on the term "Welfare Work" made its appearance. Industrial Betterment stands for the perfection of the plant, including improved hygiene and sanitation; it does not necessarily include club houses, athletics, educational and recreational movements; welfare work deals with these problems, but unfortunately is often received by the workmen with suspicion and dislike—a true workman does not like to be patronized. It now seems to me that neither of these phrases adequately connotes the coöperative spirit which should exist between capital and labor, a mutual relationship which is best expressed by the term "Mutuality." It is therefore the work of the social engineer, the exponent of a new profession necessitated by the complexity of socio-industrial relations, to apply to the solution of the special social or industrial problem under advisement, world experience in life and labor.

INDEX

Lightning Source UK Ltd.
Milton Keynes UK
UKHW020639270922
409514UK00005B/280

9 781376 53366